EXAMINATION
OF THE PATIENT

EXAMINATION OF THE PATIENT
A Text for Nursing and Allied Health Personnel

Lawrence B. Hobson, M.D., Ph.D.

Deputy Assistant Chief Medical Director
for Research and Development, Veterans Administration

McGRAW-HILL BOOK COMPANY
A Blakiston Publication

New York   St. Louis   San Francisco   Auckland   Düsseldorf   Johannesburg
Kuala Lumpur   London   Mexico   Montreal   New Delhi   Panama   Paris   São Paulo
Singapore   Sydney   Tokyo   Toronto

EXAMINATION OF THE PATIENT

1234567890KPKP798765

Library of Congress Cataloging in Publication Data

Hobson, Lawrence B.
    Examination of the patient.

    "A Blakiston publication."
    1. Physical diagnosis. 2. Nurses and nursing.
I. Title. [DNLM: 1. Physical examination. W3 205
H684e]
RC76.H66   616.07'5'024613   74-18087
ISBN 0-07-029112-8

This book was set in Times Roman by Black Dot, Inc. The editors were Cathy Dilworth and David Damstra; the cover was designed by Pencils Portfolio, Inc.; the production supervisor was Dennis J. Conroy. The drawings were done by EDA Technical Group, Inc.
Kingsport Press, Inc., was printer and binder.

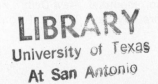

CONTENTS

PREFACE

As specially trained personnel assume expanded roles in patient care, they are expected to take medical histories and perform physical examinations. This textbook is specifically designed to introduce nonmedical students to the skills of *examining patients.*

Physical diagnosis courses in medical schools require prior intensive study of anatomy, physiology, and pathology. The textbooks present history taking and physical examination as an application of the medical students' detailed knowledge and, as the course name implies, the students are being trained to diagnose disease by means of the examination.

Nursing and allied health students with less intensive basic training can approach history taking and physical examination as a more practical, applied skill used to collect data concerning the patient. They learn to *detect,* to *define* or characterize, and to *describe* abnormal changes. Medical students learn simultaneously to *diagnose* disease; nonmedical students need not.

The educational needs of nursing and allied health students vary more than those of medical students, depending upon their future functions. The students may be trained to deliver primary patient care, a role which requires considerable knowledge and experience and hence a rather prolonged course in the examination of patients. Work in a more restricted field may require shorter, less intensive general training, with concentration in some specific area of examination. This textbook is arranged to provide the flexibility needed for these nursing and allied health courses.

Flexibility is reflected in the book's three interrelated parts:

Part 1, *Basic Examination of Patients,* is in itself an abbreviated but complete presentation of a simplified patient examination. It considers history taking as a simple, routine set of questions triggered by each complaint and followed by a standard questionnaire to elicit the history apart from the present illness. The physical examination concentrates on establishing a working idea of normal findings as a base for detecting the abnormal and omits the more difficult maneuvers. Written and verbal reporting of the findings is presented in both traditional and problem-oriented formats.

Part 2, *Advanced Examination of Patients,* extends and builds upon the work in Part 1. History taking includes detailed questions prompted by specific symptoms. The physical examination introduces more detailed consideration of the findings, more complicated maneuvers, such as ophthalmoscopy, and more emphasis on abnormalities. Special reporting is discussed and one chapter is devoted to patient examinations in surgical and medical emergencies.

Part 3, *Basis for Findings in Health and Disease,* selectively presents gross anatomy as it relates to the physical examination. It is chiefly topographic and regional, with a discussion of normal variations by age, sex, race, and other factors. Physiology is treated primarily as it is reflected in the history and physical examination; it deals with the functions of systems and organs. Pathology is discussed in terms of the general changes produced by disease and not in specific detail.

Part 1 alone can be used, for example, to train personnel for intensive care units, equipping them to detect and partially describe abnormalities even unrelated to the primary disease. If desired, sections of Part 2 can be added to give greater proficiency in specific areas.

Part 3 may serve as introductory material for Parts 1 or 2, may be used simultaneously with them, or may follow the other parts. Better-prepared students can omit Part 3 entirely. This flexible arrangement is facilitated by textual cross-references.

This book, then, is designed to give the student the basic information he needs when he examines patients. His practical work in examining people will provide the necessary skill.

Lawrence B. Hobson

TO THE INSTRUCTOR

A   *Examination of patients can be learned only by experience* and learned well only under the close supervision of an experienced teacher. A textbook can arrange, augment, and explain experience, but the students must examine real, live people. Throughout the text, exercises are clearly identified to guide the class in getting this experience.

B   An experienced instructor can lecture to forty or more students. Exercises, however, are best conducted in groups of four students, each group working under a tutor. This tutor demonstrates techniques, corrects errors, and insists upon repetition until each student performs satisfactorily.

C   All students should begin with the work in Part 1 where the exercises require the students to examine one another. This serves two purposes: It allows errors, corrections, and repetitions without embarrassing the students in the presence of a patient, and it presents the students with normal findings in the physical examination.

D   Instructors and tutors should provide as many opportunities as possible for students to examine normal people of both sexes and all ages. Similarly, students should examine normal body parts as well as abnormalities in patients. The emphasis in Part 1, carried over into Part 2, is on learning the *range of normal findings.*

E   Students using only Part 1 can have abnormal findings demonstrated to them. The instructor and tutor must remember that the student's aim is to detect abnormalities rather than to characterize them precisely.

F   Students using Part 2 should examine patients both to detect abnormalities unaided and to characterize these findings accurately. The instructor and tutor should concentrate on signs and symptoms as information—data—rather than as components in a diagnosis.

G   Tutors must expect students to be slow in eliciting the medical history and in doing the physical examination. Speed should increase only when the student gains expertise and hence need not hurry to be quick. Patients selected for the class should have relatively simple histories, as definite signs as possible, and ample patience.

H   In conducting the full course for primary-care personnel, the instructor may complete Part 1 with instruction in simpler techniques before proceeding to Part 2. Alternatively, he can begin with Part 1 but introduce Part 2 work at the completion of each section, as indicated by references in the text.

I   The instructor can assign relevant sections of Part 3 (as indicated by text references) before each class session as background material. Alternatively, Part 3 can introduce the course, serving as a quick review before beginning Part 1.

J   A student who has completed only Part 1 in a brief course can proceed later to Part 2. It is essential, however, that the student have a willing and knowledgeable preceptor if the advanced work is undertaken as on-the-job training.

Lawrence B. Hobson

EXAMINATION
OF THE PATIENT

Part One

Basic Examination
of Patients

Chapter 1

The Medical History

1-1 FUNCTION AND FORM OF THE HISTORY

Parts of the Patient Examination   New patients are examined to detect and characterize their abnormalities. This initial examination is the cornerstone of diagnosis and treatment. Subsequent examinations during the course of a disease serve essentially the same purposes—to detect changes in the patient and his illness and to guide further treatment.

The examination of a patient includes three parts that are separate but related—the *medical history,* the *physical examination,* and *ancillary procedures.*

The examiner usually proceeds in that order. He questions the patient first, examines him next, and orders or performs other diagnostic procedures last. To be sure, this order may have to be changed and one part may be omitted or delayed, but it is usually preferable to question, to examine, and only then to use other aids.

All three procedures aim at discovering abnormalities, but to do this one must make comparisons. Something is abnormal only if it differs from the *normal,* and no two "normal" human beings are identical. At the outset, this will present you with your greatest difficulty—you must learn the boundaries of normality. For that reason, you must begin by examining people who are normal. As you gain experience you will develop valid concepts of *normal limits.*

Memory is short and a busy person soon forgets details. Then too, any examiner must be able to give his results to another person precisely, clearly, and concisely. The medical profession has therefore developed rather efficient ways to record and to report the results of each patient's examination. You must learn how to present such information in an orderly fashion.

To some degree this involves learning a new vocabulary. The terms are sometimes long and difficult, but they have the virtue of being more precise—less apt to be misunderstood—than common words. For example, a *symptom* is what a patient experiences or feels and may be highly subjective. A *sign* is what someone else—usually the examiner—observes, and it is objective; that is, another trained person can observe the same thing. Other data such as hemoglobin values, venous pressure readings, or electrocardiographic results are more vaguely lumped as "findings."

The medical history, then, chiefly elicits symptoms, the physical examination yields signs, and ancillary procedures contribute findings to the diagnosis. These constitute the clinical *data* about the patient. Of the three, the medical history is in many respects the most important. It not only provides vital information but the act of taking a history establishes the subsequent relationship between the patient and the examiner.

Examiner and Patient   The relationship between a patient and you as an examiner is a highly confidential one. Usually the patient is willing, even anxious, to discuss his present troubles and past history fully and frankly. He will be truthful in most instances as long as he trusts you.

The patient is generally ready to accept you on first contact. Whether he continues to trust and confide in you depends to the greatest extent on what you do and how you do it. And a patient forms his first impression as you take the medical history. If you question your patient in a calm, confident manner with courteous, friendly interest and obviously accept him and his story, you can almost always win his trust.

The interview has two sides—the patient's and the examiner's. While confiding his troubles, the patient is trying to help you understand them and also judging you. On the other side, you are rapidly evaluating the patient—in terms of intelligence, dependability as a reporter, personality and, to some degree, just how sick he really is. You are also trying to put your patient at ease and to increase his confidence in you. More obviously, you are discovering what your patient has experienced in the course of his illness as well as what his life has been like apart from the present illness.

Parts of the Medical History The story of the illness and of the patient's past is the medical history. It is the starting point toward a diagnosis, and a skilled physician often arrives at a diagnosis—at least a tentative one—as he elicits the history. To be sure, physicians bring wide knowledge to the examining room and use it to improve their efficiency. But even they have to follow some orderly plan to avoid overlooking pertinent information.

A nonmedical examiner must be even more systematic. At the outset you will have to memorize the components of a medical history and even the questions needed to elicit them. With practice, you will recall components and questions without difficulty, but initially you may need a reminder with you.

The history has four chief parts and a number of subdivisions:

1 Introductory Data
    a Date of the examination
    b Patient information: name, age, sex, race, marital status, occupation, origin or birthplace
    c Source and reliability of the history: usually the patient, a relative, and/or a prior medical record
    d Summary of patient's previous contacts with examiner's medical facility, including prior hospitalization and ambulatory care
2 Chief Complaint
3 Present Illness
4 Background Information
    a Past history
    b Family history
    c Review of systems
    d Personal or social history

Procedure During Interview The parts are usually recorded in this order, but the interview follows a different one. Usually you introduce yourself and, unless you have it already, ask the patient's name. If you do not have the name, it is wise to write it down immediately.

The patient, however, is more interested in telling you his troubles than in giving you his age, marital status, or occupation. The logical, courteous, and natural question for you to ask is something like "What is bothering you?" or "What caused you to come here?" The reply is almost always the *chief complaint,* and you should jot it down in the patient's own words. The questioning then leads naturally into the *present illness,* a description of the patient's current troubles. Usually you ask about the *background information* after the present illness.

Much of the *introductory data* comes out during questioning about the present illness and background information. You should write it down as you hear it. You can ask later for anything else except the *reliability of the source.* This is completed last of all, when you have the best grounds for an opinion.

Writing the History   At first it is easier to make notes as the patient talks and then write the entire history later. Although experienced examiners may find it more efficient to write in final form all the history except the present illness, even they often uncover bits of the present illness while asking about background information and can describe the current illness coherently only after asking all the questions.

Medical histories are recorded in several forms (see Section 3-2). However, one principle holds regardless of the form: always write the present illness chronologically; that is, begin with what happened first and proceed in the order of events up to the present moment. This sensible and time-tested rule makes it almost impossible to write *as* the patient gives you his unorganized and sometimes jumbled account.

Even jotting notes requires some practice, especially since patients react badly when an examiner keeps his head down. It is important to *talk with* your patient, and this means that your eyes must meet his frequently. This is especially true if the patient seems nervous, ashamed, hostile, evasive, or dishonest. You *are* interested in your patient and should make him feel your interest.

1-2 FUNDAMENTAL QUESTIONS ABOUT SYMPTOMS

Chief Complaint and Present Illness   Most patients feel that some one symptom is more important than any others they may have. This symptom is, of course, the chief complaint, and you should record it as a direct quote. You then ask the duration of the symptom and record that. This chief complaint provides the best lead for questions about the present illness.

Often a single question, such as "How has it affected you?" or "Could you tell me more about it?" will prompt a spontaneous and unaided description of the chief complaint. The patient may even give a fairly complete account of his present illness. Usually he will need some guidance in the form of questions which center around his main problem.

As questioning about the chief complaint proceeds, several things happen. The patient answers what you ask, volunteers other information, and sometimes begins to ramble. You must at some point ask about any additional symptoms that are mentioned. Such a symptom may not impress the patient but still prove more important than the chief complaint. It is always safer to explore every symptom.

A patient usually volunteers information out of order, skipping about in time and from symptom to symptom. This is disturbing to the examiner, who is trying to follow an orderly arrangement of questions. But as long as the information bears on the patient's medical situation, it is valuable even if out of order. You can always make a note and ask for more details later.

The truly talkative rambler presents a greater problem. Such a patient will waste valuable time on trivial and unrelated matters, perhaps revealing a great deal about his personality but very little about his illness. There are more efficient ways to evaluate his personality.

Generally it is advisable to let a patient describe his troubles in his own way, but you must learn to guide the interview, get the information you need, and tactfully stop any nonproductive rambling. With all this to accomplish, you will find that taking a good medical history is an intense intellectual activity.

Systematic Questioning Experienced *physicians* approach a patient with an extensive knowledge of disease, shortcuts learned by talking to many patients, and an efficient technique for obtaining pertinent information. They spend little time in profitless questioning and so can obtain an excellent history quickly. They can even make the procedure seem simple and easy.

This may be the best method, but it requires experience and expertise. And there are other ways to take an adequate history. You will find that a method demanding limited medical knowledge and one less apt to confuse you is best at the start.

At the outset you must question thoroughly—symptom by symptom—beginning with the chief complaint. You will use essentially the same questions for each symptom and you must remember that each symptom has its *onset, course,* and *present situation.* For each of these there is a group of questions, and you should memorize them. The exact wording of each question can—and indeed must—vary from patient to patient and from symptom to symptom. What is important is the *meaning* of each question.

Basically you should ask each question, but some cannot be answered if the informant has no information. You then omit them. This usually arises when someone other than the patient is being interviewed.

Some questions make no sense for specific symptoms and should be skipped. It is usually pointless, for example, if the patient complains that she is pregnant, to ask "What were you doing when your trouble began?"

Common sense will help you to avoid such a silly query, but in general it is better to ask rather than omit questions.

Basic Questions   Here then are the questions:

Onset of Symptom

When? When did the symptom (or incident) occur? Is this the first time it has occurred? If not, when did it first occur? How often has it recurred?

What? Exactly what did the patient experience or an observer notice? Did it appear suddenly or gradually? How did the patient feel in general? What other symptoms did the patient have then or before?

Where? What part of the body was first affected? What other parts of the body were later affected by the symptom?

Why? What does the patient think brought on the symptom? Where was the patient when the symptom began or recurred? What was he doing?

Who? Was anyone associated with the patient similarly affected?

Course

How? How has the symptom changed since it first appeared? Has it grown worse or better? Has it changed rapidly or slowly? Has it grown steadily worse or better or has it improved and worsened repeatedly?

When? When, after its appearance, did the symptom change?

Why? What has made the symptom worse? What, including treatment, has made it better or failed to do so?

What else? What other symptoms have appeared? Where, when, and why?

Present Situation

What? Exactly what is the symptom like now? How does the patient feel in general? What other symptoms does he have?

Where? What parts of the body are now affected by the symptom?

Why? Has the patient recently done or taken anything to account for the present situation?

Use of Questions   The questions are used in the interview which follows. The examiner obviously changes the wording and omits questions which have been spontaneously answered earlier. Of course, he avoids asking pointless questions to which there are no answers and refrains from interrupting volunteered information if it is pertinent.

Following the interview you will find notes that the examiner made during the interview—notes that help him write the chief complaint and present illness. The examiner will continue his examination by getting the background information about the patient.

A 45-year-old woman reports that she has a "cough."

Onset

When?

    Q (Examiner) When did this cough begin?
    A (Patient) I think it began about Tuesday.
    Q Well, was that Tuesday of this week, say three days ago?
    A Yes, three days ago.
    Q Is this the first time you've had a cough?
    A Oh, no. I get a cough about three or four times a year and usually it doesn't go away by itself and that's why I came here today.
    Q These coughs you get, when did you first get them?
    A I don't know. I must have been about twenty, I guess. Anyway, it was about the time I met John and we became engaged and—

What?

    Q Excuse me, but I'd like to ask you—What are these attacks of coughing like? How do they affect you?
    A Well, sometimes I have a cold first. Sometimes I don't. Then I begin to cough and it gets worse and I start to spit up—
    Q Excuse me, do you mean vomit?
    A No, no. I just cough up spit and then a little later I cough again. Sometimes I cough all night and then I can't sleep or anything.
    Q Do you feel sick or anything with these attacks of coughing?
    A Not really, but I get damned tired—and tired of them. Sometimes it goes on for a week or two.

Where?

    Q You said sometimes you had a cold before the cough. Do you ever have any other trouble before or with the cough?
    A Well, sometimes my sides and my stomach ache after I cough a lot.
    Q Show me where you ache.
    A Well, along here. (Runs hands down sides of thorax.) And here. (Moves hands across upper abdomen to midline.) But I'm not aching now.
    Q You don't have any other trouble with these attacks?
    A Well, like I told you, I get so I can't sleep from the cough.

Why?

    Q Yes, I remember. Do you know of anything you do that brings on these attacks of coughing?
    A Yeah, sometimes I have a cold, sometimes I don't. When I've got an attack—like now—I get so I can't talk or laugh without coughing. I—then after a few days I get hoarse—from coughing so much, I guess. Anyway, I don't know what causes me to get these coughs. Maybe you can find out because if you—

Who?

    Q Perhaps we can. Now when you get an attack are you the only

person who is sick or do other people around you—oh, your family or friends—have coughs and so on?
A   Sometimes when I have colds I catch them from my kids or give mine to my husband.
Q   Do they cough like you do?
A   No, they're lucky. They may hack a little but like I always say, it always has to be me that—

Course

How?

Q   Sure, I know, But let's talk about this attack you're having now. Is it just like the others?
A   Yeah, just like the others when they start.
Q   And—this attack—is the cough getting better or worse?
A   It's still getting worse. Otherwise I couldn't talk to you so long or at least you wouldn't listen so long or—
Q   Is the cough getting worse rapidly?
A   No, I wouldn't say so. It just builds up and builds up.

Why?

Q   Have you taken or done anything that makes it better or worse?
A   Have I taken anything? Look—two days ago I swallowed a whole bottle of cough syrup that I bought at the drug store. Maybe it eased me a little bit but not much. Sometimes the doctor has given me some kind of medicine that knocks me out all night when I cough. I've got some home but I haven't taken any yet.
Q   But you don't know anything that has made the cough worse?
A   Sure—talking, smoking—I haven't given that up this attack yet but usually I do. I can't walk fast or climb stairs without hacking my lungs out.

What else?

Q   Is anything else bothering you now—in this attack—besides the cough?
A   Like I said, I don't ache yet and I slept some last night, but I get tired of spitting all the time or else swallowing the spit.

Present Situation

What?

Q   How would you describe your cough right now—this minute?
A   I don't know what you mean.
Q   Well, is it bad, really bad, or what?
A   Oh, I'd say about average. Not like I was going to lose my toenails or anything.

Where?

Q   And right now you don't feel bad any other way, any other place?

    A   Yeah, come to think of it, I got a bunion on my right foot and—
    Q   We'll come back to that later. But the cough isn't associated with anything else?
    A   Well, it's associated with me and I wish it wouldn't be.

Why?

    Q   But today have you done anything that makes the cough better or worse?
    A   Sure, talking so much to you makes it worse.

The examiner's notes:

Cough   3 d, gets 3–4 times each yr since age 20; some start with colds, not all; sputum, can't sleep (sleeping medicine); lasts 1–2 wk; side chest, upper abd. ache after cough; worse talking, laughing
Hoarseness from cough   no known cause of cough; no family coughs
Pres. cough worsening gradually   cough syrup 2 d ago little help; no sleeping medicine; talking, smoking made worse; walking, climbing; cough now med. severe (pt.), little sputum
Bunion

EXERCISES

1   Work in pairs—one student-patient, one student-examiner. The student-patient will remember her last illness—common cold, menstrual cramps, even sore feet or sunburn—and answer questions about it. The student-examiner will elicit the chief complaint, present illness, and introductory data, making notes as he does. Remember, the impression the examiner makes is important. Try to make it as professional as possible. After the first history is done, reverse roles.
2   Elicit a partial history—chief complaint, present illness, and introductory data—from a patient whom someone else has already examined. Compare the information that you obtained with that in the chart. Pay close attention to the patient's response to you as an examiner.

See also Sections 4-1 and 4-2.

1-3 BACKGROUND HISTORY

At this point in the examination, the examiner knows a good deal about what is bothering the patient now and something about the sort of person he is. The patient should be feeling more confident about the examiner and somewhat relieved that a sympathetic person has listened attentively to his story.

    Your impression of the patient and the patient's attitude toward you are important when the questioning about the background information begins. Some patients will find further questions rather unrelated to their problems and will resent them. It is your job to overcome any resistance. Only when the patient is too ill to continue or time demands it should part of the history be postponed.

The order in which the components of the *background history* are elicited and recorded varies in practice. You should use the one current in your hospital, clinic, or office, and it is wise not to shift to another unless absolutely necessary. In many places, a printed history form is used both to cue the questions and to record the answers.

Your questions are apt to be direct as you seek the background information. The patient will not resent this if you elicited the present illness properly. Strive for reasonably brief, informative answers. Otherwise the examination can become so long as to exhaust both you and the patient.

Past History   The patient will find it natural to be asked about earlier ills after his present troubles have been discussed. From them you can lead into other information without an obvious, mechanical change of subject. It may be best to memorize the standard questions; but to make the interview smooth, you will have to alter the wording as you go.

The following subjects will be covered, although not necessarily in this order:

General health and weight record
Childhood diseases
Adult diseases
Injuries
Operations
Immunization record
Past and present medications
Summary of previous hospital admissions

For infants and children, you should add:

Birth information
Mother's obstetrical record

The essential questions in brief form are then:

General Health and Weight Record

Has your health generally been good?

Was it getting worse before you became ill this time?
Have you gained or lost weight during the past year? How much?
When did you begin to lose or gain? Was it intentional?
For infants and children, has the growth and weight gain been
normal? When did any unusual growth or gain begin?

Childhood Diseases   Ask for them by name:

Measles
German measles
Chickenpox
Mumps
Whooping cough
Scarlet fever
Rheumatic fever
Diphtheria
Meningitis
Poliomyelitis

How old were you when you had it?

Adult Diseases   Ask for each by name:

Influenza
Pneumonia
Tuberculosis
Typhoid fever

When did you have it? Any other disease with fever?

Injuries

Were you ever seriously injured? How? When?
Have you'ever had any broken bones?
Any severe burns? A gunshot wound? When?
Have you ever been knocked out? When? For how long?

Operations

What operations have you had? When? Where?

Immunizations   Especially for children; ask for each by name:

Diphtheria
Tetanus

Whooping cough
Smallpox
Poliomyelitis
Typhoid fever
Influenza
Others

When did you last have each?

Medication

Are you taking medicines now? What are they, or what are they for?
How long have you been taking them?
Have you ever had a bad reaction to any medicine? What one? When
was it?
Has a doctor ever warned you not to take a certain kind of medicine?
What kind? Why? When?

Birth Information   For infants and small children:

How long was the pregnancy before the patient was born? Was it a
normal pregnancy?
What was wrong about it?
Was the birth normal? What complications occurred? Was the baby
normal and well after birth? What was wrong?

Mother's Obstetrical Record   For infants and small children:

How many pregnancies has the mother had?
How many babies born? How many children now living?
Where does the patient come in the order of pregnancies and births?
Did the mother nurse the patient? For how long?

Family History   You can pass from the patient's health record to
that of the family quite comfortably. The *family history* consists basically
of two parts: (1) condition of relatives and (2) diseases with "familial
tendencies." Again, direct questions can be used. It is well to emphasize
that you are seeking information about "blood relations," not relatives by
marriage.

Condition of Relatives   Ask the following questions individually
about mother, father, brothers, sisters, children (offspring).

Is he (or she) living or dead?

How old is he (or she)? How old was he (or she) at time of death?
What is the individual's present state of health?
What was the cause of death?

Familial Diseases

Do you know of any disease that runs in your family? Who has had
it?
For each of the following diseases ask: Has any blood relative had it?
Who?

Hay fever, asthma, or eczema
High blood pressure
Heart disease
Kidney disease
Arthritis
Tuberculosis
Diabetes
Cancer
Migraine
Epilepsy
Insanity

Review of Systems   Questioning under *review of systems* can—and
sometimes should—be long and exhaustive. Patients should not be
hurried because they need time to remember. Some information you elicit
will belong in the present illness and should be reported there. You need
not record it twice, but it is wise to put a note "See PI" after the heading
where it is elicited.
 The questions are asked in a set order, body system by body system.
You must remember the order, and an easy way to do so is to go more or
less from top to bottom of the body.
 The answers to the questions will be symptoms or diseases. For each
you must at least determine when it occurred and whether it had lasting
effects. In other words you must ask:

When did you have this?
Did you recover or did it disappear so that you were well again?
What lasting effects did it have?

Here then are the basic questions:

Head   Have you had headaches? Dizziness? Unconsciousness?
Convulsions?

Eyes   Have your eyes ever given you trouble? How? How long have you worn glasses? For what trouble?

Ears   How is your hearing? Have you ever had earache? Mastoid trouble? Ringing or other sounds in your ears?

Nose   Do you have frequent colds? Sinus trouble? Nosebleeds? Sore throats?

Mouth   Have you had trouble with your teeth? Gums? Tonsils?

Lungs   Have you had trouble breathing? Have you ever had wheezing? Pain in your chest? Tuberculosis? Pleurisy? A cough lasting a month or longer? When did you last have a chest x-ray? What was the result?

Heart   Have you been told that you have heart trouble? High blood pressure? Low blood pressure? Have you been breathless when you were lying flat? Have you had palpitations? Have your ankles swelled? Have your lips turned bluish? Have you had an electrocardiogram? When? What was the result?

Digestive System   Have you had pain in the abdomen? Loss of appetite? Nausea? Vomiting? Frequent indigestion? Jaundice? Constipation? Diarrhea? Bloody vomiting? Blood in your stools? Black or tarry stools? Hemorrhoids? Hernia? Have you ever been told that you had liver trouble? Hepatitis? Cirrhosis? Gallbladder trouble? Ulcers? Colitis?

Kidneys and Bladder   Have you ever had kidney trouble? Nephritis? Kidney stone? Prostate trouble (for men)? When you urinate, have you had trouble starting or stopping the stream? Dribbling? Burning? Bloody urine? Very dark urine?

Reproductive Tract   Male: Have you had pain or swelling in the scrotum or testes? Sores on the penis? Pus from the penis? Difficulty in getting or sustaining an erection? Premature ejaculation? How often do you have sexual intercourse? With whom? Have you had syphilis, gonorrhea, or any other venereal disease?

Female: How old were you when your periods began? Have they been regular? How often and of what duration? When did your last period begin? Have your periods been unusually heavy or light? Have you bled between periods? Have your periods been painful?

Is sexual intercourse painful? How often do you have intercourse? With whom? What contraceptive do you use?

Have you had any whitish discharge? Sores on your sex organs? Have you had syphilis, gonorrhea, or any other venereal disease?

Skin   Have you had any trouble with your skin? Eruptions? Acne?

Itching? Hives? Has your hair changed texture? Become thinner? Have your nails changed?

Bones and Joints   Have you ever had arthritis or rheumatism of the hands, feet, arms, legs, hips, or back? Are you stiff in the morning? Have you had a slipped or ruptured disc? Sciatica? Varicose veins?

Nervous System   Have you had a nervous breakdown? Trouble thinking straight? Difficulty remembering things? Trouble sleeping? Depressed feelings? Any serious mental illness?

Blood   Have you had anemia? Uncontrolled bleeding? Extensive bruising? Have you ever had a blood transfusion? Any reaction? What is your blood type?

Endocrine System   Have you taken hormones? Oral contraceptive pills? Do you stand cold unusually well? Do you tolerate heat better than most? Are you unusually active and jittery? Has your appetite changed? How? Do you urinate more frequently than most people? Do you drink more liquids than most?

Personal or Social History   The *personal history* is less specifically medical than the other components, but it contributes directly to understanding the patient who has the problem. Because it does not deal with his problem, the patient may be somewhat more resistant to questioning unless you have already won his complete cooperation. It is often easier to elicit the personal history as the last item.

You are trying to complete your picture of the patient as he has lived and is living. Once again, a systematic approach makes it less likely that information will be omitted, so that it is well to trace a course from birth to the present.

Birth, Residences, and Childhood   Where were you born? What countries did your ancestors come from? Where have you lived during your life? Have you traveled outside the country? Where? How far did you go in school? Why did you stop?

Military Service   Did you serve in the Army, Navy, Air Force, etc.? What were the dates? Where were you stationed? Were you wounded or ill?

Occupations   What kind of work have you done during your life? What are you doing now? Do you enjoy it? How many hours do you work a week?

Marital Status   Are you married? Divorced? Separated? Widowed? What were the dates of your marriage? Divorce? Separation? Did you remarry? When?

How old is your spouse? Is he (she) well? What is his (her) trouble? How many children have you and your spouse had? What are their ages? Are they well? If dead, what was the cause? What miscarriages or abortions were there? When?

Environment   Where do you live? Who lives with you? What kind of house or apartment do you have? Are you crowded? Do you get along well at home? What kind of transportation do you use? What do you rate as the major difficulty in your life? What worries you the most?

Habits   How many hours do you sleep? Soundly? Do you eat regular meals? Do you eat meat, fowl, or fish every day? How many times a week? Do you eat an egg daily—as such or in cooked foods? Do you eat fresh fruits and/or vegetables—as salads, for instance? Do you get a glass of milk daily, including milk in cooked foods? How many cups of coffee do you drink daily? Cups of tea? Beers? Glasses of whiskey, gin, etc.?

What do you smoke and how much daily? What home remedies or vitamins do you take? Do you use marijuana, sleeping pills, pep-up pills, heroin, cocaine, or other drugs? How often and how much? Have you ever used them? When?

What hobbies do you have? What social activities? What exercise do you get?

Run through for me what you do on your usual weekday from the time you get up right around the clock until you get up the next morning.

By the time you have finished questioning and observing the patient in so much detail, you should have formed a good idea of the kind of person he is. You should now be ready to evaluate the patient's reliability as an informant and to describe his personality. If you have handled the interview properly, the patient should be prepared to cooperate with you even to the extent of submitting to unpleasant procedures. You will have "established rapport."

EXERCISES

1   Work in pairs—one student-patient, one student-examiner. During the first session, the examiner will elicit the past history and the family history. Students will then switch roles. In the second session, the review of systems and personal history are similarly taken. In these exercises, the student-examiners should use the lists of questions, but they should know the lists well enough to inquire naturally and easily. The student-patients should note their own reactions to the questions, especially those dealing with sexual and family matters. Try to imagine the impact these would have if they "caught you unawares." Then try to formulate plans to introduce these questions as

naturally as possible in a matter-of-fact way and without seeming to pry. This will involve planning the questions leading up to the sensitive ones.

2   Elicit the past history and review of systems from a patient, preferably one where these are already recorded. Plan carefully your approach and initial contact with the patient, since you will not have the advantage of having established rapport by eliciting the present illness. Compare your information with that in the chart. Pay close attention to the patient's response to you as an examiner.

3   Repeat the exercise by eliciting the family history and the personal or social history.

4   After you have completed the above, elicit a complete history—introductory data, chief complaint, present illness, and background information—from a patient. The patient had best have an acute illness, be fairly young, not seriously ill, and cooperative. Make notes as you question but do not attempt to write up your results. At the end consider what you know of the patient as a person, how well you can describe the patient's problems, and how he reacted to you. Try to identify any "rough spots" in the interview and plan how you can avoid them in the future.

See also Section 4-3.

1-4 INTERIM OR REVISIT HISTORY

Revisit History   Most patients will be examined—at least briefly—several times after the initial contact. Hospitalized patients are seen daily, clinic patients return for revisits, and those at home are visited more than once. On each occasion new information is sought, but not by asking all the questions of the initial interview over again.

You will try to do three things on a revisit: (1) obtain information about the patient's course, (2) find out about any new problem, and (3) maintain rapport.

You accomplish all three in part by asking questions, by taking a *revisit* or *progress history* if you have seen the patient before. The questions are logical ones and—properly asked—show your interest in the patient. Again, you must remember them so that you do not omit some essential point, but you rephrase them naturally.

How are you today?
Is your (symptom, whatever that is) better? Worse? Unchanged?
Has the treatment (medicine, appliance, operation, or physical therapy) helped? How?
Tell me how you are taking your medicine (using your appliance, etc.).
Has something else occurred to disturb you since I saw you last? What is it?

Has the treatment (medicine, appliance, or operation) caused you any trouble?
What was that?

A "yes" in response to any of the last three questions leads to eliciting a history of the symptom exactly as in the present illness. Invariably some patients reintroduce the same symptoms they discussed earlier. When this occurs, questioning can be rather brief, since all that is needed is the present situation.

Interim History   Patients treated satisfactorily and discharged from care may have a recurrence of the same difficulty or present some new problem. This can occur months or years later. Under these circumstances it is necessary to elicit an *interim history,* which is a modified initial history.

Various institutions have different rules concerning the interim history, but in general a patient who returns within a year has a revisit examination. If he returns more than a year later but within 5 years or so, he has an interim examination. The initial examination is repeated if he has not been seen for a longer period.

The interim history begins as does the initial history and elicits the introductory data, chief complaint, and present illness. It then determines only how the background information has changed.

You will find this easy to do with the previous record in your hand. Some remark such as "Now, I'd like to see whether your situation has changed since you were here last" prepares the patient for what is coming.

You obviously repeat the questions about general health and the weight record, omitting childhood diseases, injuries, operations, immunizations, and medications. It is well to remind the patient several times that you are interested in what has happened since his last visit. Birth information will not have changed, but a child's mother should be asked about any further pregnancies.

The family history can usually be covered by asking about relatives who were alive during the initial examination and whether any family members have become ill during the interval. You are interested primarily in familial diseases, of course.

The review of systems requires more attention. You can run through the questions rather quickly, asking especially about the status of problems identified in the initial examination. If there was no difficulty with the eyes, ears, nose, mouth, or skin, you can ask such single question as "Have you had any trouble with your eyes during this time?" Patients usually identify problems in these systems quite readily. It is much safer, however, to repeat the more detailed questions about the lungs, heart, digestive system, kidneys and bladder, reproductive tract, bones and joints, nervous system, blood, and endocrine system.

The personal or social history can omit the information about birth and childhood but usually warrants a question about foreign travel and residency. Obviously, you will ask about changes in occupation, marital status, environment, habits, and the daily routine.

A final question is: Why have you not been to see us since your last visit?

If the patient has been under the medical care of someone else, you can ask: Would you tell me his name (or their names)? Why are you returning to us now?

It should be obvious why it pays to read the prior record before seeing a patient for a revisit or interim examination. This will be true even if you wrote the earlier record. Do not be surprised, however, if the patient now remembers things somewhat differently. Human memory is fallible and it does no good to chide the patient for "changing his story."

EXERCISES

1 Read over the initial history and revisit or progress notes of two or three patients who have been seen repeatedly. Ignore the physical examinations, diagnoses, laboratory findings, and treatment for the present. As you read, plan what you would ask on a revisit examination and what you would cover in the background information if you had to obtain an interim history. It would be well to make brief notes to yourself as you plan.

2 Obtain a revisit history on a patient whom someone has seen the day before and on one who has been seen a week or so earlier. By now you may find that the patients accept you readily and that you can question them smoothly and confidently. If they do not, try again with the same patients another day.

Chapter 2

The Physical Examination

The physical examination of a patient depends upon the examiner's own senses. Instruments assist those senses much as artificial light helps one to see in a dim place. Training your senses and increasing your awareness of sensations are more important than learning to use the instruments properly. A really skilled examiner can discover most signs without instruments; he just does a better, more efficient examination with them.

The most commonly used instruments are the following:

Watch with a second hand
Stethoscope
Flashlight
Tongue depressor
Sphygmomanometer—the "blood pressure apparatus"
Reflex hammer
Rubber gloves—for rectal and vaginal examinations
Thermometer
Scales for weighing the patient

These are adequate for basic examinations. For infants and children it is well to add:

Otoscope—the lighted instrument for examining the ears

Other instruments have more advanced and specialized uses. The stethoscope, flashlight, sphygmomanometer, and otoscope are easily damaged and need some care.

You should carefully select your *stethoscope* and have it fitted, since it must be comfortable to use. It consists of several parts: earpieces, rubber tubing (with or without a Y-shaped connector), and the chest piece. The earpieces require the "fitting." They must sit snugly but comfortably in the ears, held there firmly but gently. Stethoscopes have a spring that can be bent to increase or decrease the pressure of the earpieces. It is even more important that the earpieces be positioned so that the holes in them point directly at your eardrums. The bends in the metal tubing can be changed to accomplish this, since the direction differs slightly from person to person. A knowledgeable equipment salesman can make the necessary adjustments.

There are two standard designs for chest pieces—the *bell* and the *diaphragm*. One head may hold both. Since each has its uses, it is wise to have both. Even the length of the rubber tubing influences the performance of the stethoscope. If too long or too short, it changes the sound's properties and makes the stethoscope mechanically awkward as well. The overall length from earpiece to chest piece is usually about 2 ft.

You should buy a stethoscope and small flashlight before beginning to learn the techniques of physical examination. You will need a sphygmomanometer, otoscope, and rubber reflex hammer as well unless they are already available. Tongue depressors, rubber gloves, thermometers, and scales are usually provided.

2-1 FUNCTION AND FORM OF THE PHYSICAL EXAMINATION

A physical examination, like a medical history, aims primarily at detecting and characterizing anything abnormal about the patient. Unlike the history, it seeks to establish the signs of disease, the observed rather than the reported evidence of something wrong. To do this you use sight, touch, and hearing; your sense of smell may contribute as well.

The trained examiner uses these senses systematically. Even the order in which he proceeds to probe any part is usually the same. This order is:

Inspection
Palpation

Percussion
Auscultation

Inspection is the visual examination of a part—say the front of the chest. It embraces whatever the examiner can see: deformities, pulsations, the manner of breathing, scars, and so on.

Palpation is examination by feeling with the fingers or hands. Besides exploring masses, it includes determining tenderness: feeling the grating of a broken bone; the fine, regular, rapid trembling sensation called a *thrill* as blood flows past an obstruction; and the rough vibration from an airway with thick mucus in it.

Percussion is examination by rapping or tapping, the usual "chest thumping." It gives information by both the sense of hearing and that of touch. Basically it detects what is filled with air or gas—the lungs for instance—and what is not, such as the blood-filled heart.

Auscultation is examination by listening either with or without the stethoscope. It really includes hearing the patient cough as well as listening to the beating of his heart. In practice, however, the term "auscultation" is used to mean listening to sounds that are within the body.

Smell frequently is used during any of these steps. A foul wound will intrude its odor unbidden, or you may ask the patient to breathe in your face deliberately so that you can smell his breath.

From now on you will learn to use inspection, palpation, percussion, and auscultation—as well as smell—to detect abnormalities. You will have to learn first, of course, what the normal person usually shows at each step of the examination. You begin, therefore, by examining your classmates as examples of normal adults.

2-2 METHODS OF PHYSICAL EXAMINATION

The physical examination begins the moment the examiner first sees or hears the patient. The initial inspection includes the patient's posture, expression, state of clothing or bedclothing and—if the patient walks into view—gait. Palpation begins when you gauge the patient's grip as you shake his hand or feel his arm as you help him into a chair. The physical examination really continues throughout the taking of a medical history and only becomes more particular during the "physical."

You have been meeting and evaluating people all your life. You already have, in other words, part of the experience you need to do a physical examination. There is, however, a difference in your motives when meeting a social acquaintance as opposed to examining a patient. In a social setting, you are quite justified in trying to judge what a new acquaintance will mean to you personally. In a clinical setting, however, your evaluation is for the patient's benefit. You are not concerned with whether the patient will be pleasant to know but whether and how he is ill. A happy expression on a patient's face means most because it indicates the absence of suffering.

Beginning the Examination   The physical examination cannot be well done with the patient clothed, so he is asked to undress at the end of the history. Usually you will have to show him how to put on the examining gown or cape and sheet, before you leave him to disrobe.

It is a good idea to wash your hands *before* you begin your examination, especially if the patient can see you do it. It will be obvious that this act is for the *patient's* benefit. If you then wash again during or after the examination, it will look less as though it were for *your* benefit. In any event, your hands and nails should be clean.

The examiner usually begins by obtaining the "vital signs"—the temperature, pulse, and respiration rate, or TPR. The patient should be weighed while clothed, either before or after examination, unless there is a scale in the examining room for weighing him stripped.

Systematic Examination   Examiners follow a predetermined order of examination to avoid omissions. You can work out one for yourself that wastes as little time as possible and then stick to it. One common sequence closely parallels that in the review of systems.

With the patient seated on the edge of the examining table:

Head and neck
Hands, arms, shoulders
Anterior chest of men
Knee jerks
Blood pressure

With the patient sitting up, his legs on table:

Back
Back of chest

With patient lying:

Blood pressure
Anterior chest and breasts of women
Abdomen
Legs
Genitals and rectum

In more detailed examinations, other parts are worked into this sequence.

Conditions During the Examination The entire examination can—and sometimes must—be carried out with the patient lying on the examining table or bed. It is customary for the examiner to be at the patient's right side.

Throughout the examination the patient is kept covered except for the parts being examined. The room should be as quiet and private as possible. In other words, the examiner should avoid embarrassing the patient and be able to concentrate on the examination.

At first, you may find it helpful to use a checklist and to make notes during your physical examinations. Later this will be unnecessary unless you must delay writing the results.

At the beginning, one small matter makes trouble: You must keep clearly in mind which is the patient's right side and which is his left. This sounds easy, but in going from the patient's front to back, raising one leg as he sits facing you and the same while he lies down, you may become confused.

EXERCISES

1 Inspect the examining room or area that you will use. Find where the examining gowns or capes and sheets are kept, how they should be put on, and what to do with them after the examination. Learn where the thermometers, sphygmomanometer, otoscope, scale, tongue depressors, rubber gloves, and the jelly for them are kept. Note where you can write unobtrusively during the examination, where the waste can is, and where you can wash your hands. Locate disposable tissues, which a patient may need.
2 Recall and describe the posture and gait of a healthy child, an adult, a pregnant woman, and an elderly person. Describe from memory how the posture and gait are changed in a person with back pain, one with a severe stomachache, one who is blind, and someone who is drunk.
3 Recall and describe the face of a person in severe pain, one who is chronically ill, who is frightened, worried, or embarrassed.
4 Describe the handshake of a 5-year-old, a young athlete, a frightened or anxious person, a timid woman, and an 80-year-old.

2-3 EXAMINATION OF NORMAL PERSONS: GENERAL APPEARANCE, SKIN, PULSE AND BLOOD PRESSURE

The physical examination can involve many maneuvers and detect many signs of disease. Certain parts of it are generally useful—basic—and will uncover most of the evidence. This chapter introduces these basic portions and Chapter 5 discusses more detailed examinations.

Since you will be awkward at first, you will have to practice on your classmates and serve as a model for them. You will also begin to develop your concepts of what is normal in the adult; later you will extend this experience to older and younger persons. Roommates, if willing, also provide models, and the more you practice the better.

General Appearance All that you have seen and heard of the person contributes to your appraisal of his general appearance. Specifically you should notice the patient's posture and gait, facial expression, handshake, and speech and should evaluate his alertness, neatness and cleanliness, and cooperativeness. The patient's emotional state and ability to cooperate will usually be obvious. You can detect any gross evidences of disease or other difficulty, such as coughing, breathlessness, hoarseness, deformity, tremor, or paralysis. You must also evaluate his physical development and state of nutrition.

In the usual examination these observations are made piecemeal, some with the patient clothed, some after he is disrobed. It is well, however, to start learning by making the observations all together on your classmate.

EXERCISES

1 The student-models strip to their underclothes—shorts for men, panties and bra for women. The student-examiner observes the student-model standing quietly and then requests further actions to answer the following questions:

Is he well developed? Of normal size and proportions? Is the muscular development normal?

Does he appear of normal weight? Thin or emaciated? Plump or obese?

Does he appear about his stated age? Older? Younger?

Does he stand erect but at ease? Is the stance slouched or rigid?

Does his back curve slightly backward at shoulder level and forward at the waist?

Are these curves exaggerated or flattened?

Is the backbone, as shown by the groove over it, straight? Does it curve sideways in a slight S shape when he stands erect?

Are there any obvious deformities?

Does he walk easily and naturally, moving his arms freely? Is there any limping, awkward movement, or unsteadiness?

Does he sit down and get up easily?

Does he seem healthy and have good skin color?

What is his facial expression? Relaxed? Tense? Anxious? Suspicious? Deadpan?

When he shakes hands, is his grip firm? Limp? Fleeting? Too hard? Does his hand tremble? Is it cold and sweaty? Hot and dry? Unusually soft? Hard and callused?

Does your patient-model appear alert? Clean? Cooperative? Evasive? Is he clowning?

Is his voice firm and resonant and his enunciation clear? Is his voice hoarse or trembling?

Does he cough? Wheeze? Get out of breath easily?

There is no need to memorize these questions. They are designed to show you what to look for and will come to you naturally if you remember only to observe the person closely.

2 Repeat the exercise with one or more classmates. As you repeat the observations try to make them automatically and quickly without the list of questions. Then see whether you can answer them all after a brief observation.

Skin   Examination of the skin includes the entire body surface and requires good illumination. It usually is carried out piecemeal as part of the inspection of each body region. Thus the face, arms, and hands are seen first, the scalp and neck when these regions are examined, the back next, and so on. The patient need not be completely uncovered at any one time.

Inspection, as usual, is the first part of the examination. The examiner looks at the general *pigmentation,* seeking out any heavily pigmented or *depigmented* areas or evidence of tanning. He notes the character and distribution of the body and facial hair. The eyelids, palms, soles, and parts of the genital organs are truly hairless. The rest of the body is covered with short hairs. The *hirsute* (hairy) person simply has darker, thicker body hair than most. *Hirsutism* in a man means little; it is worth noting in a woman or child.

The skin surface normally is somewhat moist and glistens where it is oily, especially in areas such as the nose. You may notice excessive sweating, particularly in a relatively cool examining room, or may find the widespread, transient, small raised bumps of "gooseflesh" if the patient is really chilled.

Having completed the general inspection of an area, you then observe more closely whether there are any scars or *lesions,* circumscribed areas of abnormality or disease. These lesions may be small, flat, red spots called *macules;* raised pimples or *papules;* small collections of pus called *pustules;* or small blisters called *vesicles.* You may find scratched areas or *excoriations,* scraped areas called *abrasions,* or open, pitted sores called *ulcers.*

The lesion may be dry. It may "weep" or *exude* liquid. It may be bleeding, scabbed, or crusted with dry *exudate.* There may be small collections of fine, netlike veins without other changes.

The skin may flake or *scale;* it may "peel" (*exfoliation*). You may see a raised mass or *tumor* in the skin itself. There may be a bruise, called an *ecchymosis*, or very small areas of bleeding into the skin called *petechiae*. Between the toes there may be cracks or *fissures*. There are other lesions, but these are the most common.

Palpation of the skin begins with a determination of its texture. This varies over the body from extremely thin and fine, as on the eyelids, to the thick, coarse skin of the palms, soles, and upper back. Areas of abnormally thick, tough skin occur as *calluses*.

The texture also includes firmness which is akin to fullness or plumpness of the skin itself. Such good *turgor* contrasts with the slack skin of starvation, *dehydration*, or old age, and with the woody hardness of *induration*.

Palpation also reveals whether the skin is normally warm or unusually hot or cold. The back of the examiner's finger or hand is more sensitive to temperature than are the tips of the fingers and the palms. Since the skin cools when uncovered or heats with exercise and the temperature varies from region to region, it requires some experience to determine what is normal.

The eye may be unable to distinguish a slightly raised from a flat area, and palpating across a lesion with the fingertip lightly may be necessary to determine *elevation*. Palpating more firmly will determine *tenderness* and can also help establish the size of a skin tumor. When the tumor moves with the skin rather than remaining fixed as the skin moves over it, it is good evidence that it is in the skin.

The size of skin lesions should be estimated carefully or—better still—measured. The metric system is used most widely, but even an approximation such as "the size of a dime" is better than nothing.

EXERCISES

1   With the student-model undressed and draped for examination, the student-examiner inspects and palpates the skin. Pay particular attention to the normal variations in color, temperature, oiliness, and texture over the body. Compare the palm, back, abdomen, buttocks, anterior thigh, and eyelid. Notice also the differences in distribution of the fat in and under the skin. Compare the hair texture and color. Carefully examine any lesions and identify them by the terms used.

2   Compare the skin of a woman and a man on the palm, shoulder, outer forearm, and inner forearm. Note the difference between the sexes in skin and hair texture, thickness, and fat layer.

3   Compare the skin pigmentation of a redhead, blond, brunette, and black. Determine whether there is any variation in texture, turgor, or oiliness of the normal skin in individuals with different degrees of pigmentation.

4   Compare the normal skin of a young child or baby and of an elderly person as to texture, turgor, thickness, moisture, and oiliness. Note also any difference in the hairs on the arms.

See Section 5-1.

Pulse and Blood Pressure   The heart, of course, forces blood outward through the arteries with each beat. Each thrust momentarily raises the pressure in every artery, and to "take the pulse" is simply to palpate that thrust. It is possible to see the pulse, especially in the neck, but palpation yields much more information.

You may already know how to feel the pulse at the wrist just below the base of the thumb and probably at the temple or in the neck as well. It is important to count the beats for the *pulse rate,* but palpation tells the experienced examiner much more.

Pulse Rate and Rhythm   It is well to begin palpation of the pulse by counting the beats per minute to determine the rate. Generally any rate below 60 beats per minute is considered slow; any above 100 beats per minute abnormally fast for resting adults. Since exertion speeds the heart, it is advisable to have the patient sit or lie quietly for several minutes before counting.

The pulse rate also changes with age. The normal range of pulse rates for children is:

Age	Pulse rate, beats per min.
At birth	70–170
After delivery	120–140
1 year old	80–140
2 years old	80–130
3 years old	80–120
4 years old	70–115

The pulse normally is regular or rhythmic, but irregularities or *arrhythmias* occur. The second observation, then, is the *rhythm* as determined by feeling the regular interval between beats. Arrhythmic beats may be felt as you count the pulse. It is well, however, to feel for them without counting while you are learning.

Character of the Pulse   The remainder of the examination requires better positioning of the palpating fingers than when detecting rate and rhythm because you must feel *amplitude* or force of the beat and the *tension* between the beats. It is best to use two fingers exactly placed over the artery. As you relax the pressure of your fingers, the pulsations will seem to stop. When you press again, the pulsations will reappear; and if you increase your pressure even more, they will diminish again and fade out.

The *difference* between the pressure required to just feel the beat and the greater pressure to obliterate it is the amplitude of the pulse. The amplitude is great if the difference between these pressures is great.

The *amount* of pressure (not the difference) you must exert to obliterate the beat is the tension. If the obliterating pressure is relatively slight, the tension is low; if it is considerable, the tension is high.

It will require practice and experience to gauge amplitude and tension. You gain useful information, however, and the examination requires no instruments.

Blood Pressure You measure the blood pressure with instruments—the sphygmomanometer and the stethoscope. The former consists of an inflatable cuff made to fasten about the upper arm, a bulb to inflate it, and a gauge which indicates the pressure in the cuff. After fastening the cuff, you should rest the patient's forearm on a surface with the palm up and the elbow nearly straightened. You then palpate the inside of the elbow for the pulse there. It is about two-thirds of the arm's width from the outer side and can be felt where the skin crease crosses that point.

The chest piece—bell or diaphragm—is placed over that pulse and held firmly but without much pressure. You will hear nothing. You then inflate the cuff to about 260 mm of mercury. If you hear the heartbeat at that pressure, you inflate the cuff above the point at which the sound disappears. Watching the gauge, you release the pressure in the cuff slowly, listening carefully as it falls. You must read the gauge at the precise moment that the thump of the heartbeat is first heard. Still watching the gauge, you gradually reduce the pressure again and read the pressure when the thumping just disappears. The first of these readings is the *systolic* pressure and the second is the *diastolic* pressure. The difference between these two is the *pulse pressure.*

Sometimes the sound of the pulse fades sharply as the pressure falls but does not disappear completely until the cuff is deflated further. In that event you read the gauge at the sudden fall and again when the sound disappears. Both are considered *diastolic* readings, and this double reading may be a normal finding.

Recording the Blood Pressure To record the blood pressure, the systolic pressure is written followed by a slash (which is read as "over") and then the diastolic pressure, thus: BP 130/74. This is read as "Blood pressure 130 over 74," where 130 mm of mercury is the systolic pressure and 74 mm of mercury the diastolic.

A double diastolic reading is recorded in the same way except that the higher of the two is recorded first, followed by a comma and the lower diastolic pressure, thus: BP 130/74,52. This is read as "Blood pressure 130 over 74 and 52."

It is usually helpful to indicate in which arm the blood pressure was measured: LA for the left arm, RA for the right. Sometimes the leg is used and shown as LL or RL. To this the patient's posture may be added: L for lying, St for standing, and S for sitting. Thus BP 146/88 RAS is read "Blood pressure 146 over 88 in the right arm with the patient sitting." The pulse pressure at this reading is 58 (146 minus 88).

Precautions   Exertion increases the blood pressure, and so does tension or anxiety. You should be certain that the patient is comfortable, relaxed, and at ease when you make your measurement. It is well to have him remain quiet for several minutes before the reading.

Several precautions make the measurement easier and more accurate. The patient need not undress but the arm should be bare to the shoulder and there should be no tight clothing such as a pushed or rolled-up sleeve. The lower edge of the blood pressure cuff should be 2 or 3 inches above the skin crease, with the center of the inflatable part along the inner side of the upper arm.

If the pulse sounds cannot be heard, feel for the pulse at the wrist while you decrease the pressure in the cuff. The reading at which you first feel the beat is the systolic reading. This is usually several mm of mercury below the systolic pressure obtained by auscultation, and the diastolic pressure cannot be measured by palpation.

The ordinary cuff (12 cm wide) will bulge and give a false high reading on a thick or fat arm. There are special wide cuffs for such circumstances; but if one is not available, you can wrap a small towel or folded pillow slip firmly around the cuff already in place. The wrapping should extend at least an inch above and below the cuff. Three or four safety pins along the edge of the wrapping will hold it in place, but you must take care not to stick them through the rubber bag of the cuff.

Pediatric cuffs come in smaller sizes. The smaller the arm, the narrower the cuff must be.

EXERCISES

1 Count the pulse rate and determine whether the rhythm is regular while your subject is seated quietly. Note the amplitude and tension of the pulse. Have the subject climb a flight of stairs or jog in place for 1 min. Count the pulse, note the rhythm, and determine whether the amplitude or tension has changed immediately after the exertion. How long does it take for the pulse rate to return to its prior level?
2 Palpate the pulse in the temple just above the outer ends of the eyebrows and in the neck at either side of the Adam's apple. Remember to use only as much pressure as necessary for the examination.
3 While you feel the pulse, have the subject take a deep breath and then "bear

down" as though to move the bowels. What happens to the rate, rhythm, amplitude, and tension? This is actually called a *normal arrhythmia* (really a change of rate), and it may be felt in some people as they breathe normally. It should not be taken as a sign of disease.

4 Measure the blood pressure of a classmate while he is sitting quietly, lying down, and standing. Measure it in both right and left arms, writing it down with the position and arm shown. Determine the systolic pressure by palpation and then by auscultation so that you can compare the readings.

5 Feel the pulse while the cuff pressure is about midway between systolic and diastolic readings. Note especially the amplitude of the pulse. Inflate above the systolic reading. What happens to the tension?

6 Take the blood pressure in the right arm with the subject seated. Tell him to clench his left fist tightly and push hard with it against the tabletop. Record the blood pressure before, during, and just after this action.

7 With the cuff in place but the gauge detached, have the subject walk briskly 20 ft or so. Reattach the gauge and record the blood pressure just after the exertion.

8 Determine the systolic pressure, set the pressure in the cuff 10 to 20 mm of mercury above this, and—while still listening—prick the subject with a pin. Try it again with the pressure 40 to 50 mm of mercury above the systolic reading.

9 Inflate the cuff above the systolic level and leave it there for 1 min by your watch. Note the color of the forearm and fingertips and ask the subject what sensations he has. Deflate the cuff and wait a few minutes. Inflate the cuff to about halfway between the systolic and diastolic pressures for 2 min and repeat the observations. This may help explain why you should learn to take the blood pressure smoothly and quickly. (See Section 5-1.)

2-4 HEAD AND NECK

Skull and Scalp Inspection of the face will show any deformities, and having the patient open his mouth wide will exaggerate any defect of the jaws. Inspection of the scalp includes the hair distribution and color. If the patient is wearing a wig or hairpiece, it should be removed. Tinted or dyed hair usually shows its true color next to the scalp but away from the part, which is frequently "touched up." Separating the hair so that the scalp shows where the growth is thickest will show the hair's natural color. The hair, rolled between the fingers, can be felt as fine or coarse.

Skull You should palpate the skull beneath the scalp to detect any bony irregularities, masses, softened areas, or tenderness. Infants less than 2 months old have two *fontanels,* or soft spots, where the separate platelike bones have not yet fused to form the single skull (see Figure 2-1). The smaller *posterior* or back fontanel lies in the midline just where the top of the skull curves downward toward the neck. It closes before the larger *anterior* or front fontanel, which is on top of the skull in the midline

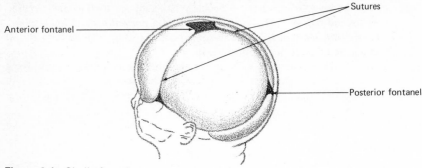

Figure 2-1 Skull of newborn.

and toward but well above the forehead. This often remains palpable until the age of 2. You can usually feel a slight ridge connecting these two areas up to 6 months of age or even later.

In young infants ridges may also run down along the sides of the skull from each fontanel. Another runs from the anterior fontanel down the middle of the forehead. These normal ridges are the *sutures* where the skull plates will knit together into one bone. Adults may retain these normal, palpable ridges long after the sutures have knit.

The fontanels are palpably soft and the anterior one may pulsate slightly as the heart beats. When the baby cries, you may see or feel the fontanel bulge with each forceful *expiration.* It collapses again as the baby sucks in its breath in *inspiration.*

See Section 5-2.

Ears   The basic examination of the ears begins with a crude test of hearing. This often involves holding a watch near the ear and moving it away until it is no longer heard. If your own hearing is normal, you can then compare this to your own hearing similarly tested.

Inspection may include only the outer ear and the canal leading inward from it. Any pus, blood, crusting, or clotting can be seen in those parts.

You will usually inspect within the canal when examining children and even adults. This requires the use of an *otoscope,* an instrument with a *speculum* or funnel-shaped part to fit into the *external auditory canal* and with a light source. Most otoscopes have a lens to magnify what is seen. Specula come in several sizes; select the one that just fits comfortably into the auditory canal and then secure it to the otoscope head.

The canal can be examined more easily if the external ear is pulled firmly away from the head, toward the top and back of the head. You must pull hard enough to straighten the slightly curved auditory canal.

With the otoscope light on and aimed down the speculum, gently introduce the tip of the speculum into the canal, pointing the tip slightly forward and downward. It is never wise to use force or to move the speculum forward into the canal unless you can see it open ahead of the tip. The normal canal contains some dark brownish or orange wax called *cerumen* along its walls. Not infrequently there is enough wax to block—partially or completely—the canal, so that you can see nothing. A cerumen plug cannot be pushed aside and you will hurt the patient if you force it inward with the speculum. It must be removed if an otoscopic examination is essential.

If there is no cerumen plug, the tip of the speculum should pass easily a little way along the smooth red canal walls until the eardrum, or *tympanic membrane,* comes into view. It is normally a glistening pearly or pinkish disc which bows inward away from you very slightly except for a whitish ridge running from its center to its upper forward edge. You get a complete view of this membrane by gently angling the tip of the speculum rather than trying to push it inward (see Figure 5-1).

The ear can be examined with the otoscope in an adult who is sitting, standing, or lying. Usually the last is easiest unless the ear is about the level of your eye. A struggling child presents more of a problem, especially since you can damage the canal or tympanic membrane if a sudden lunge by the patient jams the speculum inward. You may need someone to help you by holding the child and his head. You then hold the otoscope so that you can prop two fingers of the hand grasping it against the child's skull. The instrument will then move with his head.

EXERCISES

1 Examine the skull and scalp of several of your classmates. Pay particular attention to the color, texture, density, and distribution of the scalp hair. Palpate the skull carefully to see whether you can detect the closed suture lines at any point.
2 If possible, examine the skull of an infant of 6 months or so. Gently palpate the sutures and fontanels.
3 Examine the ears of your classmates. If you use the otoscope, try it with and without the lens. Do not try to remove any cerumen. Pay particular attention to the angle at which you best see the tympanic membrane. Note its color, contour, and sheen.

Eyes Complete examination of the eyes requires complicated equipment, but the more basic parts can be done with a flashlight. Vision can be tested roughly, for example, by having the patient read newsprint at about 15 in. Each eye is tested separately as the patient is asked to cover first one eye and then the other (with his hand). It is well to test without glasses and then with them if the patient uses them. If the vision is really bad, you can ask the patient to count the number of fingers you hold up, testing each eye separately.

In examining the eye itself, the lids should be inspected first to notice whether they droop unnaturally and blink at a normal rate. You scan the margins of the lids for evidence of crusting or pus and then pull the lower lid gently downward to expose the shining, red, moist membrane called the *conjunctiva*. This membrane also covers the white of the eye or *sclera*. The color of the conjunctiva on the lower lid is important and you should also notice whether it is smooth. The color of the sclera should also be noted. It varies somewhat between normal individuals. The fine vessels ordinarily are not very prominent. When networks of them can be seen, the sclera is said to be *injected*.

With the patient looking straight ahead, a quick glance will tell whether the eyes are steady or whether they wobble, and whether one eye turns inward, outward, upward, or downward. Another glance from the side of the patient will show whether the eyeballs are unusually prominent or somewhat retracted. There is a wide range of normal in the position of the eyeballs and you will have to develop experience in judging it.

To test the eye movements, you hold up a finger or a lighted flashlight and ask the patient to follow it with his eyes. Many times you will have to remind the patient again and again to keep looking at your movement and not to turn his head.

You watch the patient's eyes and, with your hand about 2 ft in front of the patient's face, move your finger or light smoothly and fairly rapidly to the right, then to the left (or the reverse). You stop your hand when the eyes reach the extreme gaze to the right or left. At that point you pause and look closely at the eyes. Normally the eyeballs should both follow your hand smoothly and together, not one lagging behind the other. Beginning with your hand in the center position again, you swing it straight upward and then straight downward, always watching the eyes.

To test how the eyes *converge* or come together, you move your hand directly from the front of the patient's face to 3 or 4 ft away and then advance it toward his nose, still watching the eyes. These will "cross" or turn inward together until your finger or light is near the nose when one eye stops moving or swings outward. This usually occurs at less than six inches.

Now turn your attention to the clear, glasslike *cornea*, the colored *iris* behind it, and the black *pupil* in the center. Note whether the cornea is clear and glistening, whether the iris has a fairly uniformly distributed color, and whether there is any blood or pus in the watery liquid behind the cornea. Compare the size of the two pupils, which should be the same, and then check whether each pupil is round with smooth margins or irregular.

If the room is light, darken it for a moment, turn on your flashlight, and sweep the beam from the side of each eye into the pupil. It should have *dilated* or gotten larger in the dark and briskly *contracted* as the light entered it. This reaction should be about the same in each eye. You will notice that both pupils contract no matter which eye is lighted, but both should be tested. This test, incidentally, will always detect the most perfect artificial eye.

A substitute test is used if the room cannot be darkened, but it is less satisfactory. Cover with your hands both the patient's eyes for a moment and then quickly uncover one eye while you watch the pupil. After replacing that hand for a moment, quickly uncover the other eye.

Sometimes the normally black pupil will appear whitish either in the room's light or in the flashlight's beam. This almost always means that the eye has an opaque *cataract* in the *lens* behind the pupil. If the pupil flashes red in the flashlight's beam, it is a normal finding.

EXERCISES

1 Estimate roughly the vision of your classmates, checking the two eyes separately.
2 Check the eyelids, conjunctiva, sclera, and prominence of your classmates' eyes. Pay particular attention to the redness of the conjunctiva, the color and blood vessels of the sclera.
3 Determine the range of eye movements of a classmate, noting the point at which convergence is lost. Carry out the maneuver several times until the movements of your hand are smooth, natural, and fairly rapid.
4 Examine the cornea, iris, and pupils of a classmate, including the pupils' reactions to light. Look at enough normal pupils in several intensities of light to form a good idea of the size under various conditions.

See Section 5-2.

Nose   The simple examination of the nose includes examination of the nostrils for watery liquid and thick *mucus* and for a discharge containing blood or pus. Any crusts or scabs at the edge of the nostrils should also be noted.

Then ask the patient to tip his head back slightly and place the fingers of your hand on the subject's forehead so that you can raise the tip of his nose with your thumb. Shining the flashlight up one nostril, you can see the *nasal septum,* a firm partition dividing the two sides of the *nasal cavity.* It should lie in the midline but often *deviates* or bulges to the right or left. The septum and indeed the entire chamber is lined with a moist, pink, shiny *mucous membrane.* If the nasal tip is reasonably flexible and the nostril fairly large, the front end of the *inferior turbinate* can be seen—the lower of two or three curved bony plates that protrude from the side of each nasal cavity and almost reach the septum. This turbinate normally is covered with pink and moist mucous membrane (see Figure 2-2).

After inspecting both sides of the nose, hold one nostril closed and ask the patient to blow gently through it. Then repeat the maneuver with the other nostril to test for any *obstruction.* With experience you can tell from the flow of air and the effort the patient makes in exhaling whether one or both sides of the nose are partially or completely obstructed. The maneuver, of course, does not reveal the cause of the obstruction.

Mouth and Pharynx Inspection of the mouth begins with the lips, where you note the color and search for any crusts or ulcers. You also look for redness and *fissures* or "cracking," especially at the outer angles of the lips.

The patient is asked to open his mouth wide, but not so wide as possible, and to keep his tongue in. You use a tongue depressor in one hand and a flashlight in the other. With the tongue depressor, push the inner side of one cheek outward so that you see the mucous membrane there. Then sweep the tongue depressor over the lower lip to depress it, exposing its mucous membrane. Examine the inside of the other cheek as you did the first, then tip back the patient's head and inspect the *hard palate,* the bony roof of the mouth. You are looking for any lesions on the normally smooth, pink, and shiny mucous membrane.

You inspect the teeth and gums next, using the tongue depressor to push the cheeks, tongue, and upper and lower lips out of the way. Watch for lesions on the gums and for missing, broken, or grossly decayed teeth. Any loose teeth can be identified by trying to "wobble" them with the tongue depressor or a finger.

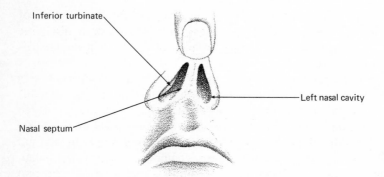

Inferior turbinate

Left nasal cavity

Nasal septum

Figure 2-2 Nose seen through nares.

If the patient has false teeth, note this and ask the patient to remove them so that the mucous membrane and gums can be inspected. The teeth can then be replaced immediately.

Lesions on mucous membranes are similar to those on the skin except that the thin, moist membrane tends to break down and form an ulcer rather than to show a pustule or vesicle. The ulcer usually has a ragged, whitish bed with a slightly raised, reddened border.

To examine the tongue, ask the patient to stick it out. The upper surface is covered with hundreds of tiny projections which normally give it a "velvety" look. These projections may be long, so as to produce a *hairy tongue,* or much reduced in size and number on a *smooth tongue.* The sides and tip normally are smooth and deserve special attention, since ulcers of the tongue usually appear there.

Ask the patient to put the tip of his tongue on the roof of his mouth. This exposes the mucous membrane under the tongue (see Figure 2-3). The thin partition fastening the tongue to the floor of the mouth is the *frenulum.* On either side of it, near the floor, is the opening of one *salivary duct* in a tiny red hillock of tissue. You may see saliva welling up from this duct.

Examination of the back of the mouth and *pharynx* or throat requires some cooperation from the patient. This can be difficult with children. To make the examination easy, the patient must open his mouth wide, keeping the tongue relaxed and in the floor of the mouth. If the tongue is rigid, the depressor will shove it backward and gag the patient. The depressor should encounter little resistance as it is pushed downward on the center of the tongue and then on either side of the midline.

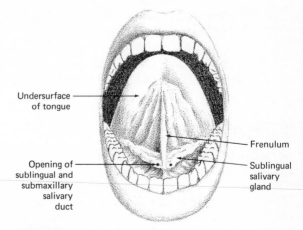

Figure 2-3 Area under the tongue.

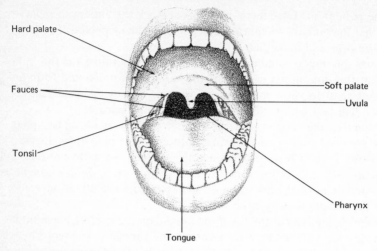

Figure 2-4 Mouth and pharynx.

The posterior or back boundary of the mouth is made up of the base of the tongue below, the *soft palate* above, and a sweeping arc of tense tissue, the *fauces,* on either side (see Figure 2-4). The soft palate is somewhat floppy when relaxed and moves upward when the patient says "ah." From its center hangs a limp, fingerlike *uvula.*

The fauces really consist of two folds, one behind the other, on either side. Between these two is the *tonsil,* a rather pebbled, brownish or pinkish cushion of tissue.

The pharynx lies behind the fauces, and between them you can see its posterior wall. This usually is pink and smooth, though it is commonly somewhat yellowish or red and pebbled with small, smooth nodules in smokers. This appearance is called *granular.*

You can inspect these areas by using the tongue depressor to expose them to view. With the depressor in the center of the tongue, have the patient say "ah" so that you can see whether the soft palate moves well. This also exposes more of the posterior pharyngeal wall to inspection.

EXERCISES

1   Examine the noses of several classmates. Try to see the tip of the inferior turbinate and its relation to the nasal septum. Test the nose for obstruction, having the subject vary the force with which he exhales. Listen or feel for the force of the airstream and watch him to judge how forcibly he is exhaling.

2   Examine the mouths and pharynges of several classmates. Pay attention to the surface of the tongue, to the appearance of the tonsils, and to the posterior

pharynx. If one has had his tonsils out, note how this changes the appearance of the fauces.
3   Use the tongue depressor properly to expose the pharynx. Then have the subject hold his tongue firm and try again. Note how well the pharynx is exposed as well as your subject's reaction to the maneuver. When you are comfortable using the depressor, ask the subject to open his mouth and then pass the depressor straight back until it gently bumps the posterior pharyngeal wall. Note the result.

See Section 5-2.

Neck   The neck is a compact but complex region. Its examination begins with inspection of the skin. You then ask the patient to tilt his head as far forward as possible, then backward as far as possible; to rotate it as far to the right and to the left as he can without moving his shoulders; and finally to tilt it to the right and to the left. These maneuvers determine the *range of active motion.*

The examiner can take the patient's head in his hands and carry out the same movements while the patient relaxes completely. This determines the *range of passive motion.* You should not carry out these maneuvers, of course, on a patient with injuries about the head, neck, or upper back.

You palpate the side of the neck to detect any masses, which are often enlarged *lymph nodes.* These nodes occur in chains or groups, one of which lies just behind and below the angle of the jaw. To palpate them, you tilt the patient's head slightly backward and away from the side to be examined. You then rather firmly run your fingertips backward and forward just below the angle of the jaw.

As you do this, you can feel, behind the angle of the jaw, a column of muscle running from just behind the ear downward and forward to the collarbone. The *anterior chain* of lymph nodes runs downward just behind this muscle in its middle half. The *posterior chain* lies farther back behind it.

You then continue palpation for the nodes by sweeping your fingertips downward just behind the muscle. The fingertips are later moved backward and forward behind the lower half of the muscle.

Normal lymph nodes cannot be palpated, but there are other normal irregularities which can be. It is important, therefore, that you carefully palpate normal necks so that you will not mistake the normal structures.

The balance of the neck should be palpated for tumors. At first you will find the same difficulty in doing this, so you should be familiar with the feel of the normal structures. The most prominent of these is the *larynx,* voice box, or Adam's apple. You can feel it easily as an irregular, hard object in the midline of the neck. Continuing down from it into the chest is the *trachea* or windpipe. It is best palpated when the patient's head is thrown back. By pressing firmly and deeply on either side of the larynx, you can feel the pulse of the *carotid artery* running up to the head.

Back   A simple examination of the back can be carried out with the patient sitting. By inspecting and palpating downward along the processes of the spine, you can detect any gross *curvature* and tenderness. The curvature may be an S-shaped curve when the spine deviates to the side, a bowing backward, an increased curvature forward, or a combination of these.

When one leg is shorter than the other, the spine will curve as long as the patient stands flat-footed. This will disappear when he sits. The movements of the spine are also best seen with the patient standing. You ask him to bend as far forward as he can, then backward while you provide support by placing your hand on the small of his back. You ask the patient to bend from one side to the other and finally to rotate his shoulders to right and left while standing erect. It is best to anchor the *pelvis* or hipbones with your hands so that the rotation is in the spine and not the hips. You should observe carefully for curvature as the patient bends forward, since this may make the change more obvious.

The skin of the back is important, especially if the patient is wasted and has been long abed. You can roll him to one side to look in the region of the buttocks, the shoulder blades, and the spinous processes. You may find a reddened or somewhat purple area where the part presses the bed. This discoloration can progress to form a large ulcer—the *bed sore.*

The back of an infant has quite a different shape, with the spine almost straight. As the child walks and grows, the spine becomes more and more adult in contour.

EXERCISES

1   Examine the necks of your classmates, paying particular attention to the area where the lymph nodes occur.
2   Find the carotid pulse and trace it upward and downward as far as you can. Be careful not to press it so hard that you *occlude* or block it.
3   Examine the back of a classmate, paying particular attention to the shape and flexibility of the spine.
4   Have the subject raise one heel about 1 in off the floor so that he stands on the ball of that foot and the full sole of the other. What happens to the shape of the spine? Place one hand on each hipbone, keeping the palms down and resting the base of each index finger on the bone. Does this make it evident that one leg is now "longer" than the other?

5 If possible, examine the back of an infant who is being held upright, back toward you, by grasping the child under the arms.
6 If possible, examine the back of a healthy elderly person, paying particular attention to the flexibility of the spine. You can use palpation without having the subject undress.

See Section 5-2.

2-5 THE CHEST

The chest begins at the root of the neck and continues down to the *diaphragm,* a pistonlike sheet of muscle across the entire body about the level of the lower end of the breastbone. The chest walls have a skeleton of twelve ribs on either side attached posteriorly to twelve *vertebrae* or backbones. Anteriorly, ten of these ribs attach to the *sternum* or breastbone; the two lowest ribs have free anterior tips. Between the ribs are sheets of muscle, and attaching to them are muscles of the neck, shoulders, arms, back, and abdomen, many involved in the movements of *respiration.*

Respiration   When a person *inspires,* the diaphragm contracts or shortens. This pulls it downward, changing it from an upward-bulging

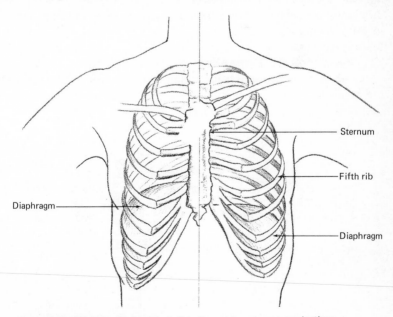

Figure 2-5   Thorax. Right side (left in figure) in extreme expiration; left side in full inspiration.

dome toward a flat sheet shape. The muscles of the chest wall also contract, lifting the ribs and rotating them outward with the attachments to the vertebrae acting as pivots. The sternum then has to move upward and outward (see Figure 2-5).

To *expire* quietly, a person simply relaxes the muscles. The contents of the abdomen push the diaphragm up into a dome shape again and the rib cage collapses downward and inward. In forced expiration, some of the muscles between the ribs help pull them down and inward, aided in this by muscles deep in the back. The muscles of the abdominal walls contract and force the abdominal contents upward to bulge the diaphragm more forcefully.

Lungs   Within the chest or *thorax* lie the two *lungs,* the right divided into three separate parts or *lobes,* the left into two. The trachea enters the thorax from above, and at about midchest it divides into the left and right *bronchi* (see Figure 2-6). From the right bronchus, secondary bronchi open into the *right upper lobe,* the *right middle lobe,* and the *right lower lobe.* Similarly, the left bronchus sends secondary bronchi to the *left upper lobe* and *left lower lobe.* Each lobe with its bronchus is discrete, separate from its neighbors.

Further subdivisions of the lung within the lobes are less discrete, but into each part go finer and finer branches from the bronchus. The smallest branches are called *bronchioles,* and from these open tiny, air-filled *sacs* or *alveoli* (see Figure 2-7).

Variations in Respiration   As the chest expands during inspiration, air rushes down the trachea and bronchi until it enters the air sacs.

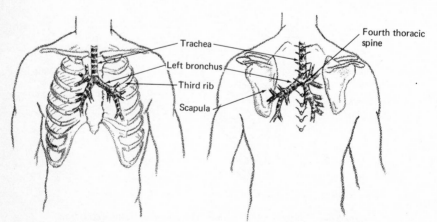

Figure 2-6   Trachea and bronchi.

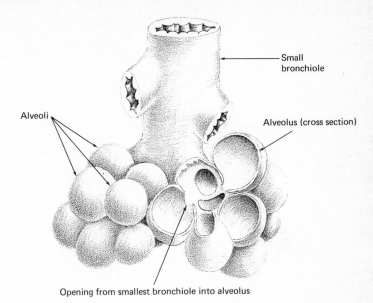

Small
bronchiole

Alveoli

Alveolus (cross section)

Opening from smallest bronchiole into alveolus

Figure 2-7   Bronchioles and alveoli.

During expiration, the air retraces this route. Ordinarily respiration—inspiration plus expiration—is repeated fourteen to eighteen times per minute for an adult resting and at ease. Infants normally breathe more rapidly, with a respiration rate as high as forty in the newborn. Young children may breathe more than twenty times per minute even when quiet.

It is common experience that exertion increases the respiratory rate and breathing becomes deep as well as rapid. Fever, pain, and anxiety will speed respiration as well, but inspiration is usually not so deep and may be quite shallow. You should note whether rapid breathing is deep or shallow and whether it is *labored,* with evidence of the neck muscles contracting, or quiet.

A cough is an explosive expiration which clears the trachea and bronchi of mucus or other material in them. A sigh is simply a slow, deep inspiration and expiration. A yawn is a slow inspiration with the mouth wide open.

Heart and Great Blood Vessels   The heart occupies most of the chest outside the lungs. It lies just above the diaphragm near the anterior chest wall, behind the sternum and extending beyond it to the left farther than to the right. The great *veins* bring the blood to the heart, and two large *arteries* carry the blood from it.

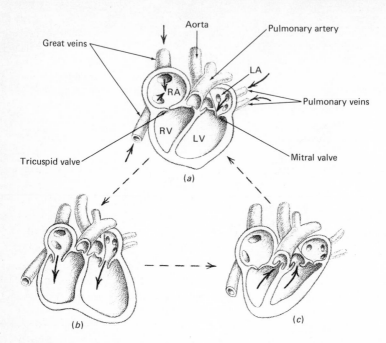

Figure 2-8 Cardiac cycle (diagrammatic). (*a*) Atria and ventricles in diastole; blood entering from great veins and pulmonary veins; aortic and pulmonic valves closed. (*b*) Atria in systole, ventricles in diastole; tricuspid and mitral valves open. (*c*) Ventricles in systole, atria in diastole; aortic and pulmonic valves open; tricuspid and mitral valves closed.
RA, right atrium; RV, right ventricle; LA, left atrium; LV, left ventricle.

The heart is essentially a double sac of muscle with no direct communication between its right and left *chambers.* Each side in turn has two chambers, but these are connected with one another through a large opening. The one chamber, the *atrium* or *auricle,* has thin muscular walls; the other, the *ventricle,* has muscular walls several times as thick (see Figure 2-8).

Circulation   Blood coming from the lungs by way of the *pulmonary veins* flows into the *left atrium* while its muscular wall is relaxed or "in diastole." When this wall contracts "in *systole,*" the *left ventricle* is in diastole with relaxed walls ready to receive the blood. The atrial contraction forces the blood through the open *mitral valve* into the ventricle. This valve has two thin but tough leaves which passively flap back out of the way to let the blood flow from the atrium.

When it is filled, the ventricle goes into systole; that is, its wall contracts. The pressure promptly flaps shut the leaves of the mitral valve so that the blood cannot escape back into the atrium. At the same time another valve, this with three leaves and called the *aortic valve,* is pushed open by the blood as it is forced into the body's main artery, the *aorta.*

The aorta leads the blood through smaller and smaller *arteries* until it reaches the microscopic blood vessels called *capillaries.* Tiny *veins* collect the blood from the capillaries and join other veins until they form one of two great veins—one from the top, the other from the bottom of the body—leading into the heart.

These veins empty the blood into the *right atrium* during atrial diastole. Atrial systole then forces this blood into the *right ventricle,* which is in diastole. The opening from the right atrium into the right ventricle is guarded by the *tricuspid valve,* so called because it has three leaves. It functions on the right, as does the mitral on the left side of the heart. As the right ventricle contracts during systole, the pressure closes the tricuspid valve and pushes open the three-leafed *pulmonary valve* leading into the *pulmonary artery.* When the ventricle enters diastole and the pressure within it falls, the pulmonary valve, like the aortic valve, is snapped shut by the pressure in the great arteries.

The pulmonary· artery, by way of smaller and smaller branches, delivers its blood to the capillaries of the lung and nowhere else. From these pulmonary capillaries the pulmonary veins carry blood back again to the left atrium (see Figure 2-9).

Heartbeat   The normal heart beats rhythmically and has a regular cycle of activity. In this the right and left sides of the heart act almost simultaneously or *synchronously.* This is true even though the blood cannot pass directly from one side to the other.

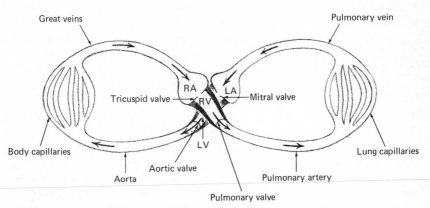

Figure 2-9 Diagram of circulation. RA, RV, right atrium and ventricle; LA, LV, left atrium and ventricle.

The cycle runs as follows: (1) right and left atria in diastole with the right and left ventricles relaxing; (2) both atria contracting, opening the tricuspid and mitral valves with the ventricles relaxed in diastole; (3) ventricles contracting as the atria relax, closing the tricuspid and mitral valves and opening the pulmonary and aortic valves; (4) ventricles relaxing in diastole so that the pulmonary and aortic valves snap shut; (5) both atria and ventricles relaxed until the two atria again contract as the cycle repeats (see Figure 2-8).

The heart valves snap shut with some force and, being tough but thin, they vibrate. Vibration produces sounds, and the sounds of the valves closing are heard by an examiner during auscultation as the *heart sounds.*

EXERCISES

1 Define the limits of the thorax. As seen during examination, should the right and left sides be symmetrical? Is the internal arrangement of the organs symmetrical? Why or why not?

2 Describe the act of quiet respiration, naming the structures involved. How does this differ from forced or strenuous respiration? What substance fills the lungs normally?

3 Trace the flow of blood through the heart, body, and lungs beginning with a drop in the great toe and ending its circuit there. Why has the circulation been described as a figure-eight loop?

4 Define systole and diastole. What occurs in the chamber of an atrium during diastole? During systole? What occurs to the muscular wall of the ventricle during diastole? During systole? Review the movements of the valves during ventricular diastole and systole.

Inspection of the Chest   Examination of the chest begins with inspection. This of course includes the skin, but specifically it begins with an evaluation of the rate, depth, and effort of respiration. You should count the rate, especially if it appears unusually slow, fast, or irregular. It is easy to judge whether the patient is drawing each breath to about the usual depth—whether the breaths are shallow or unusually deep. It is also a simple matter to recognize quiet respiration and to detect labored or forced respiration which actively uses the neck and abdominal muscles. It is important to note whether the patient is straining during inspiration, expiration, or both. This is also a good point at which to note whether the lips or nail beds are bluish or *cyanotic.*

The next step is to evaluate the *symmetry* of the thorax. In evaluating this, the comparative heights of the two shoulders provide a lead, as does the shape of the spine. The relative size of the two sides of the chest can often be best judged if the patient is viewed from the side. At the same time, it is well to note whether one side moves more in respiration than does the other.

Inspection will also disclose whether the chest is of a size appropriate to the patient's build. Again, a side view is best for determining the depth of the chest or *anterior-posterior diameter* from the sternum to the back. You can also judge from the side how well the chest expands when the patient takes a deep breath.

Here palpation will help if you stand behind a seated patient or at the head of one lying down. You can place your hands over his shoulders with palms down on either side of the anterior chest wall. Your thumbs should rest on the upper part of his sternum, with your fingers spread so that the little fingers reach downward and to the side. You will feel your fingers rise upward and outward during inspiration, even without forced respiration.

During your inspection you should note any deformities or masses. You should palpate these as well, especially to determine whether a mass is hard or soft and whether you can move it with the skin, under it, or not at all. At the same time, any *pulsations* that occur away from the region of the heart should be noted. Such pulsations are most apt to be on the anterior chest wall and are best seen from the side or with side lighting.

The region over the heart, or *precordium,* normally shows the pulsation of the heart. You will have to lift a large breast upward to see this, and a fat chest wall obscures it. You can see it best with the patient sitting up or even leaning forward. Even when easily seen, the normal pulsation is over an area only about the size of a dime or a quarter. It looks like a brisk heave, almost like a tap from within. You should note whenever the *precordial pulsation* can be seen over a larger area or when it is anything other than a single brief thrust for each heartbeat. In infants and young children with thin chest walls, however, the normal pulsation looks stronger and more diffuse.

The center of the precordial pulsation indicates a point called the *PMI* or *point of maximal impulse* of the heart (see Figure 2-10). This varies in position with posture and body build, but normally it lies on or inside the *MCL* or *midclavicular line.* This is an imaginary line dropped straight down from the center of the *clavicle* or collarbone. To locate this center, feel for the inner end of the clavicle where it joins the sternum. You can find this end by moving the patient's left shoulder forward as you palpate the joint. The outer end is located by palpating along the front edge of the clavicle until a bony notch is felt at the shoulder. Halfway between this notch and the joint with the sternum is the center of the clavicle. In men the MCL will usually pass through the nipple area.

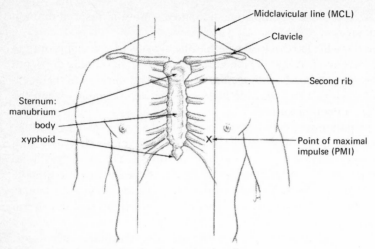

Figure 2-10 Landmarks of anterior chest wall.

EXERCISES

1 Examine by inspection the thoraxes of your classmates. Locate the MCL whether or not you can see the precordial pulsation. Inspect that pulsation with the subject (*a*) standing or sitting and (*b*) lying down.
2 Count the subject's respirations for 1 minute: then have him run upstairs or engage in some other activity that produces breathlessness. Count the respirations for 30 seconds immediately and again at 2-minute intervals until they return to the original rate. Also note the depth and effort of respiration immediately after the exertion.
3 Repeat the observations, but instead of using an exercise, have the subject hold his breath as long as he can.
4 Compare by inspection and palpation the relative chest wall movement of your subject during quiet breathing, shallow breathing, maximal breathing, coughing, and sighing.

Palpation of the Chest Palpation of the chest aids inspection of the skin and of any deformities. It also helps identify *landmarks,* as in locating the MCL.

On the posterior thoracic wall the most prominent landmarks are the tips of the *vertebral spines,* running down the center of the back, and the *scapula* or shoulder blade on either side (see Figure 2-11). It is easy to palpate the lower tip or *pole* of the roughly triangular scapula and then to run the fingers up along the *medial* edge nearest the spine. At about the level of the shoulder joint, there is a crosswise or *transverse* ridge, the

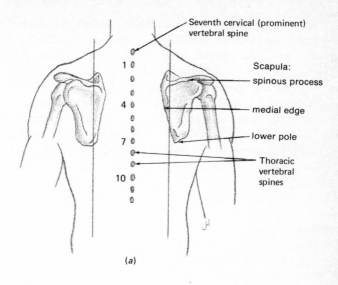

Seventh cervical (prominent) vertebral spine

Scapula:
spinous process

medial edge

lower pole

Thoracic vertebral spines

1

4

7

10

(a)

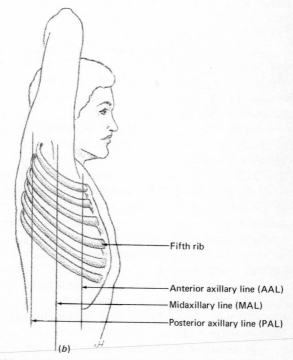

Fifth rib

Anterior axillary line (AAL)

Midaxillary line (MAL)

Posterior axillary line (PAL)

(b)

Figure 2-11 Landmarks of (a) posterior and (b) lateral chest walls.

spinous process of the scapula. It may feel as though it were the top of the bone, but in fact it is not. The location of signs on the posterior thorax can be described roughly in relation to the spine, the lower pole of the scapula, and the scapula's spinous process.

On the *lateral* or side aspect of the thorax the most commonly used landmarks can be seen. The *axilla* or armpit has an anterior fold of skin when the arm is slightly raised. An imaginary line dropped straight down from this is the *anterior axillary line* or *AAL*. An imaginary line dropped from the center of the axilla is the *midaxillary line* or *MAL*. The *posterior axillary line* is less used but corresponds to the anterior axillary line.

Breast   The human breast consists largely of fat except in pregnant or nursing women. Men and children have a small amount of *glandular tissue* just under the nipple. The mature woman has glandular tissue, capable of forming milk, throughout the breast. This glandular tissue is active during pregnancy and *lactation* or milk formation, when it fills most of the enlarged breasts.

Palpation of the breasts is carried out chiefly to detect tumors and begins with the patient seated. The nipple area and the breast immediately behind it are palpated between the thumb and forefinger for tenderness, tumors, or discharge from the nipple.

After examining both nipple areas, ask the patient to lie down with her arms at her sides. A small pillow under the shoulder of the side to be examined helps the breast to spread more evenly over the chest wall. If you have no pillow, you can hold the patient in position by slipping a hand under her shoulder.

Palpation is best carried out with a firm but gentle stroking movement of the four fingers—palm down—held flat against the chest wall. You begin at the midaxillary line on the level of the top of the breast, well above the nipple. Your fingers then move toward the sternum, feeling the tissue beneath them. The sweep is repeated from the MAL to the center of the breast, each time with the fingers below their previous level. The palpation then is repeated, stroking from the sternum laterally so that the entire breast is examined.

It is well to ask the patient to raise her arm while you repeat the palpation, especially if the breast is large. Afterward you lower the arm almost completely and slide your fingers up along the chest wall deep into the axilla. Fingertip palpation there will detect enlarged lymph nodes, but you will have to palpate normal axillae in order not to mistake normal structures for nodes.

An identical examination is then carried out on the opposite breast and axilla. You should note any masses, any tenderness, and the *consistency* of the breast. This consistency changes from that of fatty tissue to a firmer, "granular" feel in pregnancy and lactation. The breast tissue feels "lumpy" at these times, especially in thin women.

The breasts of many normal women become tender in the few days before each *menstrual period.* Such breasts usually feel "shotty" or granular at that time.

Respiratory Signs Palpation of the chest for changes in the lungs, trachea, and bronchi is essentially feeling for events inside the chest wall. This is possible because air transmits vibrations and these vibrations can be felt. It is best to press firmly on the chest wall with your palm, just at the base of your fingers, or with the side of your hand just below the little finger.

The rattling of mucus within the trachea or bronchi produces palpable vibrations. They are usually felt best between the scapular poles and the spine but sometimes above or below that point. You should ask the patient to breathe slowly and deeply while you palpate. You may have to press so firmly that you must support a weak patient with one hand on the chest while you palpate the back with the other.

Voiced sounds, unlike whispered ones, are produced by the vibrating vocal cords in the larynx. The vibration is carried downward as well as upward and outward, because there is a continuous body of air down the trachea and bronchi into the air sacs that make up most of the lung. At the outer boundary of the lung these vocal vibrations are strong enough to be felt through the chest wall unless it is very fat. The deeper voices of men cause stronger vibrations than do the higher voices of women. Children generally have thin chest walls and so transmit the vibrations strongly.

Anything that increases the distance between the vibrating air sacs and the palpating hand will weaken or completely suppress the sensation felt. Not only fat in the wall but air or liquid inside the chest cavity but outside the lung can interfere. So too can anything that blocks a bronchus.

The palpable vibrations produced by speech are called *vocal fremitus.* Fremitus varies in intensity from top to bottom of the chest, but it is normally as strong on one side as on the other except, of course, where the heart blocks it.

You can best palpate vocal fremitus with the palm or side of your hand, and your examination must be systematic. You ask the patient to say "ninety-nine" in a reasonably loud voice and to repeat it at the same level of sound. Patients tend to use a weaker and weaker voice unless reminded. Each time the patient pauses, you can shift the palpating hand.

Starting at the top of the chest, you palpate first one side and then the corresponding area on the opposite side. You move your hand downward and repeat the symmetrical palpation. The aim is to compare the fremitus on the two sides over the back, front, and lateral chest walls. It is fruitless, however, to try over a woman's breasts or when the patient cannot speak loudly enough to produce palpable vibrations. Infants and small children have such thin chest walls and such small chests that changes on one side are practically undetectable.

Cardiac Signs You palpate the precordium to detect or verify the PMI, the point of maximal impulse. For this purpose your fingertips are best. You will need to press fairly firmly, especially if the chest wall is thick.

Normally you will feel a rather small, localized area which thrusts sharply as a single tap against your finger with each heartbeat. You must find the PMI and determine whether the thrusting sensation extends over a larger area; for example, whether you feel it in more than one *intercostal space* between the ribs. You should determine whether the PMI lies toward the sternum, "inside the midclavicular line," at the MCL, outside the MCL, or even at the anterior axillary line. It sometimes lies outside the AAL if the heart is very large.

If you have difficulty feeling the PMI, you may have to palpate with the patient sitting and leaning forward slightly. You may have to move a large, pendulous breast upward as well.

EXERCISES

1   With a skin-marking pencil or ballpoint pen, mark on the subject's chest wall the midclavicular line, the anterior axillary line, and the midaxillary line. Similarly, sketch the lower pole of one scapula, its medial edge, and the spinous processes. Have the subject move his arm while you palpate the scapular pole. Is it fixed in place? Is the medial edge fixed?
2   Palpate the subject's breasts and axillae. This should be done for practice even though the subject is a man. If possible, examine a woman's breasts and axillae. It will be necessary to palpate normal breasts to learn the range of normal consistency.
3   Palpate the larynx with the fingertips, the base of the fingers, and the side of the hand while the subject says "ninety-nine." Vibrations should be felt easily, and you can compare the relative sensitivity of the parts of your hand to vocal fremitus.
4   Examine the chests of several subjects for vocal fremitus, having each subject speak in a reasonably loud, uniform voice. On one subject, repeat the examination with the subject speaking in a soft voice, in a high-pitched, squeaky voice, and in as low-pitched a rumble as possible—both reasonably loud. Can you detect the differences in vocal fremitus in various parts of the thorax? What voice type gives the most pronounced fremitus? How far down the back and lateral chest wall can you feel the fremitus?
5   Palpate the precordium for fremitus. Compare this to the corresponding area on the right side. Have the subject lie on his right side, back toward you, and

examine his back for vocal fremitus. Is it symmetrical? Repeat with the subject on his left side.

6 Locate and characterize the PMI by palpation. Feel the pulse in the neck while palpating the PMI. Is the impulse synchronous in the two sites? Repeat using the pulse at the wrist and the PMI.

7 Press your fingertips against the middle of your own forehead with increasing pressure. Pay particular attention to any sensation of pulsation. Can you, at some rather firm pressure, feel a "pulse"? This is an artificial pulse introduced by the pulsations within your own fingertips. You can verify this by feeling your own PMI while you experience the "artificial pulse." The rate in the two will be identical. Are they synchronous?

See Section 5-3.

Percussion of the Chest Percussion, like palpation, requires "educated hands." You receive information by feeling as well as hearing when you use your fingers in a special way. Percussion depends upon vibrations but, unlike fremitus, the vibrations are produced by the examiner. If you tap on an object you set it in motion, at least immediately under the point where you strike it. If the object is solid and you tap it lightly, the vibrations will be too weak to be heard or felt. If the object contains liquid and has thin walls, there will be no sound other than the knock of impact, although you may feel a sort of surging pulsation. If the wall is reasonably thin and the vessel contains only a gas, such as air, your tap will produce both sound and a palpable vibration. If the wall is taut as well as thin, the sound will be higher-pitched and the vibrations will last longer.

The chest wall is thin enough to vibrate and the normal chest contains air in the lungs. *Properly* struck, the wall produces both sound and palpable vibration.

To strike the wall properly you must deliver a brisk, sharp tap and move the striking fingertip away again. Your finger will damp or deaden the vibrations if it remains in firm contact. Besides being brisk, your blow must deliver the correct force. Strike too lightly and you cannot hear or feel the vibrations. Strike too hard and you mask slight but significant changes in the vibrations. To make matters more complicated, you must strike harder in some places than in others.

Percussion Technique In the usual percussion the examiner does not strike the chest wall; he hits his own finger. This technique is used because the struck finger, held lightly against the chest, feels the vibrations without damping them and because it is easier to deliver a blow of known force in this way. You must, however, use the *struck* finger as well as the *striking* finger in a precise way. You can practice this by percussing a tabletop or a flat-topped, empty can. The description here is for a right-handed person. A left-handed examiner can easily reverse the hands.

The left hand is held palm down over the surface with the fingers slightly spread and the thumb comfortably out at the side. Only the middle finger touches the surface, and that finger only from its first joint to the end. By pressing down, which is necessary anyway, the fingertip is "bent backward" so that it makes proper contact and the remainder of the finger does not touch. This struck finger will be hit between the first joint and the nail (see Figure 2-12).

The right hand is held partly closed, the ring and little fingers curled loosely in toward the palm. The first finger and thumb are extended comfortably and relaxed, so they usually curve slightly. The middle finger is the striking finger and its position is important. It must come straight down on the struck finger at right angles to it. This means that it must be bent more than the first and less than the ring and little fingers. It is the only one held rigid.

In delivering the tap, the right wrist makes the movement. It swings the striking finger in a smooth arc, usually through about 2 in, so that the tip—not the finger's pulp—hits the struck finger. It comes down swiftly and bounces back up immediately into its original position.

You must both listen and feel for the result of each tap. You will be sensing the *pitch* of the vibrations, how strong they are, how musical they

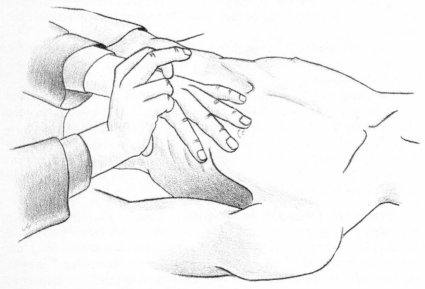

Figure 2-12   Position of hands during percussion.

are, and how long they last. These qualities let you distinguish between *resonance, dullness, flatness,* and *tympany.* It is easier to recognize these by experience than by description.

EXERCISES

1 Practice percussion using a tabletop, a freestanding blackboard, or a closed, flat-topped, air-filled container (an empty tobacco can with a plastic top will do). Try striking slowly, then briskly. Try leaving the striking finger down after it hits. Try raising the struck finger onto its tip before the blow. Try leaving the struck finger lying loosely on the table when it is hit. Can you feel as well as hear the vibrations? What do the various changes you tried do to the vibrations?

2 Percuss your subject just below the scapular pole, practicing until you get a clear, consistent sound and feel. Then try the various changes given above.

3 The following are to give you experience in the qualities discriminated by percussion. You should be certain that you percuss properly before you leave each. Try to discriminate the differences in pitch, strength, duration, and musical nature.

　　a *Resonance.* Percuss below the right or left clavicle. Percuss below the scapular pole.

　　b *Dullness.* Percuss the precordium anywhere between the PMI and the sternum.

　　c *Flatness.* Percuss the front of the thigh.

　　d *Tympany.* Percuss about 2 in below the PMI. Percuss the side of the cheek with the jaw slightly slack, the mouth slightly open, and the lips somewhat pursed.

4 When you feel that you can distinguish the quality of each area above, percuss the following and give the quality of the result:

> Over the sternum
> Side of the neck
> Right midaxillary line about nipple level
> Over the larynx with the mouth open
> On the clavicle
> Just above the right lower rib in the midaxillary line

　　Percussion Procedure In examining the chest by percussion, a systematic procedure is as important as in palpation, and for the same reason. Comparison of one side with the other makes the examination more accurate.

　　You had best begin with the back. The patient should sit with head bent forward and arms crossed. You percuss first at the level of the shoulders. As you move downward, you start at each level near the spine and, after comparing it with the corresponding spot on the opposite side, place the struck finger about 2 in farther out. At each level this continues until dullness replaces resonance or until you reach the anterior axillary line.

You should pay close attention to the sound and feel at each point, thinking in terms of relative resonance or dullness. The chest is not uniformly resonant and the two sides may differ and still be normal. A right-handed tennis player will have a somewhat less resonant right than left upper chest, for example, because his shoulder muscles are heavier and thicker on that side. You will have to learn to take such normal variations into account.

When you reach the bottom of the lungs, percussion reveals dullness. Percussing from above downward, you can outline the level of the movable diaphragm by finding the level of dullness. If the patient takes a deep breath and then holds it as you percuss, you can determine the extreme *descent* of the diaphragm. Percussion while the subject holds his breath after exhaling detects the extreme *ascent.* The distance between these two extremes is the *diaphragmatic excursion.* In practice it is measured on each side but only up and down a line midway between the spine and the posterior axillary line.

Percussion of the anterior chest wall is somewhat more complicated because the heart must be outlined, and its presence destroys the symmetry. It is easier to detect the change from resonance to dullness than the reverse. For that reason most examiners percuss from the anterior axillary line toward the sternum when outlining the heart.

The patient sits upright or lies flat with arms at sides. The percussion of the lungs begins just above the clavicles, comparing right and left sides. The comparison continues below the clavicles and then progressively downward. At first you percuss only the resonant areas, comparing those outside the *cardiac dullness.* The bottom of the right lung should be percussed as it was on the back of the chest. Here the boundary is the *upper border of the liver,* which lies just below the diaphragm on that side. If you percuss the same way just to the left of the cardiac dullness, the percussion note usually goes from resonant to tympanitic. Here the stomach lies just under the diaphragm and is tympanitic because— normally— its upper end contains an air bubble under tension.

It is easier to percuss the heart with the patient lying down, especially if a woman is being examined. You must move the breast tissue from the point you are percussing insofar as this is possible.

Percussion for cardiac dullness can begin just below the clavicle. You place the struck finger *across* the space between the ribs each time you move it, so that it always lies parallel to the sternum. The striking finger comes down just between the ribs.

To outline the heart, your percussion is light and brisk, just strong

enough to yield distinct resonance over the lung. A change to relative dullness as you approach the sternum marks the border of
cardiac dullness (see Figure 2-13). No attempt is made to compare right
to left side, and usually the entire left border is percussed before the
right.

Percussion proceeds downward in each *intercostal space* between
the ribs. If you palpate the upper end of the sternum carefully, you will
feel a notch at the top between the clavicles. A flat anterior surface facing
slightly upward lies just below this and ends in an angle. Here you can feel
the sternum bend, so that its surface faces forward. If you place one
finger on either side of this angle and palpate outward, you will find each
finger in an intercostal space with a rib between your fingers. This rib is
the second one. The upper finger is in the *first* intercostal space, or ICS 1,
the lower is in the *second,* the one just *below* the second rib. You can
palpate each space outward and by counting downward can identify the
third, fourth, and fifth intercostal spaces. These spaces are the landmarks
by which you locate the vertical position over the heart.

Percuss the border in the first, second, third, fourth, and fifth left
intercostal spaces. Normally it lies about 1 to 1 $^1/_2$ in from the middle of
the sternum in the ICS 1. Below this it swings outward to the vicinity of
the PMI in the ICS 5.

On the right you can accurately percuss from the ICS 1 through the
ICS 4 (or occasionally the ICS 5) before liver dullness interferes. The

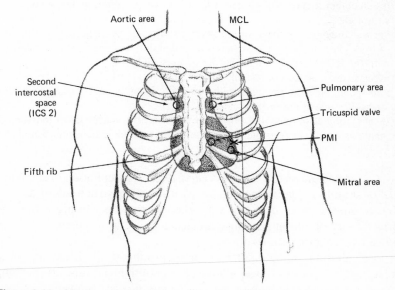

Figure 2-13 Anterior chest wall. Area of cardiac dullness shaded.
Valve areas circled.

border, however, normally is within 1 $1/2$ in of the midline and so is very near the sternal border.

Proper percussion detects the size, shape, and location of the heart. These vary even in normal people. Small people have relatively small hearts. Taller, "stringier" people with narrow chests have *vertical* hearts with left borders nearer the sternum. Squat people with broad, short chests have left borders farther to the left. A deep breath or an overdistended chest pushes lung in front of the heart along its left border and so makes the border of cardiac dullness lie closer to the sternum.

EXERCISES

1 Examine the back of the chest wall in several normal subjects, paying close attention to the percussion notes throughout. Determine the diaphragmatic excursions in each, using a ballpoint pen to mark the extremes. In measuring the distance between the marks, use the metric scale and give the distance to the nearest centimeter (cm).

2 With one subject, percuss the chest below the level of the scapular pole. Have the subject exhale as completely as he can and percuss again. Then have the subject inhale as completely as possible and repeat the percussion at the same point. Can you detect any change in resonance?

3 Percuss the back of the chest wall with a subject sitting in the usual position. Repeat this with the subject lying on his left side and then on his right. What happens to the relative resonance of the two sides? Repeat this often enough to remember it. You will sooner or later have to examine a patient who cannot sit upright.

4 Percuss the anterior chest wall of several subjects, paying particular attention to the right side in the area where precordial dullness prevents a comparison with the left. Mark the upper border of liver dullness.

5 Percuss the cardiac borders of several subjects, marking the border in each interspace. Measure the distance horizontally from the midsternal line in each interspace, using the metric scale.

6 In one subject percuss the border in the left fifth space. Have the subject inhale as deeply as possible and locate the border while the subject holds his breath.

Auscultation of the Chest *The Lungs* Auscultation of the lungs detects sounds made by moving air as it meets obstructions to its free flow. In speech, the vocal cords are the obstructions. In breathing, the normal walls of the air passages obstruct the flow to some degree. In disease, other obstructions appear.

Auscultation detects other sounds produced by breathing in a diseased state. The chest wall is lined by a smooth membrane and the lung is covered by a continuation of this same *pleura.* Between the two membranes is the *pleural space,* normally a potential rather than a real space. Normally too, the pleura of the lung slips noiselessly over pleura lining the chest. The pleura, however, can become rough when diseased. Its movements during breathing then produce a *friction rub* which can be heard.

If fluid and air are present together within the pleural space, they behave much like water and air in a jar. That is, any sudden movement— like shaking—produces a slapping sound.

Any sound produced in the larynx, trachea, bronchi, or air sacs must pass through lung tissue and the chest wall to be heard at the thoracic surface. This not only muffles the sound but modifies its quality. It is not surprising, therefore, that the sounds heard by auscultation vary at different points on the normal chest and under various conditions.

Auscultation in its simplest form concentrates on evaluating the *breath sounds,* detecting abnormal sounds called *rales* and *rhonchi,* and locating friction rubs. Rales and rhonchi are usually signs of disease, noises due to changes in the lungs or air passages.

BREATH SOUNDS   The breath sounds can be heard with each respiration. They are described as *vesicular, bronchovesicular,* and *bronchial.* Vesicular breath sounds can be described as soft and rustling. They have been likened to the rustling of silk. More important, they are audible only during inspiration, when air is rushing into the air sacs. Bronchial breath sounds are harsher, higher-pitched, and heard during both inspiration and expiration with about equal intensity. Bronchovesicular breath sounds resemble vesicular sounds during inspiration and bronchial sounds during expiration.

BREATHING DURING AUSCULTATION   As with percussion, you can best learn the normal variations of breath sounds by experience. You will, however, need to have your subject breathe in a standardized way in order to reduce the variations introduced by different types of breathing. You cannot listen well through any clothing, so your subject must be stripped to the waist or wearing an examining gown which can be moved away from the part you are auscultating. The patient should be sitting.

You instruct the patient to breathe through his mouth fairly deeply. You cannot hear well if he breathes too lightly, and he will become dizzy if he breathes too deeply and too rapidly. The patient must not grunt, groan, gargle, or snore, as some people tend to do when breathing deeply. He should breathe fairly slowly and you should be able to move the chest piece of your stethoscope between breaths.

Either the bell or the diaphragm may be used and both should be tried. Whichever you use, you must hold the chest piece firmly in place; any slippage will cause noise as it rubs the skin. Any rubbing of the rubber tubing similarly causes confusing noise.

EXERCISES

1 With your subject seated and breathing in the standardized fashion, listen with
   both diaphragm and bell at the indicated areas until you can recognize the
   breath sounds by name. Be sure that you listen both during inspiration and
   expiration.
   a Vesicular breath sounds: above the clavicle and posteriorly above the
      diaphragm
   b Bronchovesicular: in the second right intercostal space near the sternum
   c Bronchial: just above the top of the sternum
2 In the same manner examine the following areas and name the type of breath
   sounds heard in each:
   a About midway between the pole and the spinous process of the scapula,
      but near the vertebrae
   b In the midaxillary line above the diaphragm
   c Above the liver dullness on the right anterior chest wall
   d At the base of the neck just above the shoulder
   e High up in the axilla
3 With the subject breathing as instructed, listen first to inspiration only in the
   following areas. This is difficult because you must train yourself to ignore the
   phase you are not listening to. It may help if, at first, you lift your chest piece
   slightly just at the end of the phase you want to hear and press it down again
   when that phase begins. Eventually, however, you should be able to listen
   differentially to either phase with your stethoscope in place.
   a As before, between the scapula and spine
   b Above the liver dullness
   c Above the sternum
      Then compare inspiration alone in those three areas, and after that
   compare expiration alone in those three areas.
4 If you have not inadvertently done so already, move the chest piece over the
   skin as you listen to the breath sounds. Rub the rubber tubing with your fingers
   and rub it with cloth as you listen to the chest. Listen to the breath sounds
   through a layer of cloth. Listen to them through a hairy chest or by laying a
   thin strand of hair across the chest under the stethoscope. Can you recognize
   these *extraneous,* outside sounds? Repeat until you can identify them immediately. Otherwise they may confuse you later.

   AUSCULTATION PROCEDURE   Auscultation of the lungs proceeds as
systematically as palpation and percussion. With the patient seated and
breathing as instructed, begin high on the back, comparing identical areas
on the right and left, moving from the spine outward and then from above
downward. It is well to listen to two or more respirations each time before
shifting your chest piece. If the patient becomes too tired, interrupt the
procedure for a few moments. Otherwise examine the posterior and
lateral chest walls in one continuing auscultation.
   On the anterior wall of the chest, start above the clavicles and

proceed downward, always comparing right and left except where the heart interferes.

During this auscultation, consciously listen for the characteristics of the breath sounds as vesicular, bronchovesicular, or bronchial and for the relative duration of the inspiratory and expiratory sounds. Listen as well for any unusual sounds heard in rhythm with the breathing; ignore the regular beating of the heart and concentrate on association with inspiration or expiration.

EXERCISES

1 Auscultate the lungs of as many subjects as time allows. Consciously listen throughout for variations in the breath sounds.
2 On one subject, after auscultation with standardized breathing, repeat the examination with quiet, shallow breathing, then with very deep breathing. Pay particular attention to any changes in the characteristics of the breath sounds. What is the effect of the deep breathing on the subject?
3 Try auscultation while a subject does the following:
   a Grunts lightly with each expiration
   b Holds the lips so that he whistles slightly with each expiration and, if possible, inspiration
   c Snores slightly with each inspiration
   d Rattles or gargles in his throat with each expiration
   e Groans faintly
      Unconscious patients may do any or all of these. It may be necessary to auscultate their chests, and you must allow for these extraneous sounds without considering them abnormal.
4 Auscultate the back of the chest without a stethoscope, pressing your ear to the skin. How does what you hear differ from the breath sounds through a stethoscope?
5 If possible, auscultate a few areas on an obese subject and on a very thin one. Does the thicker chest wall change the character, as opposed to the intensity, of the breath sounds?

See Section 5-3.

The Heart Auscultation of the heart concentrates on four principal precordial areas. These are the spots where the sounds of the four sets of heart valves are most distinctly heard. They are the *mitral area* at the heart's *apex* or tip at about the PMI or the left border of dullness in the fifth intercostal space, the *tricuspid area* in the fifth space just to the left of the sternum, the *aortic area* in the second space to the right of the sternum, and the *pulmonary area* in the second space to the left of the sternum.

The normal *heart sounds* are two for each beat, and these two differ in relative intensity depending on the area. The sounds resemble the phrase "lubb dup" repeated over and over. If the heart rate is below about eighty, it is easy to hear a longer pause between each phrase than between the "lubb" and the "dup." The "lubb" is the first heart sound or S_1, the "dup" is the second heart sound or S_2. The longer pause between S_2 and S_1 is diastole, the shorter pause between S_1 and S_2 is systole, when the ventricles are contracting.

You recall that the mitral and tricuspid valves close when the ventricles contract. The first heart sound (S_1) is produced by their snapping shut. As you would expect, S_1 then is usually louder in the mitral and tricuspid areas than it is in the aortic and pulmonary areas. The second sound (S_2) is produced by the aortic and pulmonic valves closing at the end of ventricular systole and, as expected, is relatively louder in the aortic and pulmonary areas.

Each heart sound heard in each area and at other points over the precordium has characteristic *intensity, duration, pitch,* and *quality.* These properties also vary depending upon many factors within the normal range. These include the work load on the heart, the thickness of the chest wall, and the exact position of the heart within the chest. It is important, therefore, to auscultate as many normal hearts as possible to develop your concepts of normal limits.

RATE AND RHYTHM   The heart sounds also have characteristic time relations. The normal rate and rhythm vary, as do the rate and rhythm determined by palpation of the pulse. The intervals between S_1–S_2 and S_2–S_1 also vary, most strikingly with a change in rate.

It is even more important in examining the heart than in auscultating the lungs to listen differentially. You should be able to listen to S_1 and ignore the remainder of the sounds, to hear S_2 and shut out the rest. You must also be able to listen to the *diastolic pause* between S_2 and S_1 without hearing the rest, and similarly to concentrate on the shorter *systolic interval* between S_1 and S_2.

When the rate is rapid, as with a young child, it may be difficult to distinguish between S_1 and S_2 and hence between diastole and systole. One aid is to feel the thrust of the pulse with systole while you listen. The apex is the best place to palpate, but the carotid artery in the neck will do. The wrist is too far from the heart to help. The sound just about the start of the thrust is S_1. S_2 comes just after the thrust at the PMI, just before its end in the neck.

OTHER SOUNDS   In addition to listening to the rate, rhythm, and characteristics of the heart sounds, the examiner must detect any other sounds in rhythm with the heart. These sounds include *murmurs* ranging from soft, blowing to loud, rumbling noises. There are also *cardiac rubs,* which often sound like squeaky shoe leather. There may be *extra heart sounds* that resemble S_1 or S_2 but occur in addition to them.

To hear all these details it is best to have the patient lie flat on his back, arms at his sides, and with no interfering clothing. The patient should breathe lightly; if normal respiration interferes, you should ask the patient to hold his breath after he takes a relatively shallow breath. If the sounds are too faint to be heard easily, you can have the patient sit up, leaning slightly forward. This throws the heart against the anterior chest wall.

AUSCULTATION PROCEDURE   Auscultation begins in the aortic area. You must first identify S_1 and S_2, listening to each. You should listen to the two pauses as well. The rhythm will usually be readily evident. If not, you should determine what it is.

Auscultation then proceeds in order across to the pulmonary area, down to the tricuspid area, and out to the mitral area. At each area you should listen to S_1, S_2, and the two intervals. After you have completed all these areas, you can listen more briefly to the rest of the precordial area, principally to detect any rub. Of course, you should note any murmur, as well as the point at which it is loudest and where else it can be heard over the chest. Usually it will be distinctly loudest in or very near one of the valve areas.

EXERCISES

1   Auscultate the heart of your subject, listening in one area until you can distinctly isolate S_1, S_2, diastolic pause, and systolic interval. No one except yourself can tell at this point how well you succeed. If you tire before you accomplish this isolation, rest and try again.

2   When you can isolate the sounds, compare S_1 in the aortic, pulmonic, tricuspid, and mitral areas as to loudness, duration, pitch, and quality. Repeat with S_2. Where is S_1 loudest? S_2?

3   Compare S_1 with S_2 in each of the four areas. Compare the duration of the diastolic with the systolic interval.

4   Auscultate the hearts of three or more subjects. Do the heart sounds vary from person to person?

5   With one subject, auscultate the heart while he is lying on his back, sitting upright, and then leaning forward slightly. In one position try listening while the subject holds his breath in full inhalation and in full expiration.

6   Have the subject do five sit-ups and then lie back. Auscultate the heart, concentrating on identifying S_1 and S_2. Note the change in each sound in the vigorously beating heart and as it returns to normal rate. Repeat the exercise several times until you are sure that you can recognize and characterize S_1 and S_2 and the diastolic and systolic intervals in the fairly rapid heart. When the

heart rate increases, what happens to the relative duration of the diastolic and systolic intervals?

7 Listen carefully to S_2 in the pulmonic area while the subject breathes quietly or somewhat more deeply than usual. As the patient inspires, you may hear S_2 become two sounds with a brief interval between them. It sounds a little like "lubb duppup." During expiration S_2 becomes a single sound again. This is called *physiological splitting of S_2*. It is normal but can be confused with some signs of disease.

See Section 5-3.

2-6 ABDOMEN

The abdomen contains most of the internal organs or *viscera*. It, like the chest, is a closed cavity, but its walls are chiefly muscle. Above, it is capped by the diaphragm and lies partially within the lower part of the rib cage. Below, it is enclosed within the bony pelvis. The vertebral column helps form the posterior wall, and this *lumbar* spine bows forward into the abdomen.

A common scheme for locating areas in the abdomen uses the *umbilicus* or navel as the chief landmark. An imaginary line is drawn across the abdomen through the umbilicus and another is drawn vertically through it. These divide the abdomen into *quadrants* or quarters: the right upper quadrant (RUQ), left upper quadrant (LUQ), right lower quadrant (RLQ), and left lower quadrant (LLQ) (see Figure 2-14).

Within the RUQ and normally covered by the right lower ribs is the *liver*, with its *gallbladder*. In the LUQ lie the *stomach, pancreas,* and *spleen*. The kidneys are at the back of the abdomen on either side of the spine, within the upper quadrants. The *colon* or large intestine begins in the RLQ, rises along the side of the abdomen up behind the liver, where it turns across the upper abdomen and bends downward behind the spleen to descend along the left side. In the LLQ it turns again to the midline, where it descends once more to form the *rectum* in the posterior part of the lower pelvis. The *urinary bladder* usually lies on the anterior wall of the lower pelvis; when distended with urine, however, it can rise above the bony pelvic rim.

The nonpregnant internal sex organs of the female are within the pelvis. During pregnancy the enlarged *uterus* or womb rises above the rim until it fills the middle anterior part of the abdomen.

Otherwise the greater part of the abdomen is filled with the *small intestine,* which coils and folds as it runs from the lower end of the stomach to the start of the colon in the RLQ. Near this point a small blind pouch, the *appendix,* hangs from the start of the colon.

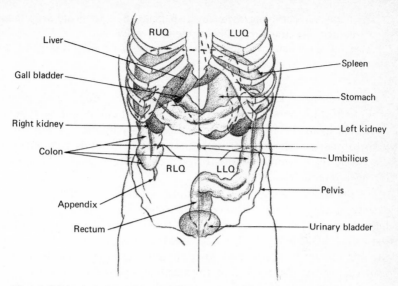

Figure 2-14 Anterior abdominal wall with landmarks, quadrants and principal viscera. RUQ, right upper quadrant; LUQ, left upper quadrant; RLQ, right lower quadrant; LLQ, left lower quadrant.

Normally it may be impossible to feel any of these viscera by palpating the abdomen. The stomach and large and small intestines are too soft to be defined; the liver and spleen are tucked up under the ribs; the bladder and uterus are concealed by the pelvis. The kidneys are also largely under the ribs.

The intestines can, however, be heard. They contain some gas as well as digesting food; since these are moved along together, the moving gas can vibrate. This produces *bowel sounds.*

EXERCISES

1 With the subject lying on his back, outline by percussion the diaphragm on right and left. Palpate the lower rib cage, which houses the upper abdomen. Then palpate the contours of the bony pelvic rim. Have the subject raise his head to tense the anterior abdominal muscles. Feel along the large muscle near the midline from the lower sternum and ribs to the pelvis. This muscle is not a smooth strap; rather, it is interrupted by cross bands, so that it feels as though it were one muscle below another. These segments and bands can be confusing in palpating the abdomen, especially in lean, muscular men. The discrete segments can be mistaken for deeper masses or organs.

2 Trace out the boundaries of the quadrants. What are the principal viscera lying in each? In the pelvis?

3 With the patient lying face down, palpate the ribs posteriorly below the
diaphragm. Continue palpation of the bony pelvis and note the deep forward
curve of the spine, which thrusts the vertebrae forward into the abdominal
cavity.

Inspection Examination of the abdomen begins with inspection,
looking first at the skin and any scars. The patient should be lying on his
back, his head raised slightly by a pillow. If palpation is difficult, it will
help to position the patient with his knees bent, body relaxed, and feet
placed on the examining table. Inspection, however, should be done with
his legs extended.

You should inspect the abdominal surface from the side as well as
above, noting the general contours and size. Any local swelling is
important. By asking the patient to raise his head, you may be able to see
the abdominal muscle and to accentuate any local swelling. If you watch
the umbilicus carefully and look at any scars, you may see a mass
protrude as the patient strains to raise his head.

You may occasionally see intestinal movement in a normal but very
thin patient who is relaxed. The abdominal wall may rock slightly with
each heartbeat. In the later stages of pregnancy, you may see *fetal*
movements as the baby shifts within the large uterus.

Palpation of the Wall Palpation begins by determining the thickness of the fat layer on the abdominal wall. You can pinch up the skin
gently in the center of either lower quadrant to get an impression of the
thickness. Next follows downward palpation to test the muscles. Normally they offer firm but not unyielding resistance. If the muscles feel too
rigid as you palpate, it will help to have the patient raise his knees. If the
abdominal wall seems very relaxed, test the result of having the patient
raise his head.

Tenderness Palpation for tenderness follows evaluation of the
wall and is done systematically. First, you should exert firm but not deep
pressure starting in the RLQ, passing from it to the RUQ, and then
proceeding to the LUQ and LLQ. Finally, the region about the umbilicus
is palpated. You can do this with one hand, your elbow held low,
preferably on a level with the patient's abdomen. It is best to keep all your
fingers straight and to deliver the pressure with the palm surface of all the
fingers. If one spot is tender, rock your hand up so that you are feeling
with your fingertips.

After this *superficial* or fairly light palpation, the circuit of the
quadrants can be repeated with deep palpation. In this much firmer
pressure is used. If the abdomen is tense, you can press on your palpating

fingers with those of your opposite hand. You may find it more satisfactory to distract a generally tense patient by asking him some unrelated, inconsequential questions. You must guard, however, against being distracted yourself.

When the patient has complained about localized pain in the abdomen, you should begin palpation in the quadrant farthest removed from the pain. Generally you will need gentleness and reassurance, and you may have to omit deep palpations, especially if palpation at distant points produces pain in the area which already hurts.

Feeling the Liver   Palpation of the organs also proceeds systematically, beginning with the liver in the RUQ. Before palpating, you check the *upper* border of liver dullness by percussion. Normal persons, especially long, thin people, may have a liver edge that is palpable below the rib margin on deep inspiration. It is not, however, easy to feel.

To do so, you stand on the patient's right, placing your left hand in the "small of his back" behind the liver and raising it upward. The patient may try to "help" you, but you must get him to relax and let you do the lifting. This pushes the liver toward the anterior abdominal wall, where you will feel it.

The palpation itself is done by placing your right hand, palm down and fingers together, some 2 in below the lower rib margin, about in the MCL. Some examiners prefer to point the fingertips at the ribs and others to hold the fingers parallel to them. As you exert light pressure inward, instruct the patient to breathe deeply and slowly through his mouth. You may feel the liver edge lightly tap your fingers at full inspiration.

If you do not feel the liver, press a little more firmly and have the patient inhale deeply again. This is repeated once or twice more, each time pressing a little more deeply. If you do not feel the liver edge "flip" or ride over your fingers, place your hand $1/2$ in closer to the ribs and repeat the maneuver. You can move it up to about an inch below the margin for a last try.

Two errors are apt to interfere: one is pushing your fingers upward to meet the liver, the other is palpating too deeply. Normally the "flip" will occur rather superficially if at all.

Feeling the Spleen   The spleen normally cannot be felt, but it should be sought in the LUQ. Its palpation is essentially similar to that of the liver. Standing at the patient's right, you lift his left side with your left hand. Placing your right hand about 2 in below the ribs but outside the MCL, palpate during deep, slow inhalation. Then try again deeper and higher. Occasionally a normal spleen can be felt tapping the finger just above the rib margin. In disease the spleen may be very large and its lower edge may be felt almost down to the pelvis. If you suspect this, you begin palpating in the LLQ.

Feeling the Urinary Bladder and Pregnancy   If there is a history of inability to urinate or if pregnancy of 3 or more months is suspected, you should palpate rather deeply from the umbilicus to the pelvic rim in the midline. You would expect to feel a firm, rounded organ on firm or deep palpation.

Feeling the Kidneys   Having palpated for organs toward the front of the abdomen, you can now seek the kidneys. The first maneuver is to palpate for *costovertebral angle* tenderness. This angle lies where the twelfth or bottom rib joins the spine, a landmark easy to feel with the patient lying on his back. Using one or two fingers, test first with firm pressure, then by a quick, deep movement of the fingers so that they "bounce" the region of the angle.

To palpate the kidney, the left hand is placed in the small of the back, and the right hand, palm down, is pressed firmly toward it. The fingers should be just above the level of the umbilicus. Ask the patient to inhale as before, and you may feel the firm, rounded lower pole of the kidney pushed down by the diaphragm. It may just bump or slightly separate your hands.

You must, of course, palpate both sides, but the right kidney lies somewhat lower than the left. You are thus more likely to feel the right one.

Palpation for Masses   Having completed the search for the liver, spleen, bladder, uterus, and kidneys, the examiner's next task is to palpate for any other detectable masses. In a thin person with relaxed abdominal walls, you may feel the spine and the pulsing lower aorta which runs just in front of it. Also, the colon can be felt in either the RLQ or LLQ if it contains hard *feces* or stool. Usually feces can be moved upward or downward, and when displaced, they tend to remain in the new position.

You should carefully palpate any mass to determine its apparent size and shape, its consistency as hard or soft, the regularity or lumpiness of its surface, its movability, and its movement with deep respiration. You must palpate deeply as well as near the anterior abdominal wall, but always slowly and gently.

Percussion of the Abdomen   Percussion of the abdomen assists and extends palpation. It depends primarily upon the tympany of gas-filled viscera—the distended stomach and intestines—and the relative resonance of the normal gas-containing intestines.

The same technique is used over the abdomen as over the chest except that only the anterior and side walls are percussed. Also, percussion is directed chiefly to the organs or masses that were palpated. It is well to percuss in the region of the umbilicus. A rather dullish resonance there is normal; a marked resonance or tympany often means a small intestine distended with gas. The colon contains gas, and you may find an almost tympanitic note near the lateral edges of the lower quadrants. A tumor mass in these areas may yield a flat note.

It is well to percuss the lower border of the liver even if you do not find it by palpation. In percussing from below upward, the note changes at the liver's edge from resonant to dull.

The spleen produces a dull note if normal but can sound flat if abnormally large. The upper border of the spleen is sharply heard as the lower border of tympany caused by the gas bubble in the stomach. To percuss the spleen, first find the *gastric* or stomach tympany below the left diaphragm. Percussing downward, there is normally a small area of splenic dullness. If the note is flat or the dullness is larger than the palm of your hand, you should suspect a large and probably palpable spleen.

Percussing from the umbilicus down will demonstrate a shift from resonance to dullness at the upper edge of a distended bladder. Normally resonance persists to the pelvic rim.

Auscultation of the Abdomen   Auscultation detects normal bowel sounds from the small intestine even when they are not audible without the stethoscope. Normally the tinkling bowel sounds occur about five to thirty times each minute in the area about the umbilicus. If few or none are heard because the intestine is not active, a sharp, downward, bouncing movement of the hand holding the chest piece will normally stimulate several bursts of sounds. When this fails to produce sounds, you should try one or two more areas. A *silent abdomen* with these maneuvers is a sign of disease in many instances.

By about the fifth month of pregnancy, the fetus is large enough to make audible heart sounds. They are faint and rapid at first and have been described as sounding like a watch heard through a pillow. Later in pregnancy they become louder but remain rapid. They are heard over the palpable uterus and are rather sharply localized. They are, of course, an absolute sign of pregnancy.

EXERCISES

1   Examine the abdomens of several subjects, one with a thin and another with a thick wall if possible. Palpation is the most important and difficult part of the examination and most examiners prefer to use percussion immediately after

they palpate for an organ; thus, palpate for the liver, then percuss; palpate for the spleen, then percuss it. Normal organs are so difficult to feel that it is easy to delude yourself. It is well, therefore, to have the instructor confirm your findings immediately.

2 In one subject try palpation, percussion, and auscultation with the subject relaxed. Repeat these while he tenses his abdomen. Which parts of the examination are least changed by these tense muscles?

3 When your own abdomen is deeply palpated, what sensations do you feel? Have the examiner make the movements of deep palpation slowly and gently, then briskly but with the same force. What differences do you as the subject notice between these two approaches?

See Section 5-4.

2-7 GENITALS AND RECTUM

Male Genitals and Inguinal Region Examination of the *genitals* uses inspection and palpation only. In the male, the *penis* is inspected, and the foreskin or *prepuce* must be drawn back if the patient is not *circumcised. Circumcision* is the removal of the prepuce, usually in infancy. You are looking primarily for lesions, usually ulcers, on the prepuce, on the reddish *glans,* and on the *body* of the penis. You should spread wide the opening or *meatus* at the tip, since an ulcer may be just inside (see Figure 2-15). As a final maneuver, you can ask the patient to "strip" the penis by holding it at the base between a finger on the underside and his thumb on top and then moving them to the meatus. This will "milk" any pus or discharge out through the meatus.

You inspect the *scrotum,* primarily for lesions, by stretching it out. The palpation which follows should be systematic. You first feel each oval, firm *testis,* which should move freely within the scrotum. Its contour should be smooth and regular except on the posterior side. Here is a firm, elongated body, the *epididymis,* larger at the top of the testis and narrowing slightly as it extends down the posterior surface. From the top of the testis, the *spermatic cord* can be felt extending upward and toward the abdomen. It contains blood vessels as well as the tube, the *vas deferens,* leading sperm from the testis. You can trace the cord upward into the groove of the groin (see Figure 8-22).

In this palpation you should note any irregularity of the testis, any mass in the scrotum, or any loss of the smooth contours of the spermatic cord. The scrotal contents are normally somewhat tender to palpation, but you should note any unusual tenderness. The testis may be unusually large, small, or absent.

After palpating the contents of one side of the scrotum, you similarly examine the other. You then inspect and palpate the *inguinal region* or groin for enlarged *lymph nodes.* To feel these, you run your fingertips a short distance up either side of the ridge which extends from near the base of the penis toward the top of the hipbone. Often you can feel a few "shotty," nontender nodes just below this ridge in one or both groins. Large or tender nodes are signs of disease.

Male Anus and Rectum   Examination of the rectum begins with inspection of the *anus.* To carry this out, you can place the patient in one of several positions. The two most common are with the patient standing and bent forward over the examining table or lying on his side, the lower leg extended and the upper bent so that the foot rests on the lower knee. In the latter posture, he may lie on the side you find most convenient.

You then put on a rubber or plastic glove, keeping a tube of lubricant at hand. To expose the anus, the cheeks of the buttocks are spread apart. The reddish brown mucosa appears somewhat puckered but should not have any raw *fissures* or cracks, ulcers, or dark-red protruding bodies which are distended veins or *hemorrhoids.* There may be small, loose, saclike structures of skin or mucosa which are *hemorrhoidal tags,* the remnants of healed hemorrhoids.

You then ask the patient to "bear down as though he were going to move his bowels." Normally this only causes the anus to bulge slightly, but it may cause it to *prolapse* or "turn inside out." Or it may expose a hemorrhoid that was otherwise invisible.

To palpate the anus and rectum, lubricate your gloved index finger well and lay the pulp, not the extreme tip, of that finger on the anus. You ask the patient to "bear down" again, and as he does, you bend the finger so that the tip rolls into the anal opening. As the finger advances, the ring of muscle about the anus should tighten but there should be no pain.

The tip of the finger as you advance it along the anterior wall of the rectum will encounter the *prostate gland,* one of the internal male sex organs (see Figure 2-15). It lies in front of the anterior wall and bulges slightly into the rectum. It is somewhat smaller than a testis, is firm and somewhat rubbery, and has a smooth surface. This palpable surface feels somewhat flattened, with a shallow groove separating it into right and left *lobes* of equal size. Pressure should produce only discomfort, not pain. You should note any tenderness, of course, as well as an unusually large gland or inequality in the size of the lobes, any *nodules* on the surface, any hardness, or any boggy softness.

You advance the finger as far as possible along the anterior wall above the prostate. By turning the hand and withdrawing the finger almost to the anus, you palpate the right lateral wall. Turning the hand further, you run the fingertip up the posterior wall before you turn the hand back to sweep down the left lateral wall. During this palpation, you will note

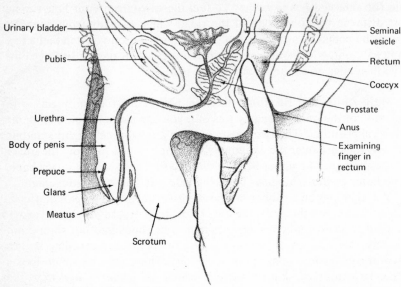

Urinary bladder

Pubis

Urethra

Body of penis

Prepuce

Glans

Meatus

Scrotum

Seminal vesicle

Rectum

Coccyx

Prostate

Anus

Examining finger in rectum

Figure 2-15 Male pelvic organs.

any tenderness; but chiefly you are feeling for any mass or *tumor*. If one is felt, you must determine its *contours*—whether smooth, rough, or grossly irregular; its consistency—whether hard, firm, soft, or easily broken; its *movability*—whether, in moving, it moves the rectal wall or whether it lies outside the rectum.

The rectum normally is surrounded by structures which are irregular enough to be confusing when first palpated. It is necessary, therefore, to palpate more than one normal rectum in order to learn the normal findings.

As a final maneuver you should insert your finger as far as you can and ask the patient to bear down. This may enable your finger to touch a tumor that is too high up to be felt in any other way.

When you withdraw your finger, there will be some feces on the glove. You should note the color and whether there is any blood. If none is seen, there are quick tests to detect the presence of "hidden" or *occult* blood in small amounts.

EXERCISES (MALE SUBJECTS)

1 Examine the penis of male subjects, preferably some circumcised. How does the glans differ in circumcised and uncircumcised subjects?
2 Examine the scrotum and its contents in several subjects, paying particular attention to the epididymis and spermatic cord. Trace the cord upward as far as you can.

3 Examine the inguinal region of several subjects for lymph nodes. Can you also palpate the *femoral pulse* on the inner part of the anterior surface, just below the landmark ridge?

4 Examine the anus and rectum in several subjects, paying particular attention to the size, symmetry, and consistency of the prostate. One lobe may be slightly larger than the other in the normal prostate, but the difference is small. Palpate carefully all walls of the rectum to become familiar with the normal irregularities. Does the wall of the rectum move over or with these irregularities?

See Sections 5-4 and 5-5.

Female External Genitals Complete examination of the female genitals includes inspection and palpation of the internal organs, the so-called *pelvic examination.* Much can be discovered, however, from inspection and palpation of the external genitals. This is the only part of the examination carried out routinely in young girls, virgins, women in advanced pregnancy, and women who have just given birth.

Most examining tables are equipped with stirrups into which the patient can slip her feet while lying on her back. Her buttocks are brought to the end of the table and the stirrups adjusted so that her knees bend at right angles or somewhat more sharply. The knees are dropped apart and the patient is draped with the examination sheet.

You can examine a woman without using stirrups, but it is more difficult. To do so the buttocks are brought within a foot of the edge of the bed or the end of the table. She rests her heels on the surface about at the outer sides of the buttocks and drops her legs apart.

You put on a rubber or plastic glove and keep some lubricant close by. With your gloved hand held fingers down and palm toward you, you place the nails of the first and middle fingers about two-thirds of the way down the heavier, outer lips or *labia majora* of the *vulva.* Your fingertips are placed against the labia while held together and then separated to spread the labia majora (see Figure 2-16). You should inspect the vulva systematically, using palpation primarily to confirm what you see.

Anteriorly in the midline is the small red *glans,* often covered wholly or in part by a fold of membrane. Extending backward from it are the thin red folds of the *labia minora,* or small lips. In the midline below the glans and sometimes rather deep is a slight prominence in the center of which is the *meatus.* Below that is the larger *introitus* or *vaginal outlet* of the birth canal. An irregular, thin membrane, the *hymen* or maidenhead, may partially cover this in virgins (see Figure 2-17).

You inspect the entire vulva beginning with the inner surfaces of the labia majora, looking for lesions which often are ulcers. You note any pus, blood, or discharge as well. You may also see cysts, nodules, or

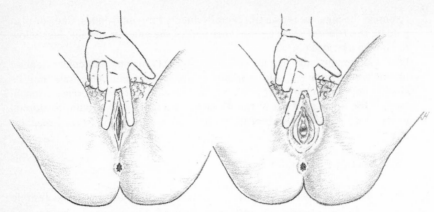

Figure 2-16 Examination of female external genitals. Placing of fingers (*a*) and spreading (*b*) to expose genitals.

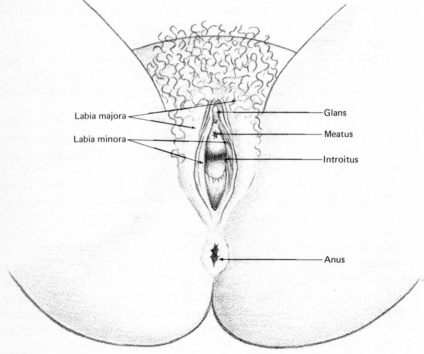

Labia majora ⎯ Glans

Labia minora ⎯ Meatus

Introitus

Anus

Figure 2-17 Vulva.

papules; especially near the meatus or introitus, there may be a red, tender nodule.

After examining the vulva, you ask the patient to "bear down."

Women who have borne many children or who have been torn during childbirth may show a pronounced bulging about the introitus, and tissue may protrude through it. This is *prolapse* of lesser or greater degree.

It is well at this point to palpate the inguinal region for lymph nodes. The maneuver is exactly as described for the male examination.

Female Anus and Rectum   Examinations of the anus and rectum in women are carried out in the same manner as in men but with the woman on her back with her knees bent. The findings are the same as well except during palpation of the anterior rectal wall. A woman, of course, has no prostate. Somewhat higher on the anterior wall, however, your fingertip will encounter a firm, rounded mass which obviously lies outside the rectum. This is the *cervix* or neck of the *uterus* (see Figure 2-18). It is firm, smooth, movable, and nontender in the nonpregnant woman or girl. During pregnancy, it enlarges and becomes softer. During early labor, it feels large and ring-shaped, with a central opening through which the baby will pass.

You may have to push down the uterus if the cervix is difficult to feel. To do this, you hook your ungloved hand over the anterior pelvic bone so that your wrist rests on it as a pivot. You can then push inward and downward to displace the uterus toward your palpating finger.

With or without abdominal pressure, you may feel a second, larger

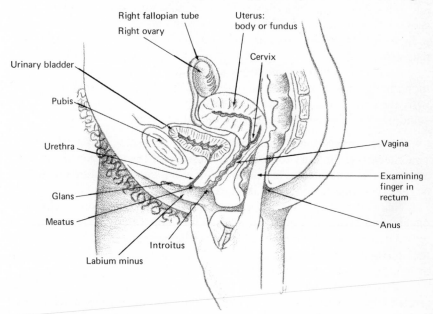

Figure 2-18   Female pelvic organs.

organ above the cervix. This is the body of the uterus when it is bent backward. In such instances it occupies an unusual position, but this by itself does not indicate the presence of disease.

EXERCISES (FEMALE SUBJECTS)

1 Examine the external genitals of several subjects. Pay particular attention to any bulging produced when the subject "bears down."
2 Examine the inguinal region in several subjects for lymph nodes. Can you also palpate the femoral pulse on the inner part of the anterior surface, just below the landmark ridge?
3 Examine the anus and rectum in several subjects, paying particular attention to the position, size, and consistency of the uterine cervix. Does abdominal pressure move the cervix or make it easier to palpate? Palpate carefully all walls of the rectum to become familiar with the normal irregularities. Does the wall move over or with these irregularities?

See Section 5-5.

2-8 EXTREMITIES

Arms and Legs Inspection and palpation of the arms and legs, aside from the skin, deal chiefly with bones, joints, muscles, lymph nodes, and blood vessels. Muscles so cover the bones that only rather gross abnormalities can be seen. Movement of the joints can be judged by inspection, but muscles and vessels are better evaluated by palpation.

As always, your examination should be systematic, first one arm, then the other, and finally a comparison of the two. You then do the same with the legs. The arms are best examined with the patient sitting or standing, the legs usually best with the patient lying.

Arms Inspection of the arms begins, of course, with the skin. Then you check the contours for any unusual angle of the upper or lower arm, elbow, wrist, and hand. An odd angle may indicate a *fracture* or broken bone, especially in a recently injured patient.

Next, the joints are inspected and palpated, beginning with the fingers and working up to the shoulders. You can quickly judge the movability of the finger joints by having the patient make a tight fist and then having him move his thumb as widely as possible. Swelling, redness, or tenderness of any finger joint should be noted.

Wrist movements are tested by asking the patient to bend his fist inward and outward as far as possible and then to roll it toward the thumb and toward the little finger. You can test passive motion by having the patient relax his wrist while you move it in the same fashion.

To examine the elbow, ask the patient to *flex* or bend his elbow as far as possible, then to *extend* or straighten it to the limit. Also ask him to *rotate* the forearm, turning the hand palm up and then palm down. Note whether the elbow is red, swollen, or tender on palpation.

To examine the shoulder joint, place one hand atop the shoulder to steady it. Otherwise the clavicle and scapula will move and obscure stiffness of the shoulder joint. Have the patient move his arm as far as possible upward, forward, backward, and out from the side. The patient should also rotate his forearm inward across the waist and outward with the elbow bent. Swelling and redness are not common signs in the shoulder, but you should palpate carefully for tenderness. Also, a hand placed across the shoulder joint while it moves may feel a sort of roughness or grating.

After the joints, examine the muscles. They should feel firm to palpation but not rigid. You can test strength by having the patient squeeze three of your fingers and then move the forearms while you try to hold them still.

Finally, ask the patient to hold his arms straight to the front, palms down and fingers spread wide. Watch for signs of unsteadiness and for *tremor* or trembling. You may be unable to see a fine tremor which you can feel by placing your fingertips lightly on the backs of the patient's fingers. Also, quickly compare the arms for any differences in contour.

Legs Examination of the legs begins with inspection of the skin and of the feet and ankles. You should note the color of the feet. At the ankles, look for swelling due to *edema* or excess water within the body. This swelling may be woody, hard, and with or without tense, thin, white or bluish skin over it. Or you may be able to indent the skin slowly with firm pressure of your finger. If so, this is *pitting edema.* If the patient has been long abed, pitting edema may disappear from the ankles and appear over the lower back.

Inspection may also show distended, bluish veins, which appear lumpy and often tortuous. These are *varicose veins* and may be tender with swelling and redness over some part of them as they snake up the lower legs.

To examine the joints, begin at the toes, looking especially for deformed ones. The ankle can be twisted around in a circle, cocked up, and bent down to test its movements. Flex the knee backward and extend it forward as far as possible. A hand laid flat on it may detect grating during movement. Also, look for swelling, redness, and tenderness.

The hip joint is examined while you hold the pelvis steady with one hand. You test the motion with the patient on his side so that he can extend his leg backward, flex it forward, and swing it as far to the side as possible. While the patient lies on his back, ask him to rotate his foot as far outward and inward as possible. Redness and swelling are uncommon, but you should palpate for tenderness around the hip joint.

In children, it is important to palpate the *femoral pulse* where the leg joins the body. You find it by pressing firmly just below the inguinal fold, slightly inside the midline of the leg.

See Section 5-6.

Reflexes   A *reflex* is an involuntary, automatic response by the body to a change or *stimulus*. The response can reveal something about the condition of the *nervous system*. There are many reflexes, but the most generally useful ones in the extremities are the *knee jerks*.

To test this reflex, seat the patient with feet hanging free or with soles resting on the floor and knees bent at right angles. The patient should be so seated that his legs are hanging or resting symmetrically. He must be relaxed and had best not watch you. You commonly tell him to look at the ceiling.

Then feel the flexed knee, at the front of which is a rounded bone, the *patella* or kneecap. Just below it is a tough cord. Farther down, this attaches to the large bone of the lower leg. To elicit the reflex, you must strike this cord below the patella.

You can strike it with your bent fingers, with the side of your hand, or, more conveniently, with a rubber-headed reflex hammer. You should tap it lightly at first. That is all that is necessary if the foot jerks forward. If it does not, strike harder. Sometimes even a fairly hard blow produces no jerk. Then you should try *reinforcing* the reflex. Ask the patient to hook together the fingers of both hands at chest level and to pull hard at them when you say "pull." As he pulls, you strike. This can produce a *reinforced knee jerk.*

If the jerk is very weak, you may feel a response that you cannot see. You do this by placing your free hand palm down across the top of the thigh, above the knee.

Eliciting the knee jerk with the patient lying on his back is essentially the same maneuver. You bend the patient's knees while he relaxes his legs. To do this, you slip one hand under his knees and lift them until they are bent to about 45°. The patient's heels, of course, remain on the table or bed. The important thing is to have both legs bent to the same angle before you strike with the hammer.

This is important because a comparison of the response at the right and left knee is valuable whether the patient is lying or seated. To call the reflexes equal or unequal, you must use the same force, strike the same way in the same spot, and carefully observe the vigor of the response.

See Section 5-7.

EXERCISES

1 Examine the arms and legs of one or more subjects. Particularly note the contours of the extremities. Put the fingers, thumbs, wrists, elbows, shoulders, ankles, knees, and hips through the full range of active motion. Then repeat as passive motion with the subject relaxed while you bear the weight of the limb.
2 Carefully feel the large muscles of the arms and legs. Do this first with the limb held normally, then with it relaxed as completely as possible, and finally with the muscles tensed. You should be able to identify these states instantaneously.
3 Palpate carefully the irregular bony surfaces at the finger and thumb joints, the wrist, elbow, shoulder, ankles, and knees. If your own joints are normal, you can always use them as a standard with which to compare the patient's.
4 Elicit the knee jerk with the subject sitting and lying. What effect does reinforcement have? Test the reflex while the subject tenses his leg muscles somewhat. What effect does this have?

2-9 PROCEDURE FOR PHYSICAL EXAMINATION

Thus far your physical examination has concentrated on normal findings. When you know the normal you can detect the abnormal, the signs of disease, deformity, or injury. Some abnormalities must be demonstrated, others you will detect for yourself. Insofar as time and facilities allow, you should continue to examine the normal parts of patients, especially when they are much older, younger, or of different sex or race than your student-subjects.

You can now plan the order in which you will do your full, systematic physical examination. At the same time you can summarize the signs that are generally found at each step. Remember, however, that there may be other, unexpected abnormalities. The summary that follows is arranged in one common order for the examination.

1 From start to end of the examination, observe *general appearance.* Look for evidence of weakness or distress, emaciation or obesity, of pain, labored breathing, coughing, or other respiratory difficulty, of poor color or too rosy a complexion. Note any unusual posture or gait, paralysis, tremor, or deformity. Note also any bizarre behavior or speech, any dullness, crying, or jitteriness.

2 During the examination note the *skin* in all regions, even though these are examined separately. Look for changes in color—general or spotty, red or otherwise. Note unusual hairiness in women and children or lack of hair in either sex. Watch for macules, papules, pustules, vesicles, excoriations, abrasions, ulcers, exudation, scaling, exfoliation, ecchymosis, petechiae, fissures, tremors, or calluses. Note also slackness of the skin or induration and scars.

3   With the patient seated, examine the *head* and *neck*, checking for bulging fontanels in infants and any unusual bumps or lumps on the skull. Note any trouble opening the jaws. Of the *ears*, note deafness, any discharge from the canal or crusting about it. Watch for bulging or retraction of the tympanic membrane, any reddening of its surface or any perforations—holes—in it.

In the *eyes*, look for blindness or poor vision, unusually pale conjunctiva, tearing, redness or yellowing of the sclera. Watch for bulging or retraction of the eyeballs, restricted or uneven eye movements, spontaneous eye movements in unconscious patients, failure of the eyes to converge. Note any cloudiness of the cornea. Note especially unequal or irregular pupils and any failure to contract and dilate as the light changes.

In the *nose*, watch for any discharge or blood and for crusts or clots; deviation of the septum to right or left; and pale, swollen inferior turbinates. Note any obstruction on one or both sides.

In the *mouth*, look for pale, fiery red, or dry lips, redness or fissuring at the outer angles, and ulcers or crusting. Within, note loose, decayed, or missing teeth, macules, ulcers, or dryness of the mucous membrane. Look for dryness, ulcers, fiery redness, or smoothness of the tongue. In the *pharynx*, look for redness, dryness, a granular appearance, ulcers, or pus, and watch for enlarged, red, or pale tonsils with pus on the surface.

In the *neck*, look for a limited range of motion, for large, tender, or nontender lymph nodes, and for tumors.

4   With the patient still seated, examine the *arms*. Begin with the *pulse* at the wrist, timing an abnormally fast or slow beat. Look for any arrhythmia, for a great amplitude—the bounding pulse—or a small one—the thready or feeble pulse; for great tension—the hard pulse; or a reduced one—the soft pulse. Follow this with measurement of the *blood pressure*, looking for unusually high or low values and for abnormally wide or narrow pulse pressure.

Check each arm for unusual contours and all joints for restricted motion, swelling, redness and tenderness, and any grating on shoulder motion. Then look for flabbiness or rigidity in the muscles and for weakness. With the arms extended, look for unsteadiness or tremor.

5   While the patient is still seated, try the *knee jerk*, watching for reduced or absent reflexes or for too brisk a response. Look especially for unequal knee jerks. You can also check the knee joints to discover limited motion, too great an extension, swelling, redness, tenderness, or grating on motion.

6   With the patient still seated, examine the *anterior chest* (in women, this can be done with the patient lying down), looking for deformities of the chest wall, increased thickness front to back, and reduced respiratory movement even when forced. Note unusually shallow, deep, rapid, or labored respiration. Check whether the lips or nails are cyanotic. Note any mass or pulsation away from the PMI and whether the PMI is unusually large or pulsates too forcefully. Checking by

palpating, note whether and how far outside the MCL the PMI lies. Palpate to detect any mucus rattling on deep inspiration and for increased or decreased vocal fremitus over the lungs.

Percuss over the *lungs* to detect dullness or heightened resonance generally or locally. Percuss the *heart* to detect an enlarged area of cardiac dullness. Auscultate the lungs to detect breath sounds that are abnormally faint or loud, that are bronchovesicular where they should be vesicular, and that show relatively too prolonged expiration or inspiration. Note any rales, rhonchi, or friction rubs as abnormal sounds occurring in rhythm with the respiration. Rales may sound like the bursting of tiny bubbles or be heard as a louder bubbling sound. Rhonchi are louder rattling, snoring, or musical wheezing sounds. Rubs sound as the name implies, sometimes grating or squeaking.

Auscultate the heart to verify an abnormal rate or rhythm. Note whether the heart sounds are unusually loud or soft and distant, whether S_2 is abnormally loud in the aortic or in the pulmonic area, one greatly exceeding the sound of the other. Note too whether S_2 is louder than S_1 in the mitral area, whether the heart sounds are slurred and "sloppy" rather than crisp and clear. Watch for extra heart sounds and especially for murmurs.

Finally, note any cardiac rub. You may have difficulty distinguishing between a rub and a murmur, but you should be able to tell a cardiac rub from one associated with the lungs. The cardiac rub occurs in rhythm with the heart sounds.

7 While the patient is sitting but with legs up on the examining table, you turn to the *back.* Look for deformities and tenderness of the spine, then for limited spinal movements. Complete your examination of the lungs, watching for the same signs that you sought on the anterior chest. In addition, check for limited diaphragmatic excursions and an unusually low or high diaphragm on one or both sides.

8 You now have the patient lie on his back. At this point you should check the blood pressure again if it was too high or too low when taken in the sitting position. You can also examine the anterior chest if you did not do so in the sitting position.

Examine the *breasts,* looking for tenderness, tumor, or discharge of the nipple areas and for tumors or tenderness in the breasts and lymph nodes in the axillae.

9 With the patient lying, examine the *abdomen,* watching for general distention and for local swellings, noting an abnormally thick, fat wall and general or localized tenderness, superficial or deep. Palpate and percuss for an abnormally large liver, spleen, kidney, or bladder. Also watch for a pregnant uterus in women of childbearing age.

Palpate all the quadrants systematically for a tumor. Finally, listen for bowel sounds—noting whether they are unusually active or absent—and for fetal heart sounds in a pregnant woman.

10 With the patient still lying, examine the *legs,* watching for abnormal contours, then checking the feet for any abnormal color or deformity. In the ankles, look for edema and for limited motion, swelling, redness, or tenderness. Also check for limited rotation at the hip joints.

Turning the patient first onto one hip then the other, check the hip for limited motion.

11 With the patient on his back again, check the femoral pulses to note whether they are too weak or whether they are unequal. With female patients, it is well to check the inguinal region for large or tender lymph nodes.

12 While the *male patient* is on his back, examine his *genitals*. Watch for lesions on the penis or scrotum and for discharge from the penis. Look for absent or small testes, irregularity of a testis, any mass in the scrotum, and peculiar contours of the spermatic cord. Watch for abnormal tenderness of the scrotal contents and, finally, check the inguinal region for large or tender lymph nodes.

The *female patient,* after examination of the legs, is positioned at the foot of the table for examination of the *external genitals.* In examining these, watch for lesions on the labia and about the meatus and introitus. Watch also for any discharge or bleeding and for nodules. Look for prolapse or poor support of the introitus.

13 You can now examine the male patient's *anus* and *rectum,* either with him on his side or standing bent over the table. Check for anal fissures, ulcers, hemorrhoids, tags, or prolapse. Then palpate the prostate, looking for enlargement, unequal lobes, unusual softness or hardness, tenderness, or nodules on the surface. Palpate the rectum for tumors, and finally check the feces on the gloved finger for blood.

In examining the *anus* and *rectum* of the female patient, look for the same signs as in the male except that you will be feeling the cervix, not a prostate. Note whether the cervix is of unusual size and consistency and whether moving it causes pain.

Obviously not every patient can have as thorough an examination as this. In an emergency, there may be no time and your examination must center first on the most urgent defect. A minor illness such as an acute sore throat may not warrant a full examination. Nevertheless, it is usually wiser and safer to look beyond the immediate problem and, particularly early in your experience, you should do a full examination whenever you can.

EXERCISES

1 Do the entire physical examination of a subject in an organized fashion. As you do, remind yourself of the signs you might find in each part. The subject can assist by asking what you are looking for in each region and maneuver.

2 As a group, examine patients selected to show specific signs. Remember that patients have feelings and are usually overly aware of what you say. You can recognize frightening words such as "tumor," "murmur," or even "rub." Avoid using them in the patient's hearing. You can always feel "something" or hear a "sound" even when you know very well what it is.

3 If it can be arranged, do the thorough physical examination of a patient with an instructor present to check you. Remember, you will encounter only normal structures or functions in most regions, but you must always recall the signs of disease you may find.

See also Chapter 7.

2-10 INTERIM OR REVISIT PHYSICAL EXAMINATION

The examination of a patient seen a few days or weeks earlier usually centers on certain signs. It is rarely necessary to do thorough examinations frequently while the patient remains in the hospital or continues in clinic or office attendance. This, of course, assumes that a good record of earlier examinations exists.

The important decision is what to examine during a revisit. You decide using two guides: (1) what signs of the original disease or problem are likely to change between visits and (2) what signs are likely to bear on any new problem. Likely changes in the original disease may be foretold from the original diagnosis and a knowledge of the course of that disease. This may be quite simple, as it is in a sprained ankle, but it may be so complex that a physician must identify the changing signs to be followed. There is rarely any point in repeatedly reexamining a leg paralyzed 5 years earlier but it is important to check the blood pressure even if it has been elevated for 5 years.

You will do a partial reexamination when you uncover a new problem while taking the patient's interim history. If he complains that last week he had a runny nose and sore throat which has led to a cough, you certainly would examine the nose, throat, neck, and lungs.

Unfortunately, many situations are more complex and the complaint may be a poor lead in itself. A headache may be due to many causes and examination of the head usually reveals little. Unless you are quite sure of your own judgment in such a situation, you must get help from a physician or make a thorough examination.

Hospitals, clinics, and doctors differ in their policies for repeating a thorough examination. Some have a rule that another full examination should be done each year. Many say that whenever a patient is readmitted to the hospital or when he returns as an outpatient after the lapse of a year, he must be thoroughly reexamined. You will have to comply with the local rules.

EXERCISES

1 The instructor will assign you the chart of a patient who has already been examined, diagnosed, and treated. Read the physical examination, the diag-

noses, and the interim notes. Discuss with the instructor what signs you should look for on reexamination. If the patient is available, do the parts of the examination required to detect these signs and discuss the results with the instructor. Such patients could have hypertension, bronchitis, or bronchial asthma, or they may be making posthospitalization visits after cholecystectomy or appendectomy.

2 The instructor will assign you a patient for revisit. Review the chart as before, but take a revisit history (see Section 1-4). Then discuss with your instructor all parts of the examination to be repeated, i.e., to follow the underlying disease and to investigate any new problem. Complete the relevant parts of the physical examination and discuss the results with your instructor. Here the patients can be more acutely ill or have a more complicated course, as in an acute respiratory infection, active rheumatoid arthritis, recurrent pyelonephritis, benign prostatic hypertrophy, recurrent pulmonary embolism, recent cerebrovascular accident without speech defect, immediate postoperative gastrectomy, cholecystitis, or appendicitis.

Chapter 3

Presentation of Clinical Information

3-1 FUNCTION AND FORM OF PRESENTATION

You presented findings from the patient's history and your physical examination when you discussed them. You have also seen how medical records are written. Now you must learn to communicate medical data—the facts of the case—in a systematic fashion.

Whether you report these data verbally or in writing, you must make your communication *accurate, complete, concise, organized,* and *understandable.* You have learned to report accurately, but completeness presents more of a problem.

Obviously you will rarely report everything that you hear and observe. A complete written report contains more details than a verbal one, however, because someone may refer to it weeks, months, or years later when you cannot answer his questions.

Conciseness, in a way, competes with completeness. It attempts to pack more information into fewer words and is one reason for the special vocabulary of medicine. One medical word often replaces an entire phrase; for example, "colic" says "sharp pain that comes and goes in waves." Medical terms, however, can mislead. The words have very specific meanings, and if you misuse one, you become inaccurate. You can check a meaning in a medical dictionary, but if you are still doubtful, you had better use common words.

Organizing a medical presentation helps you be complete and concise. It also makes the report more understandable. Medicine—like other professions—has certain customs in communicating data. If you follow the custom, a trained listener knows the order in which you will relate or write your information and is less apt to misunderstand it.

Medicine does change the organization of its presentations from time to time. At present such a change is in progress, but this should create no problem for you. You simply have to understand the difference between the *classical medical record* and the newer *problem-oriented record*. You can then use the one favored by your organization. In your presentation of the history and physical examination, the differences are really not great.

3-2 WRITTEN PRESENTATION

Some medical organizations use printed forms that indicate specific titles under which you enter each piece of information in the history and physical examination. They may provide checklists of symptoms and signs. These forms vary, but you can quickly learn to use them if you know how to write your presentation without one.

You can write a satisfactory record on plain paper, but usually you will be asked to use special sheets which identify the institution and provide a space for the patient's name and identification number. You should be certain that the name, number, and date appear on each separate sheet. Medical records must often be taken apart, and without this minimal information it may be impossible to get the sheets into their proper order again.

Initial Examination   You begin the record of an initial examination by writing the introductory data. You can use a telegraphic form such as this:

> 29-yr-old, single, white, female stenographer of Italian extraction. Source—patient, reliable.
>> Previous contacts: Pediatric clinic, 1948–1955. Tonsillitis, 1953.
>> Dermatology clinic, 1970—acne.

You will find many mysterious abbreviations in medical records.

Some, such as "yr," are standard. Many are purely local and not recognized outside the institution. Thus "S-pt., RH" may mean "Source—patient, reliable historian" in one hospital or clinic and nothing at all in another. Abbreviations save time in writing, but you should only use those that any trained person can understand. It is wise to stick to those given in standard lists of medical abbreviations.

"CC" is an accepted abbreviation for "chief complaint" at the start of a medical history, where "PI" means "present illness." Your record could then continue with

CC: "Bad cold"—2 d
PI: The patient was well until 2 d ago, when she . . .

You should remember to record the chief complaint in the patient's own words and follow it by the duration. The balance of the record is in your own words except where you use quotation marks to show that the patient said something specifically.

The present illness will be read more often than any other part of the record and deserves your special attention. You should start where the patient's illness began, even if this was years ago. You then develop the history as it occurred, earliest events first, the next second, and so on until you describe the present situation. Generally speaking, you should give the date for events that occurred long ago, but state the interval in months, weeks, days, or hours when something occurred in the recent past. Thus you can write:

In 1950 the patient first had arthritis, for which she was treated for a year. Since then she has had an attack in 1953, 1960, and 1969, always in her wrists, elbows, and especially her fingers and always disappearing with treatment in about a year. She was free of symptoms and had full use of her joints until two months ago when . . .

The present illness is the story—a true one—of the patient's illness. It should be well written and easy to read. More important however, it must be accurate, complete, and concise.

The background history follows the present illness. When you have enough experience, you can write it as the patient gives it to you and before you put together the present illness. To do this on plain paper, you simply leave enough space for the PI between the CC and the past history.

Usually the background history is written in telegraphic style, not in complete sentences, and with standard abbreviations. Otherwise you cannot complete it while the patient answers your questions. For example, you could write:

PH: Gen'l health fair. Wt constant—165 lb
CHD: measles, chicken pox—about age 5–7
ADULT DISEASES: "Pneumonia"—no details—1969
INJURIES: Broken rt upper arm—age 12
OPERATIONS: Tonsillectomy—age 9
IMMUN.: Only vaccination age 6 recalled
MEDICATIONS: None in last 2 yr. No reactions
PREVIOUS HOSP. ADMISSIONS: None

The abbreviations "PH" for "past history" and "CHD" for childhood diseases are accepted at this point in the record. "Gen'l" for general, "lb" for pounds, etc., are standard. "Pneumonia" is a quote, and the marks indicate that you really doubt the patient's accuracy.

The physical examination or PE follows the history, and the first line gives the vital signs using abbreviations. It could appear as:

PE: P64 R12 T99° BP 124/76 RAS

There follows the general appearance in complete sentences or in telegraphic style. Usually it forms a paragraph of its own and has no title. You can write:

The patient is a well-developed, well-nourished, muscular young man who does not appear ill but seems in pain when he moves his rt. arm. He is alert, cooperative, and somewhat nervous.

It is equally acceptable to write:

Well-developed and -nourished, muscular young man; does not appear ill but in pain on moving rt. arm. Alert, cooperative, somewhat nervous.

The balance of the examination is written after the general appearance in telegraphic form with abbreviations. At the outset, you will be wise to include the normal findings. This indicates that you did each part of the PE, and it helps you remember what you examined. This makes rather a long writeup, and you can indicate any abnormal finding by underlining it or by putting an "X" in the margin on the same line. This lets you locate your description quickly.

The exact order in which you describe the parts of the examination is not very important, but you should adopt one set order so that you always include each part. It is logical to group the head and neck, thorax, abdomen, genitals, and rectum in that order. Often the skin is put first, the extremities and back after the above groups.

After the history and physical examination are written, you are ready for the final part of this presentation. This is where the two current types of records differ.

The classical medical record calls for a *summary*. This is usually a paragraph or two recounting the positive finding in the history and physical examination. An example would be as follows:

A 34-yr-old white carpenter with a 10-yr history of asthma recurring every fall. He began to have difficulty breathing with much wheezing and no cough or pain 3 d ago and this has grown worse until he cannot sleep at night. He also says that he drinks a half pint of gin each day and his wife left him for this reason 1 month ago. On PE he is thin, looks ill, and has trouble breathing. His chest has increased AP diameter, diaphragm is low. Expiration is prolonged and he has rales throughout the chest. Liver is firm and down 5 cm below rib margin.

The problem-oriented record requires an identification of each problem the patient has. Each is given a number and for each is given the *subjective* (S) and *objective* (O) findings. In this situation, "subjective" means symptoms from the history and "objective" means signs from the physical examination. Together with any findings from laboratory tests, x-rays, electrocardiogram, or other examination, the subjective and objective findings constitute the *data base*. For the same patient this problem list would read:

1 Difficult breathing
   S 10-yr history of asthma recurring each fall. For 3 d, increasing difficulty in breathing with wheezing but not cough. Now cannot sleep.
   O Difficult breathing, looks ill. Increased AP diameter of chest, low diaphragm, prolonged expiration, rales throughout chest.
2 Drinking
   S Drinks half pint of gin daily. Wife left him 1 mo ago because of it.
   O Thin, looks ill.
3 Enlarged liver
   S None.
   O Liver firm, down 5 cm below rib margin.

A physician would add more to either record at this point. Specifically, he would diagnose the case at least tentatively and indicate any tests and treatment. He probably will do so when he reads your record regardless of whether it is classical or problem-oriented.

The following is the complete, initial medical record as you might write it after the examination of the patient whose history was taken in Chapter 1, Section 1-2 (page 9).

Nov. 11, 1975   VIOLET, Rose—No. 687520
45-yr-old, white, housewife of Irish extraction. Source: Pt., reliable. No previous contacts here.

CC: Cough—3 d

PI: The patient has had three or four severe attacks of coughing annually since 1950. The attacks are sometimes preceded by a cold and the cough, which lasts a week or two, is severe enough at times to prevent sleep. Her sides and upper abdomen ache after she coughs hard. She produces sputum with brief relief. During the attacks talking, laughing, exertion, or smoking makes her cough. A doctor has given her medicine in the past to stop the cough and let her sleep.

Family members may have colds when she does. None has prolonged attacks of coughing.

The present cough began 3 d ago and resembles the early phase of previous attacks. It is gradually growing worse and she obtained little relief from a drugstore cough syrup 2 d ago. She is still able to sleep and has not yet stopped smoking as she usually does. She does not feel ill but considers her cough moderately severe.

PH: Gen'l health good. Always "plump," wt. constant at 180 lb.

CHD: Recalls measles, mumps, probably German measles.

AD: None except recurrent coughs.

INJURIES: Cut left leg badly as child.

OPERATIONS: "Some kind of scraping for female trouble"—1970—Lakeside Hosp.

IMMUNIZATIONS: "All the usual kids' shots"—no details recalled. None recently.

MEDICATIONS: See PI. Aspirin 2–3 times each yr for headache. Had rash after penicillin shot—age 14–16.

PREV. ADMISSIONS: 1969—Normal delivery, 4th child.

FH: F—died age 60—"heart attack."

M—living and well—age 65.

3 brothers—ages 46, 42, 41—one has diabetes, one brother killed in Vietnam.

2 sisters—ages 43, 38—one had gallbladder operation.

Mat. grandmother and brother have diabetes, father and pat. uncle died of heart attacks.

Mat. aunt hospitalized for mental illness.

Review of Systems:

X   HEAD: Infrequent headaches, sometimes severe.

No dizziness, unconsciousness, or convulsions.

EYES: Wears glasses for reading—1 yr.

EARS: No deafness or earaches, ringing, etc.

X   NOSE: See PI. Told she might have sinus trouble about 5 yr ago—no follow-up. No nose bleeds. No sore throats except 1–2 d with colds.
MOUTH: Has had teeth filled. No trouble with gums or tonsils.
LUNGS: See PI. Only has trouble breathing while she coughs. No wheezing, tuberculosis, pleurisy. Last chest x-ray—2 yr ago—reported "OK."
HEART: No known heart trouble, high or low blood pressure, breathlessness, cyanosis, ankle swelling. Never had EKG.
DIGESTIVE: No abdominal pain, appetite loss, indigestion, vomiting, jaundice, diarrhea, or blood in stool. Constipated "all my life."
X   Hemorrhoids during pregnancies. "Maybe a little one now." No hernia, liver, or gallbladder trouble. No ulcers or colitis.
X   URINARY: Had "kidney infection" during second pregnancy—1956—no trouble since. No dribbling, burning, bloody or discolored urine.
GENITAL: Periods began age 13, usually regular, every 28–30 d for 4–5 d. Last period October 30, 1975. No unusual periods, pain, or bleeding between.
Painless intercourse, 1–3 times each week with husb. Uses diaphragm. No genital discharge or sores. Denies VD.
SKIN: Acne when young. Redness and itching under breasts in hot weather—"all my life." No hair change. Dyes hair brown—"would be gray otherwise."
X   BONES & JOINTS: No arthritis, but back aches most evenings. Has had bunion on rt foot for 4–5 yr. Has had varicose veins since 2d pregnancy.
NERVOUS SYSTEM: No mental illness or depression.
BLOOD: No anemia, bleeding, bruising. Transfused during 3d delivery —1962. Type AB, Rh pos. (she "thinks")
ENDOCRINE: Oral contraceptives—1968–71.
Normal heat tolerance, no jitteriness, appetite always large. Drinks more water than family.
SH: Born and always lived in Lakestream. Ancestors all Irish. No foreign travel. Completed HS. Clerked in store until birth of 1st child & fills in 1–2 mo every summer as clerk. Likes to work.
MARRIED. 1952. Husband—age 48—living & well, "drinks too much." 2 sons—ages 19 & 13; 2 dau.—ages 21 & 6; all well. 1 miscarriage—1958. Lives in half of old frame duplex. 7 rooms. House too small now but older dau. will marry soon. Family gets along "OK" except when husb. gets drunk & "turns nasty," usually 3–4 times annually, "mostly at weddings."
X   MAJOR DIFFICULTIES: Financial & 13-yr-old son who is rebellious, does poorly in school. Worries most about husb's. getting drunk and losing job.
SLEEPS SOUNDLY—8 hr. Eats regularly & snacks. Meat or fowl 5–7 times a week, egg 2–3 times a week. Fresh fruits or vegetable "most days." No milk drunk. Coffee 4–8 cups daily. No tea. Beer—once monthly.

X   SMOKES $1/2$–1 pack cigarettes daily. No regular medicines, vitamins.
Uses no drugs. Has no hobbies or regular exercise. Social activities are
PTA and many friends.
USUAL DAY: Up at 7 AM. Prepares, eats, and cleans up breakfast until
8–8:30 AM. "Picks up and cleans" until 9–9:30. Watches TV & "sometimes sews or irons" until 12. Prepares, eats, cleans up lunch until 1:30
("They all come in at different times"). Rests until 2:30. Shops or visits
neighbors until 4. "Watches the kids" until 6. Prepares, eats, cleans up
dinner until 7:30. Watches TV until 10:30 or 11 & goes to bed.

PE: P84 regular R16 T99.8 W194 lb BP 154/84 RAS
Well-developed, obese, middle-aged white woman who coughs often and
hard, producing no sputum. Cheerful, talkative, relaxed, does not appear
ill. Reasonably clean.

X   *SKIN:* Red, excoriated area in fold under each breast, slightly yeasty
odor. Tobacco stains on fingers, rt hand. Otherwise normal color,
texture, moisture.

HEAD & NECK:

SKULL & SCALP: Hair gray at roots. Otherwise normal.
EARS: Hears watch normally—both ears. No discharge.
EYES: Reads newsprint at 15 in with glasses, at 30 in without.
No tearing or discharge. Pupils: equal, round, react to light. Movements
normal. Conjunctivae and sclerae normal except for tannish, raised area
next to cornea on side away from nose of each eye. Cornea clear.
NOSE: No obstruction or discharge. Septum midline. Turbinates not
seen.

X   MOUTH: Normal lips & oral mucosa. Two teeth missing in upper jaw.
One lower tooth decayed. Tongue normal. Fauces and tonsils normal.
PHARYNX: Granular, deep, dusky red. Uvula red. Neck: Moves
normally. No palpable lymph nodes or tumors.
CHEST: Very thick wall. Moves normally. Breasts: Large and pendu-
lous. No masses or tenderness felt. No discharge.

X   LUNGS: Vocal fremitus reduced everywhere. Less resonance than
normal over entire thorax. Diaphragms high and descend 2 cm. Breath
sounds distant everywhere, but inspiration & expiration of usual
duration. Rhonchi heard over midchest front and back just before cough
& disappear or almost disappear after it.
HEART: PMI not palpable. Cannot percuss LBD. Sounds distant. S_2
equal in aortic & pulmonic areas. S_1 louder than S_2 in mitral area. No
murmurs.
ABDOMEN: Very thick wall (poor examination). No localized swelling.
No palpable organs, masses, or tenderness.
GENITALS: No lesions or prolapse.

X   RECTAL: Single small hemorrhoid on left side of anus. Numerous tags.
No masses or tenderness felt. Cervix normal size & consistency,
movable without pain. No blood seen on finger.
BACK: Normal contour. No tenderness.

X   *EXTREMITIES:* Symmetrical and joints move normally except that rt

   X
great toe overlaps next one and has tender bony mass at base. Small
varicose veins, not red or tender, up entire length of each calf. No ankle
edema. Knee jerks active and equal.

Summary (Classical)

45-yr-old married woman with 25-yr history of 3–4 annual attacks of
coughing, severe and lasting 1–2 wk. These are sometimes preceded by a
cold. Present cough began 3 d ago and is following usual course. Patient also
has infrequent headaches and was once told that she had sinus trouble.
She has had constipation all her life and hemorrhoids for many years. Also
she has had varicose veins for many years and a bunion on rt foot for 4–5
yr. She has been "plump" all her life and has little physical activity. She
smokes $1/2$–1 pkg. cigarettes daily. Her major worry is her husband's
occasional heavy drinking.
   On PE she weighs 194 lb and is obese; BP is 154/84. She coughs
frequently but does not appear ill, has rhonchi all over chest. Pharynx is
granular and dusky red. Also has red, excoriated skin under breasts, tannish
patches on sclerae, decayed tooth, small hemorrhoid, and small bilateral
varicose veins on both calves. Rt great toe overlaps next one and has bony
mass at base.

Summary (Problem-oriented)

1 Cough
   S 25-yr history of 3–4 annual attacks of coughing, severe and lasting 1–2
      wk. Sometimes preceded by cold. Present cough began 3 d ago and is
      following usual course. Smokes $1/2$–1 pkg. cigarettes daily.
   O Coughs frequently but does not appear ill. Rhonchi all over chest.
      Pharynx granular & dusky red.
2 Obesity
   S "Plump all her life," has little physical activity.
   O Wt. 194 lb and is obese.
3 Bunion, rt. foot
   S Bunion appeared 4–5 yr ago.
   O Rt. great toe overlaps next one and has bony mass at base.
4 Varicose veins
   S "Veins" for many yr.
   O Small bilateral varicose veins on both calves.
5 Hemorrhoids
   S Has had many yr.
   O One small hemorrhoid; no blood on glove.
6 Constipation
   S Constipated all of life.
   O Normal rectum.
7 Headaches
   S Infrequent headaches.
   O Nothing.

8 Rash
   S Redness & itching under breasts for many yr.
   O Red, excoriated skin under breasts.
9 Spots on eyes
   S Nothing.
   O Tannish patches on both sclerae.
10 Decayed tooth
   S Has had teeth filled.
   O Decayed tooth.
11 Husband drinks
   S Occasional heavy drinking.

The problem-oriented record sometimes follows a different order in recording the history, putting a *patient profile* before the CC and PI. This includes essentially the information in the SH or social history. A more uniform requirement is a separate sheet called the *problem list* and put in the front of the medical record folder or jacket. This lists, with the numbers, the summary items and the date each was first entered. For Mrs. Violet this would be:

1   Cough 11/11/75
2   Obesity 11/11/75
3   Bunion, rt. foot 11/11/75
4   Varicose veins 11/11/75
5   Hemorrhoids 11/11/75
6   Constipation 11/11/75
7   Headaches 11/11/75
8   Rash (under breasts) 11/11/75
9   Spots on eyes 11/11/75
10 Decayed tooth 11/11/75
11 Husband drinks 11/11/75

Interim Examination   The interim history and physical examination, written when the patient has not been seen for some time, follows essentially the same order as the initial record. It repeats, however, only items that could have changed. If the PI is a continuation of the previous trouble, it is headed *interval history* and picks up the story where the last note left off.

If Mrs. Violet returned 2 years after her previous visit, the record would read as follows:

Dec. 3, 1977   VIOLET, Rose—No. 687520
47-yr-old widowed housewife. Source: Pt., reliable.
PREVIOUS RECORD: Clinic visits Nov. 1975 for cough, recovered uneventfully.

CC: Recurrent cough—2 d.

INTERVAL HISTORY: The patient stopped smoking as advised here, restricted speech and activity if she had a cold or began to cough, and took prescribed expectorant cough syrup. She had only one brief episode of coughing during 1976 and one which lasted 5 d in early 1977. She developed a cold after husb.'s funeral, 4 d ago, and 2 d ago began to cough. This has not been severe and is unaccompanied by other symptoms. She returns, she says, because she needs a new cough syrup prescription.

PH: Gen'l health has continued good but wt. is still at previous level.

No interval illness, injuries, or operations (decided not to have bunion operated on as advised).

FH: M—died age 66—"stroke."

Bros. & sisters—as before.

R of S:

X HEAD: Many headaches, relieved by aspirin, during past 2 wk (husb. in hosp. & died).

MOUTH: Had decayed tooth extracted and another filled.

X GENITALS: Last menstrual period July 1976. "I'm having an easy change of life."

SKIN: Still has redness and itching under breasts despite recommended treatment, but "I wasn't very faithful."

BONES AND JOINTS: Bunion becoming painful—6 mo.

SH: MARRIAGE: Husb. died age 50—1 wk ago. "Car rolled back on him and crushed his chest." Hospitalized 1 wk before death.

CHILDREN: Older son & dau. married. Live in own homes.

Still lives in same house, adequate for present family.

Major difficulty—financial. Husb.'s employer says she will get employment compensation but it will be tight. Son & dau. may help. Younger son still does poorly in school.

Diet, habits, & daily routine changed only in that she stopped smoking 2 yr ago. During past 2 wk "Everything has been upside down." "Cried 2 d when my husb. died. Just let my daus. take care of me. Still haven't done anything."

PE: P 90 regular R 16 T99.6 W 192 lb BP 156/84 RAS

Well-developed, obese, middle-aged white woman who coughs occa-

X sionally but hard. Depressed, cries when talking of husb. but relaxed and does not seem ill.

SKIN: As before except no tobacco stains.

HEAD AND NECK: Skull and scalp: Hair gray except 4–5 in at end.

EARS, EYES, NOSE: As before.

MOUTH: As before except one tooth missing in lower jaw where

X another is decayed.

PHARYNX: Slightly granular and reddened.

NECK: As before.

X CHEST: As before except rhonchi are scattered and completely disappear with cough.

ABDOMEN: As before.
GENITALS: As before.
RECTAL: As before except no hemorrhoid.
X   EXTREMITIES: As before except base of rt. great toe is moderately tender on firm pressure.

Summary (Classical)

47-yr-old recently widowed woman with 27-yr history of recurrent coughs. She remained well since last visit 2 yr ago except for relatively mild attacks of coughing. Now returns because cough has followed cold and she needs more medication. Husb. died after accident 1 wk ago and pt. has felt depressed since. Last period 18 mo ago. Bunion has become painful. Headaches frequent since husb.'s accident. Stopped smoking 2 yr ago. Is worried about finances.

On PE still obese at 192 lb. BP unchanged. Coughs occasionally and has only scattered rhonchi. Seems depressed but relaxed. Other signs unchanged except that she has had tooth extracted and now has another decayed; hemorrhoid has disappeared; bunion has become tender; pharynx is less granular.

Summary (Problem-oriented)

1 Cough
   S Has had 2 relatively mild coughing attacks in 2 yr. Has begun coughing after cold, needs more medication. Stopped smoking.
   O Coughs occasionally. Scattered rhonchi.
2 Obesity—unchanged.
3 Bunion, rt. foot.
   S Has become painful.
   O Tender at base rt. great toe.
4 Varicose veins—unchanged.
5 Hemorrhoid—has disappeared.
6 Constipation—unchanged.
7 Headaches—frequent since husb.'s accident.
8 Rash—unchanged.
9 Spots on eyes—unchanged.
10 Decayed tooth.
   S Had decayed tooth extracted.
   O Has missing tooth but another is decayed.
11 Husb. drinks—husb. died as result of accident at work.
12 Depression
   S Has been depressed since husb.'s accident 2 wk ago.
   O Seemed depressed but relaxed.
13 Periods stopped—18 mo ago.

The problem list would be modified as follows:

      5 Hemorrhoid 11/11/75 disappeared 12/3/77

and

   11 Husband drinks 11/11/75   Died 11/30/77
   12 Depression 12/3/77
   13 Periods stopped 12/3/77

   Revisit Examination The *revisit note* written when an outpatient returns and the *progress note* when a patient is seen often in the hospital are even briefer. They describe only what has occurred since the patient was last seen and the changes that were found on the brief physical examination.

   The form of the entire note is different in the classical and in the problem-oriented record. In the classical form, all the symptoms are presented first, followed by the signs. The problem-oriented note takes up the various items on the problem list, giving the subjective and objective findings for each problem that has changed. You need include only those examined during the revisit and not necessarily in the original order. Each, however, bears the number it has on the problem list.

   Mrs. Violet's next visit would be recorded like this:

(Classical)

Dec. 10, 1977—Revisit Note

Pt. coughed for 3 d after last visit but never very hard. Has had no cough for last 4 d. Feeling somewhat less depressed and last night slept fairly soundly for 7 hr. Has filed compensation claim but has not yet made dental appointment.

   P 86 R 16 W 194 lb BP 150/80 RAS
   No longer coughing. More cheerful and talkative again.
   PHARYNX: Slightly granular but normally pink.
   LUNGS: Breath sounds still distant. Rhonchus heard one time between scapulae.

(Problem-oriented)

Dec. 10, 1977—Revisit

 1 Cough
    S Coughed 3 d after last visit. No cough for last 4 d.
    O Breath sounds still distant. Rhonchus heard one time between scapulae.
       Pharynx slightly granular but normally pink.
12 Depression
    S Feeling somewhat more cheerful and last night slept fairly soundly for 7 hr.
    O More cheerful & talkative again.
10 Decayed tooth—has not made dental appointment yet.
11 Husband—finances—has filed compensation claim.

There would be no change required in the problem list.

Signature You must always sign what you have written in a patient's record no matter how brief the note. You should type or letter your name as well if your signature is illegible, and you should give your position or title the first time you sign a note in any one chart. Records can be produced in court and your signature, name, and title are important parts of each record.

EXERCISES

1 Review two more patients' records in the institution where you will examine the next patients. Pay close attention to the form—whether a printed form or the arrangement of a written record—used to record an initial examination, a revisit, and an interval examination. Note particularly any difficulties you have understanding what is written. Do the abbreviations bother you? Can you understand any symbols used? If the record is written by a highly trained examiner, he will use words you do not know and, if he is a physician, you may find "*impressions*" and "*disposition*." These are, respectively, diagnoses to be considered and tests or treatment in a classical record. You will also find A and P in most problem-oriented records. These are "*assessment,*" which roughly corresponds to impression, and "*plan,*" the counterpart of disposition. Do not become concerned about either new words or new sections of the record.
2 Examine a patient—history and physical examination—whom you have not seen before. You may have to take the history in two sessions and do the physical examination in a third. This is better than exhausting the patient. Do not worry about being slow; speed comes with experience.
3 Similarly, perform an interval examination and a revisit examination on patients whose records you have with you. Write the appropriate notes.
4 Check, if you can, your recorded examinations against those of experienced examiners. Have you uncovered new information? Have you missed important data? Your instructor can help you here. Do not be alarmed if the patient has told you something that differs from the other examiner's report. Some patients are inconsistent and all you need do is to check with the patient again to try to establish the correct facts.

3-3 ORAL PRESENTATION

You will present detailed information about patients to other health care personnel verbally under two circumstances—either with the patient listening or with the patient absent. You must speak professionally in either situation and you must communicate accurately, completely, and concisely in an organized, understandable way.

Accuracy and *conciseness* take first place in verbal presentations.

Listeners can always ask for additional information and question you if they do not understand. You will want to be as complete and clear as possible, and organizing your report helps avoid lapses or unclear statements. You should follow the conventional order for your listener's sake and for your own.

Initial Examination   Start by giving the necessary *introductory data*. If the patient is not present, give the name, age, sex, race, marital status, and occupation. If the patient is present, introduce him by name and give his age, marital status, and occupation. You can insult both the patient and any colleagues present by giving the patient's sex and race or marital status when the patient is a child. It is not necessary to state the obvious.

In the patient's absence you might begin, "Mr. Smith is a 34-year-old, married, black sailor. He says that he has had 'a pain in the pit of his stomach' for 2 weeks. He first experienced this pain 3 years ago. . . ." In the patient's presence, you could say, "Mrs. Jones, this is Dr. Smith. Mrs. Jones is 42 and is divorced. She works as a secretary and tells me that she has a severe headache. This one began about 6 hr ago, but her first one like it occurred about 10 years ago."

You need not say "chief complaint" or "present illness." But do give them in order just after the short introductory data, as well as the duration of the chief complaint.

Keep your presentation of the present illness brief but complete. Your story should follow the chronological order, just as when you write it.

In giving the background history, stick to what may be related to the patient's present problems. This requires some judgment, and at first you would do well to include anything that could be remotely related. Ordinarily this would not include, for example, the death or health of relatives unless they have had problems like the patient's.

The physical examination is presented giving only the signs that you have found. However, you customarily begin the presentation with the pulse and blood pressure, even if they are normal. Include the temperature if it is important. Describe the general appearance if the patient is not there. You can omit it if the patient is present, mentioning only something that is not obvious or that has disappeared. For example, you can say, "She has difficulty walking" when the patient remains seated or lying down, and "He coughed occasionally when I examined him" if he is not still coughing.

You should give first the signs associated with the present illness and then any you think might be related to it. After that you can quickly

review the other abnormalities you found. It is a good idea to save until
last any sign that puzzles you unless you think it is related to the present
illness.

Here then is the presentation of Mrs. Violet's case—in her presence—on her first visit:

> Mrs. Violet, this is Dr. Smith. It will save time if I tell him about your trouble.
> Mrs. Violet is 45 and a housewife. She came to us because she has been
> coughing for 3 days. This is nothing new for her because she has had three or
> four attacks like this each year since 1950. They are sometimes severe and
> last as long as 2 weeks. Sometimes they follow a cold but not always. When
> they are bad, she can't sleep and she gets sore across her lower chest and
> upper abdomen. She sometimes gets hoarse after a few days. A doctor has
> given her medicine to stop the cough and let her sleep.
>
> This attack is like the others and is getting worse. She bought some
> cough medicine in a drugstore but it hasn't helped much. The cough isn't bad
> enough yet to make her stop smoking. She uses a half to one pack a day.
>
> She has always been healthy—except for the cough—and has always
> been heavy. She has four children—the youngest is 6—and she has some
> other things wrong—hemorrhoids, varicose veins, occasional headaches, and
> redness and itching under her breasts. She has also had a bunion on her right
> foot for 4 or 5 years.
>
> Her temperature is 99.8, her pulse 84, and her pressure 154 over 84. She
> weighs 194 lb. Her breath sounds are distant and I heard rhonchi over her
> chest and back—about here. These disappear or almost do when she coughs.
> Her pharynx is granular and dusky red. Her uvula is redder than it ought to
> be.
>
> She has one badly decayed tooth. There are red, excoriated patches
> under each breast and I found one small hemorrhoid with lots of tags. She
> does have some small varicose veins on each calf and a bunion on her right
> foot.
>
> I wish you'd look at her sclerae. She has a tannish patch on each eyeball
> next to the cornea.

Interim Examination   In presenting the interval history you have to
review all the previous information. You know it only because you have
just read the earlier record.

This is how you could present Mrs. Violet's interval record in her
absence:

> Mrs. Rose Violet is a 47-year-old white housewife, recently widowed. Her
> husband died last week after an accident. This is her second visit here—the
> first was 2 years ago—for a cough. This time she has had one for 2 days.
>
> She began having severe attacks of coughing, sometimes lasting 2
> weeks, about 27 years ago. These came three or four times each year,

sometimes following a cold, until her visit here 2 years ago. We gave her some expectorant cough syrup, told her to quit smoking and to avoid doing things that made the cough worse. She did stop smoking and has had only one attack each year. Those were pretty mild.

Four days ago she developed a cold, she says because she got chilled at her husband's funeral. For 2 days, she has been coughing but not hard. She has no more medicine and says that's why she is here.

On her last visit she was obese—and still is; complained of itching under her breasts—and still does. She had occasional headaches, but she has had quite a few of these since her husband's accident 2 weeks ago. She says that she has been depressed and is sleeping poorly.

She also complainted last time of a bunion. We advised an operation which she decided against, and now the bunion hurts. She did have a badly decayed tooth pulled. Incidentally, she had a small hemorrhoid and bilateral small varicose veins. Her last period was July of last year but she doesn't complain of any trouble.

Her temperature now is 99, her pulse 90, and her weight 194 lb. Her blood pressure is still 156 over 84. She is really obese and looks depressed. Actually she isn't coughing often or hard and does not look ill. I only heard scattered rhonchi which disappear when she coughs. Her pharynx is slightly granular and reddened.

Her bunion is tender now and she has another badly decayed tooth. She still has red, excoriated patches under each breast and varicose veins. But her hemorrhoid is gone.

Revisit Examination The revisit presentation is even briefer unless you report the case to someone who did not see her on her last visit. If you present to someone new, you have to review the whole situation much as you did for the interval record, adding the progress made.

The verbal report on Mrs. Violet's second visit presented to the person who saw her on her prior visit would go like this, assuming that the patient is present:

You remember, Dr. Jones, that Mrs. Violet came in last week because she had been coughing for 2 days and had run out of her medicine. We gave her another prescription for expectorant cough syrup.

She also was very upset by the recent death of her husband and wasn't sleeping well. We didn't give her medicine for that.

Mrs. Violet says that she did cough for 3 days after her last visit but never very hard. Also, she has been feeling more cheerful and slept fairly well last night.

She has filed a compensation claim for her husband's death but she hasn't yet made a dental appointment as we advised.

When I examined her today her pharynx was normal and her lungs sounded fine. I heard only one rhonchus between the scapulae.

Problem-oriented Presentation   All three of these verbal presentations are in the classical form. They can be given, of course, in the problem-oriented form. You simply begin with the introductory data as before, followed by the chief complaint and present illness. This, then, is followed by the signs you found in the respiratory system—the cough, changes in the pharynx and lungs. This completes problem 1. You can then continue with the patient absent:

> She has a second problem—obesity. She says that she has been plump all her life and she has very little physical activity. She really is fat. She weighs 194 lb.
> A third problem is a bunion . . . .

In this way you concisely present each problem. You need not announce what is subjective and what objective but give the history first and physical findings second for each problem.

The same arrangement of information is followed when you review the past record and bring it up to date after an interval examination. You give all the subjective data—old and new—followed by the objective data—old and new—about the first problem. Then you repeat that for each problem in turn. You can, however, omit any problem that has disappeared, for example, Mrs. Violet's hemorrhoid.

The revisit report in problem-oriented form need touch only on the problems that have changed—subjectively or objectively—since the last visit. You should include any new problems as well as any old ones that need a decision.

EXERCISES

1   Present verbally in problem-oriented form Mrs. Violet's initial examination, interval examination, and revisit report.
2   Present verbally the findings you wrote for the patients you examined in Section 3-2 (page 100). As you do so, try to make your classmates hear what you heard, see what you saw, and feel what you felt. The listeners should ask any questions that arise in their minds about your information and should make any suggestions that may help you improve your presentations. Very few people are really skillful at verbal reports until they have had some experience giving them.

See Sections 6-1 and 6-2.

Part Two

Advanced Examination of Patients

Chapter 4

Medical History

4-1 INTENSIVE QUESTIONING ABOUT SYMPTOMS

The fundamental questions discussed in Section 1-2 uncover much valuable information about a patient's illness. There is, however, much more to be learned about the symptoms. To accomplish this, you must ask detailed questions, and these vary from symptom to symptom.

Many of these detailed questions will occur to you from your general knowledge. Others you must learn. This should not involve memorizing the entire list of all questions. Rather, if possible, you should review the questions for any one symptom before seeing a patient with that symptom. The specific questions gradually will fit into a general pattern as you gain experience.

It is important to remember that these questions do not replace the fundamental ones. Generally they give detail to the "What?" inquiries. You can weave them into the general outline so that they become part of the orderly flow of information.

Patients frequently supply some or all of the information without being asked. When it is necessary to prompt them, you should alter the questions to fit the circumstances. As with the fundamental questions, it is the idea, not the wording that is important.

There follows a list of questions organized by symptoms. Chapters 9 and 10 explain the basis for many of the queries and make them easier to remember. The use of one set is illustrated at the end of the list. If you compare it with the example on page 9, you will see how the detailed questions expand the fundamental ones.

Pain Can you describe the pain? Is it aching—like a sore muscle? Sharp—like a toothache or a knife or needle? Dull—like hard pressure over a muscle? Pressing or crushing—like a heavy weight? Burning? Cramping?

Is the pain steady? Does it come and go, say like waves? Is it in flashes—like lightning?

Does it change character at times—say going from dull to sharp? Does it move around? Has it spread from where it was? Or become concentrated in one spot? Or moved from one spot to another?

Where exactly is the pain? Show me. Does it seem to be near the surface, say in the skin, or deep inside?

Does it hurt to touch or press where the pain is? Does firm pressure make the pain less? Does movement make it worse? Better?

What else makes the pain worse? Eating? Bowel movement? Urinating? Coughing? Exercise?

What eases the pain? Any particular position? Heat? Aspirin? Eating? Vomiting? Bowel movement? Urinating?

What time of day is the pain worst? At night? When you get up? About midday? When you are hungry?

Have you noticed anything that comes with the pain? Nausea? Sweating? Flashes of light? Weakness? Desire to urinate or have a bowel movement? Diarrhea?

What medicine have you had for the pain in the last 6 hr?

How would you rate the pain right now? Very slight, slight, pretty bad, bad, very bad, excruciating, the worst you can imagine?

Malaise, Weakness, Debility Do you feel generally sick or sickish all the time or does it seem worse at some times? In the morning, during the day, at night? Does the feeling become worse with exertion? When you are upset or worried?

Do you feel sickish and weak at the same time or does one come without the other?

What are you able to do? Take care of your personal needs? Clean house or go to work? Go shopping? Walk up a flight of stairs without stopping? Walk a block?

Must you lie down during the day? How often and for how long? Could you exert yourself if you had to, say if there were a fire?

Do you force yourself to be active? Do you feel that everything is too much effort? Does this feeling ever reduce you to tears?

Is the weakness worse in some part of your body? Which part? Is it always this part?

Fever Do you just feel hot and feverish? Have you taken your temperature? When and what was it? Have you been flushed? Sweaty?

Have you taken aspirin or a medicine like it? Did your fever go down? Did you sweat heavily after the medicine?

Have you had a shaking chill? Did it rattle the bed or chair you were in? Did your fever get worse or better after the chill?

Have you felt weak with the fever? After it went away? Were you nauseated or did you vomit with the fever?

Has the fever recurred? When is it highest during the day? Do you sweat heavily at night?

Have you drunk liquids freely? As much as six glasses a day?

Mental Disturbances, Dizziness, Convulsions, Coma Have you been very upset? Jittery? Emotional? Crying? What seems to upset you?

Have you had trouble sleeping at night and then wanted to sleep during the day? Have you had many dreams? Nightmares? Wild fancies or daydreams?

Have you heard voices when no one was near you? Have you seen people or things that others couldn't? Do you feel that there are outside influences controlling your actions? Have you been afraid that you are losing your mind?

Have you had trouble remembering things? Give me some examples. Do you have trouble with simple arithmetic—like adding two numbers? Do you have trouble speaking? Remembering some words?

What do you mean by "dizzy"? Do you feel lightheaded? Do you feel unsteady or stagger? Do things seem to get momentarily faint or move back away from you? Does the room spin or do you turn in it? In which direction does the room turn or do you turn in it?

What, if anything, accompanies the dizziness? Nausea? Trembling? Sighing? Noise in your ears? Have you actually fallen?

Have you lost consciousness? Did you hurt yourself as you fell unconscious? Did anyone see you? Did you have a convulsion or cry out? Did you lose control of your bladder or bowels? How did you feel when you "came to"?

Lameness, Paralysis, Deformity, Tremor Did you lose consciousness when the lameness or paralysis came on? Did you have trouble speaking at that time? Was there any headache or other pain?

Does the lameness seem to improve continually? What do you do to make up for your lost motion? Does the paralysis or deformity upset you a great deal?

Is the trembling always the same? Is it worse when you are tired? Upset? Trying to do something? Does the tremor continue when you are asleep? Do you feel stiff with the trembling? Can you stop the trembling if you try very hard? How much does it interfere with your taking care of yourself?

Disturbances of the Senses   How much can you see? Do glasses help? Can you see to read? Recognize people? Tell dark from light?

Do you have spots that persist before your eyes? Can you see things "out of the corner of your eye"?

Do you see double? All the time? With one eye covered? Do you see things around bright lights? Is there any pain in your eyes? When? More in bright or dim light?

Do you have trouble hearing high-pitched sounds, like a teakettle or telephone conversations? Can you hear low-pitched sounds well—like a man's deep voice, a bass drum, or a cow lowing? Can you hear high- or low-pitched sounds better?

Do you have a whistling or roaring sound in your ear? Which one? Describe the sound to me.

Have you ever had an infected ear or "perforated drum"? Which one?

Have you ever had "true dizziness," where the room spins around or you spin in it? Do you have difficulty balancing yourself with your eyes closed?

Have you lost sensation in some part of your body—such as losing your ability to feel pain if you stuck yourself with a pin? Do you have trouble telling exactly where your hand or foot is if you can't see it? Have you ever had peculiar sensations like ants on or under your skin, "pins and needles," or prickling sensations?

Have you lost your sense of smell? Of taste? Have you smelled unaccountable odors that others did not?

Masses, Tumors, Swellings   Is the mass getting bigger? Is it painful? Tender to the touch? Has it felt warm to the touch? Has the swelling opened and drained? What came out? Pus? Bloody fluid? Watery matter? Did the drainage relieve the pain? Do you have any other swellings? Where? Have you had an operation—even a small one—on the mass? What was the result?

Bleeding, Bruising   How much blood do you think you lost? A teaspoonful, a cupful, a pint or more? Was it hard to stop the bleeding? Did the blood spurt, well up, or ooze?

Have you ever bled from the nose or gums? Have you ever vomited blood or what looks like coffee grounds? Have you passed bloody stools or black, tarry ones? Have you had blood in your urine? Have your periods been unusually heavy or prolonged beyond 5 days? Have you bled between your periods? How much?

Do you bruise easily and even without knowing that you had injured yourself? Has a joint ever swelled up suddenly, within minutes, and painfully? Have you ever been told that you had anemia? A tendency to bleed? Does any relative bleed easily and have a hard time stopping it? Do you get severe sore throats that last a long time?

Injury, Burns, Poisoning How did the injury occur? Where? What were you doing? In what position did you land when you fell? What did you do after you were hurt? Did you lose consciousness? For how long? Did you lose much blood? How much? Do you have pain anywhere except in the main injured part?

What caused the burn? Where were you? How long ago were you burned? What was done for the burn? What medicine, if any, have you had for the pain?

What did you swallow? How much? When? Have you vomited? What came up? Was it bloody? Are you having pain in your throat? Chest? Stomach? Belly? Were other people similarly affected?

What fumes did you inhale? Where? When? For how long? Do you have trouble breathing now? Have you coughed up blood? Were other people affected?

What did you get on your skin? Over what area? When? How long did it stay on your skin? Were other people affected?

Dietary and Nutritional Disorders, Weight Gain or Loss Has your diet changed considerably from a year ago? How? Have you had much diarrhea? Constipation? Vomiting? Loss of appetite? What was your highest weight? When was that? Have you always been thinner than most people? Fatter than most?

Have you been trying to lose weight? By dieting? Under a doctor's direction? Are you taking drugs to lose weight? How rapidly have you gained weight? Lost weight? How many pounds per month?

Are your parents and grandparents fat? Very lean?

Tell me what you eat at each meal and between meals.

Stomach Trouble, Nausea, Vomiting, Jaundice Do you have heartburn? Indigestion? Much belching? What foods disagree with you?

Have you always had a queasy stomach, easily upset? Does nausea come on and stay or does it come and go in waves? Does vomiting relieve it? What else eases it?

Do you vomit everything, even water? What do you bring up? Undigested food? A thick, gruellike liquid? Thin, watery fluid? Is it greenish? Bloody? Like coffee grounds?

Does vomiting ease your pain? Make it worse?

How long has it been since you ate anything? Drank anything?

Have you ever had an x-ray of your stomach? When? What was the result?

Have you ever had jaundice, where your skin and eyeballs turned yellow? Has your urine ever been very dark brownish? Have your stools ever been whitish? Have you ever had gallbladder x-rays? When? What was the result?

Do fried or fatty foods disagree with you? What happens if you eat them?

Have you ever had liver trouble? Hepatitis? Gallbladder disease? Gallstones? Have you been closely associated with anyone who has jaundice or hepatitis? Have you had a fever within the last week or two? How much do you drink? Do you shoot heroin?

Constipation, Diarrhea, Gas Have your bowel habits changed within the last month or year? How?

Have you been constipated for a long time? Do you use laxatives? Which one? Enemas? How often? How often do you have a bowel movement if you don't take anything? Is your stool hard? Do you have to strain to pass it? Does it hurt you to pass it? Is it of normal size or a thin string? What is its color? Do you have hemorrhoids?

How long have you had diarrhea? Does it come and go? What seems to start it? Emotional upset? Certain foods? Which ones? Is your stool soft and mushy? Watery? Ever bloody? How many bowel movements do you have each day? Does eating bring on an attack of diarrhea? Immediately or later? Do you have a rush of pain before each movement? Is it relieved by the movement?

Have you had alternating constipation and diarrhea?

Have you been eating regularly? What have you eaten today?

How much liquid do you drink each day? Water? Coffee? Tea? Milk? Soup? Broth?

Does anyone living or eating with you have diarrhea?

Runny or Stuffy Nose, Sore Throat, Swellings of the Neck Is your nose always runny? When does it run? Do you sneeze with it? At other times? Do your eyes itch when your nose runs? Is the secretion thin and watery? Thick and ropy? Do you feel it dripping down into your throat? Does your head or face feel full and uncomfortable? Does the inside of your nose burn? Does it crust?

Is your nose usually stopped up? When does it get stuffy?

Do you often have a sore throat? A dry or scratchy throat? How much do you smoke?

Have you been told that you have tonsillitis or bad tonsils? When? Have you had your tonsils out?

Do you have lumps or swellings of your neck? Where? Are they painful? Tender to the touch? How long do they last? Did you have fever with them?

Cough and Breathing Problems   Has your cough changed within the past day, week, month, or year? How?

What do you cough up? Color, odor, physical state (watery, stringy, sticky), amount (a tablespoon or a cupful a day)?

Where does the sputum seem to come from? From the throat? Deep in the chest? Is it easy to cough up? Does the cough stop when sputum is raised?

When during the 24 hr do you cough most? What makes the cough worse? What makes it better?

Does it hurt to cough? Where? What is the pain's character and duration?

Have you coughed up blood or blood-flecked sputum? How much? When and how often?

Do you have a postnasal drip (sensation of something in the back of the throat)? Do you "clear your throat" often?

Do you smoke? What and how much? When did you begin? When did you stop? Why?

Do you work or have you worked in a dusty atmosphere or been exposed to chemical fumes? When and for low long?

When did you last have a chest x-ray? Why? With what results?

Have you been closely associated with anyone who has a chronic cough?

Exactly what kind of trouble do you have breathing? When does it appear? What are you doing when you have trouble?

What can you do without getting breathless? Climb how many flights? Walk how far? What else do you feel when you are breathless?

Does anything (in the air, emotional tension, posture) make the breathing worse?

What do you do to make the breathing easier?

How many pillows do you use in bed?

Do you wheeze? Do you have rattling or bubbling sounds in your chest?

Do you have pain when you breathe? What is it like? Where?

Have you ever turned blue or become unconscious when you couldn't get your breath?

Have you ever had your breathing tested? When? With what results?

Have you ever been hoarse? When? For how long? With or without pain in the throat?

Have you ever had pneumonia or bronchitis? When? How often? For how long?

(If the patient has a bluish tint—cyanosis—of the lips and/or nail beds): Have you noticed that your lips (or nails) are somewhat bluish? When did you notice it first? Has it been getting more pronounced? Rapidly or slowly?

(If the patient has clubbing of the fingertips): When did you first notice that the ends of your fingers had changed shape? Has this been getting more pronounced? Rapidly or slowly?

Heart Symptoms   Have you ever been told that you have heart trouble? A murmur? Irregular heartbeat? Liable to have a heart attack? Anything wrong with your blood pressure?

Do you have pain over your heart? What is it like? Sharp? Crushing? Aching? Burning? How long does the pain last? Does it stay in one place or travel somewhere? Where?

Do you have palpitation? Describe it. Does it start suddenly or gradually? How long does it last? How does it stop? Suddenly or by degrees? What symptoms do you have with it?

Do you have trouble breathing? When? Do you wake up breathless or wheezing? What gives you relief?

Do your ankles swell? Do they go down again? When? Do you have varicose veins?

Has your belly swelled?

Do your lips and nailbeds get bluish? When?

High or Low Blood Pressure   When were you told that your blood pressure is too high? Too low? Why was it taken then? What is the highest you know it has been?

Have you had many headaches? Describe them. Do you have nosebleeds?

Have you had any fainting attacks? Any times when you could not speak clearly? (Ask for "heart symptoms.")

Edema, Varicose Veins   Do you have varicose veins? What brought them on? Do you have hemorrhoids?

Do your ankles swell? When do they go down again? Are they soft when swollen, so that your shoe top leaves a groove? Are they hard and woody? Have you had any sore on the ankle that would not heal? Is any of this swelling red? Painful?

Have you had any puffiness of your face? Have your hands and/or arms swollen? Does this go down again?

Has your belly swollen and stayed that way for a week or more? Did you pass a great deal of urine when it went down?

Kidney and Urination Problems, Incontinence   Have you ever been told that you had kidney trouble or infected urine? Did you or do you pass bloody or smoky urine?

Have you ever had a kidney stone or colic?

Do you have pain in the small of your back? On which side? Where does the pain go? Is it sharp? Dull? Burning?

Did you have a sore throat about 3 to 6 weeks before you became ill? Has your face been puffy and pale? Have you had a fever?

Do you have burning or smarting when you urinate? Is it when you start the stream? Stop it? While the urine is flowing?

Do you have trouble starting the urine flowing? Do you have trouble stopping it? Is the stream full, with great force? Do you dribble when you try to stop urinating? Do you lose urine between times? When you laugh? Lift? Strain? Have you lost all control over your urine so that it comes unbidden?

Sore on the Genitals, Pus from the Penis   Do you have a sore on the penis (or the female organs) or nearby? Is it painful? Does it bleed? Do you have any swelling in your groin? Have you had any eruption on your skin? Describe it.

Have you had a sore throat lasting more than a month? Have you felt feverish or had a dull headache?

Male   Have you had pus from your penis? Burning when you urinated? Have you tried to treat this? How?

Female   Are you a virgin? Have you had any whitish discharge or pinkish spotting on your underwear? Burning when you urinated? Deep pain low in your belly (not cramps) when you had your period?

Both   With whom have you had sexual intercourse—male or female—in the past 2 months? Does any of them have VD? Did any have sores on the genitals? A skin rash? Fever?

Menstrual Disorders, Menopause, "Female Troubles"   Have your periods been unusually heavy or light? How many days do you flow? How many pads or tampons do you use on the first day? The second?

(And so on.) Have you passed any clots? Have you had any gushing bleeding? Has the flow smelled foul?

Have you had cramps? Do you usually have them? How long do they last? Are you tense and nervous before your periods?

Are your breasts tender before or at the start of your periods? At other times? Have you had any milk oozing from your nipples? Any blood? Any discharge?

Have you had any spotting or bleeding between periods? How often? When did you first have it? The last time?

Have you had any "whites"—a whitish discharge? Does it seem to make your sex organs burn or itch? Has it ever been pinkish? Spotted your underwear?

Are your periods regular? How long is it from the start of one period until the start of the next? When did your periods become irregular? Does the flow vary much from one period to the next? Have you had any hot flashes—when you feel waves of heat sweep over you? Did your face redden? Did you perspire with the flashes? Are you more nervous than usual? Easily upset? Somewhat depressed? Do you worry more than you used to?

Have you had any bleeding since your menopause ("change of life")? Are you taking any treatment or hormones for the "change"? What are they? How long have you taken them?

Pregnancy and Its Disorders   Why do you think that you are pregnant? When did your last period start? Have you spotted since? When?

Have you felt nauseated or vomited in the morning? Does it pass off by lunchtime?

Have your breasts changed? Have you had any unusual sensations in them? Have you felt bloated or had any unusual sensations in your abdomen? Is it getting larger? Has the baby "quickened," that is, have you felt it move? When did you first feel it? Have you "lightened"—that is, felt less pressure in your abdomen at the same time that it seemed larger? When was that?

How much did you weigh before you became pregnant?

Have you been constipated? Had varicose veins—that is, more prominent vessels on your lower legs? Have your ankles swelled? Have you had much gas or indigestion? Headache? Do you sleep well?

In earlier pregnancies, have you had any trouble? Urine trouble (albumen)? High blood pressure? Prolonged vomiting? Convulsions? Premature delivery? Abortion? Stillborn baby? Was your labor easy? How long did it last? Did the doctor "take the baby"? By operating? By instruments? By forcing you to go into labor?

How many times have you been pregnant? How many babies have you borne alive? Stillborn? Premature? How many children are alive now? How many abortions have you had? How many were miscarriages (spontaneous abortions)? How many were performed? What contraception have you used? Did you have any trouble with it?

When did your labor pains begin? How often are they coming now? Are they hard? How often were they an hour ago? Has your "bag of waters" ruptured? When? When did you eat last? Last have a bowel movement? How long did your labor last?

When did you last notice the baby moving? When did you first begin to bleed? Are you having any pains?

When was the baby born? Has the afterbirth passed? Are you bleeding now? Do you have much pain? Has the cord been tied and cut?

How is the baby? Who is with you now?

Skin Disorders, Nail and Hair Changes   What was the first thing that you noticed? Where was it? How did it change?

Has there been any itching? Any pain? Any oozing? Any bleeding? Any crusting?

When any spot disappears, does it leave a scar? Any discoloration?

Describe a typical spot. Is it raised? Warm? Does it have a blister? A collection of pus? How long does it last?

Does anyone in your family have a similar thing? Do any of your associates?

What have you done for your skin trouble? What was the result?

Has your hair changed texture? Become coarser? Finer? Has it become sparse or has it fallen out in spots? Do you dye it?

Have your nails changed? In shape? In thickness? Brittleness?

Joint Changes, Limbs, Neck, and Back   Have your joints been painful? Stiff? Reddened? Swollen? Are they tender when you press them?

Is the pain worse when you move the joint? Is this worse after the joint has been quiet and at rest for a while? Does the pain ease after you move the joint?

What joints trouble you now? Which have in the past? How long does one joint bother you before it recovers?

Are any joints stiffened up? Any completely motionless?

What time of day is the pain worst? Does weather make a difference?

Has the joint been injured? How? When?

Have you developed any bumps on your hands, fingers, or arms? On your ears? Are these tender?

Do your muscles ache? Where?

Alcohol and Drug Abuse   Do you drink every day? What and how much? Do you always drink with someone? When during the day do you have your first drink? Do you feel better when you're drinking? What do you eat during the day? When did you have your last drink?

How long have you been without a drink in the last 2 years? Are you drinking more than you did 2 years ago? Have you tried to cut down? What was the result?

How is your appetite? Have you been vomiting? Have you vomited blood? How much? Do you have hemorrhoids? Bad ones? Has your abdomen ever swollen? Have you noticed any change in your skin? What change?

When did you begin drinking? This time? And during your life? Have you ever had DTs? When?

What medicines do you take? Sleeping pills? Pickup pills? Any drugs? What one or ones? How do you take it? By mouth? By smoking? By sniffing? By needles? By vein? Under the skin?

What drug did you first use? When was that? What next? (And so on.) How much do you use a day now? Do you take more than one at once?

Do you want to stop? Why? What are you willing to do to stop?

Note   The "drug culture" has its own language, its own names for drugs, its own terms for their use and for most activities associated with them. These names vary from time to time and from place to place. The variations are not included here, but an examiner should try to seek out and learn the current terms in his locality. If he is not sure of his command of this "language," he will do as well to ask his questions in plain English and request an explanation of any term he does not really understand.

Example   A 45-year-old woman with cough. (Interview has already begun.)

Q   *(Examiner):* What are these attacks of coughing like? How do they affect you?

A   *(Patient):* Well, sometimes I have a cold first, sometimes I don't. Then I begin to cough and it gets worse and I start to spit up. . . .

Q   Excuse me, do you mean vomit?

A   No, no. I just cough up spit and then a little later I cough again. Sometimes I cough all night and then, then I can't sleep or anything.

Q   What exactly do you cough up? What's the spit like?

A   It's just spit. You know, kind of white—maybe a little yellowish.

Q   Does it have any odor?

A   Sometimes.

Q   What does it smell like?

A   I don't know exactly. It doesn't smell bad, if that's what you mean. I'd say sort of sweetish, maybe.

Q   Is it watery or sticky or what?

A   Well, it's sort of loose at first. Then it gets thick and sticky with yellowish globs. Look, I don't like to talk about this.

Q   I know, but I have to find out about it. Tell me, how much do you bring up during a day? Say, what's the most?

A   I don't know. You see, I swallow some.

Q   Sure, but would you say it's a teaspoonful, a teacupful, or more?

A   I just don't know. All day and night? (Examiner nods.) Well, I'd guess maybe half a cup.

Q   Can you say whether this spit comes from the back of your throat or deep in your chest?

A   It's from down deep all right. I really have to work at it to get it up.

Q   And when you do get it up, does that relieve your cough?

A   Not much. Maybe for a few seconds. Then I'm off again.

Q   Now think about this. When do you cough the most? At night in bed, when you get up, during the day?

A   All the time. I cough all day and all night.

Q   But when is the cough worst?

A   I don't know. It bothers me most at night. But when the attack begins it's mostly during the day, I guess.

Q   What seems to make the cough worse?

A   Well, talking does. So does laughing. I'd say anything that makes me breathe hard—like, you know, walking or working.

Q   Anything else?

A   Yeah, smoking.

Q   How much do you smoke?

A   Do you mean usually?

Q   Yes, when you're not having an attack.

A   A pack or maybe a pack and a half a day. But it don't bother me then.

Q   And now?

A   Well, generally I have to cut out the smoking when I start coughing. Like yesterday, I only smoked maybe six cigarettes.

Q   How long have you been smoking?

A   Oh, since I was 15. My mother used to tell me . . .

Q   I see. But tell me—does anything you do or take make the cough better?

A   Not much. Two days ago I took a whole bottle of cough medicine that I bought in the drugstore. Maybe it eased me a little but not much. Sometimes the doctor has given me some kind of medicine that knocks me out all night when I cough. I've got some home but I haven't taken any yet.

Q   Anything else ease you?

A   Yeah, keeping quiet and stopping smoking helps.

Q   Does it hurt you to cough?

A   Not at first—not now. But after 3 or 4 days—oh boy—my sides and my stomach ache.

Q   Show me where you ache.

A   Well, along here (runs hands down side of thorax) and here (moves hands across upper abdomen to midline).

Q   What's this pain like? Is it sharp?

A   No, it's just an ache like a sore muscle.

Q   How long does it last?

A   Until I stop coughing so much.

Q   Now think hard because this is important. Have you ever coughed up blood, even a little bit streaking the spit?

A   No, never in my life. That'd really scare me.

Q   It ought to. Do you ever have the sensation of something dripping down in the back of your throat?

A   Only when I've got a cold.

Q   Have you ever worked where there was a lot of dust or chemical fumes?

A   Sure. Every time I clean the attic good I raise a lot of dust. But it don't make me cough much.

Q   When did you do that last?

A   You would ask me that! About 2 years ago, but I should do it again because . . .

Q   Did you ever have a chest x-ray?

A   Sure, about 2 years ago. You know, those free ones they make for TB and such.

Q   What did it show?

A   Nothing, I guess. At least I got a card that said I was OK.

Q   And you've never had any other chest x-rays?

A   I didn't say that. I must have had a dozen. Some the doctor took when I had an attack. Nobody ever told me anything was wrong.

Q   Who was your doctor?

A   I've had lots of them over the years—babies and so on. The last was Dr. Smith over on Main Street about a year ago, but I didn't like him and . . .

Q   That's OK. When you have these attacks of coughing, do you have anything else that bothers you that we haven't talked about?

A   I can't think of anything.

Q   Have you had trouble breathing?

A   Just that breathing hard makes me cough more.

Q   Have you had any wheezing or rattling in your chest?

A   Sometimes a kind of crow—you know, a funny sort of whistling sound—when I cough. It goes away when I finally get the spit up.

Q   And this sound seems to be in your chest?

A   Yeah. Just about here (indicates sternum), but I don't get it often.

Q   Have you got hoarse?

A   My voice is usually sort of husky like now, but sometimes I get real hoarse after I've been coughing hard for several days. Then I have to whisper.

Q   How long does that last?

A   Only until I stop coughing or maybe a day after.

Q   Have you ever been told that you had pneumonia?

A One of those doctors one time thought I did, but he took an x-ray and then said it was only bronchitis.

Q Have you ever been around somebody—somebody in the family—who had a cough that lasted a long time?

A No.

Q Well, when you get an attack, are you the only person who is sick or do others around you—oh, your family or friends—have coughs and so on?

(Interview continues)

EXERCISES

1 Elicit the present illness of a relatively simple, common disease using the detailed questions about the symptoms. You will be told what these symptoms are before you see the patient so that you can review the questions. Examples of suitable conditions are uncomplicated peptic ulcer, urticaria, hay fever, urinary calculus. Remember to use the questions of Section 1-2 (page 8) as the basis for your interview. Write the present illness you elicit.

2 Elicit and report verbally the present illness in a similar fashion for a more complex disease such as asthma, herniated lumbar disc, severe hypertension.

4-2 DISEASE- OR PROBLEM-ORIENTED QUESTIONING

The method of eliciting the present illness used to this point demands no detailed knowledge of the conditions causing the symptoms. It is not the method usually used by experienced physicians, but you will find it preferable whenever you are unsure of the patient's disease and its manifestations.

You already have considerable knowledge about certain common diseases and problems—the common cold, sprains, hay fever, sunburn, and insect stings or bites among others. It is very important that you know what symptoms each does *not* produce. You know, for example, that the uncomplicated common cold does not cause high fever, muscular aching, severe earache, or rash. Yet measles starts with a runny nose and sneezing, as does influenza, and often middle ear infections. You know also that influenza causes fever and muscular aching, middle ear infections are painful, and measles produces a rash.

From such information you can understand how the physician approaches history taking. A mother reports that her 6-year-old has been sneezing and has had a runny nose for 2 days. The doctor thinks of a cold, of course, but also of influenza, ear infection, and measles—among some other diseases. His first questions probably will be whether the child has a fever, whether he has had an earache, has complained of aching back and leg muscles, or has any rash. He eliminates a further line of questioning about influenza with a couple of negative answers, about ear infection with a couple, and measles with a couple more. The negative answers guide him as much as the positive ones.

This type of reasoning leads the physician reporting a case history or listening to one to concentrate on "positive findings and *pertinent negatives.*" The speed with which an experienced examiner elicits a good present illness is based on his ability to seek out the *pertinent* negatives, so that within minutes he has eliminated all but a few likely diagnoses. An inexperienced examiner cannot duplicate this because he does not know what negatives are pertinent. He must therefore seek a wide variety of negative answers which together narrow the field of possibilities.

Physicians spend years learning the positive findings and pertinent negatives for the many diseases and problems that beset mankind. Many physicians spend a lifetime expanding this knowledge, although they do not always describe their activity quite that way.

Part 3, especially Chapters 9 and 10, provides the basis for learning the positive findings and pertinent negatives of some common diseases. As you learn more, you will find that the questions in Section 4-1 of this chapter begin to fall into place. You will also find it easier to remember them. At the same time you will have to guard against omitting questions that do not fit into your understanding of a given disease or group of diseases. Some questions in the lists elicit pertinent negatives for less common problems and so may be important.

The physical examination, as well as the medical history, yields positive findings and pertinent negatives. The physician seeks and uses them in much the same way that he does those in the history. To these he adds the results of the special examinations and the laboratory findings, where again *pertinent* negatives may outweigh positive findings in importance.

You can tell how well you understand a group of diseases when you report your findings to a physician. Some of the questions he asks you will seek more details of your positive findings; many will be searching for pertinent negatives. In general, the more pertinent negatives you volunteer, the fewer questions he will ask. The more restless and impatient he becomes as you report negative findings, the less pertinent they are apt to be. The more he asks the patient about apparently unrelated symptoms and the more he probes apparently distant parts of the anatomy, the more pertinent negatives he is seeking for himself.

As your own knowledge and experience grow, you will use more often disease- and problem-oriented questioning. You will also improve the efficiency with which you report the positive findings and pertinent negatives.

EXERCISES

1 Review with your tutor the present illnesses you wrote for Section 4-1 of this chapter. Underscore in blue or black the positive symptoms and with his help underscore in red the pertinent negatives.
2 On individual assignment of a common disease—such as chickenpox, simple nearsightedness, warts, muscle cramp, or (inguinal) hernia—prepare to identify the outstanding *positive* symptom or symptoms. Frame a single question about that condition which if *answered negatively* would make it an unlikely diagnosis. The question must distinguish between your assigned disease and those most likely to be confused with it. What you are doing, of course, is identifying a "pertinent negative" in the history of similar diseases.

4-3 SPECIAL PROBLEMS IN OBTAINING THE HISTORY

Eliciting a medical history usually is straightforward. Patients are commonly cooperative and frank, truthful with reasonably good memories, and not overly sensitive or embarrassed. There are, however, exceptions which range from the unconscious and unaccompanied patient to the plausible, lying malingerer. Regardless of circumstances, the examiner must learn as much as needed about each patient and his individual problems.

The Unconscious Stranger The patient who arrives unconscious and unaccompanied by anyone who knows him presents a serious challenge. You have three or four potential sources of information, however. The person who discovered him or who brought him to you can tell you where and under what circumstances he was found. His clothes and person give clues to his occupation and "station in life." Absence of a wallet and valuables or of a handbag may suggest assault and robbery. It is best to have a witness present when you search the pockets or possessions of an unconscious patient for a driver's license or other identification. These may let you call family or friends for a medical history. Finally, you can easily tell whether an unconscious person has vomited, urinated, or defecated. These are poor leads but worth recording.

Child and Parent The patient who arrives with an informant presents less of a problem. The infant or young child must rely on a parent to give the medical history, and parents usually are close observers of their children's ills. If anything, they are apt to be overconcerned and to overemphasize normal or trivial occurrences that seem slightly unusual. This is especially true with a first or only child.

The parent who accompanies an older child, especially an adolescent, both aids and hinders the taking of a history. The same is often true of a very concerned spouse or relative. Such informants may give information that the patient cannot. On the other hand, they may dominate the interview, establish an instant alliance with you, use you as a weapon to attack the patient, and block establishment of any rapport between you and your patient. The moment you sense such actions or detect even slight resentment on the patient's part, you had best get the accompanying person quickly, firmly, and tactfully out of earshot. Your best informant and the one who must trust you is the patient. The other person can always be questioned later, either alone or with the patient.

You should try not to antagonize either person. As a last resort, you can break off the interview and insist on doing the physical examination alone. You can then complete the history before you begin anything else.

The Foreign and the Deaf   A patient who speaks only a foreign language should be questioned through an interpreter. This is not difficult if you can use a health care person who speaks the patient's language. An interpreter who accompanies the patient can create confusion if he has difficulty understanding or transmitting the questions and answers. One sign of trouble is a long interpretation of a short question or answer; another is the reverse, a short interpretation of a long remark. You may have to ask the same question several ways. Your written history should then contain a note that the history was obtained through an interpreter whose accuracy you doubt.

A deaf patient who does not read lips may force you to write questions. This is a long, slow process and may have to extend over two or three visits. Obviously, the chief complaint and present illness, at least, should be elicited on the first occasion.

The Suggestible Patient   There are patients who understand the examiner's questions all too well and use them as cues to give the answers that please him. Such suggestible patients will follow any leading question and unwittingly let you obtain a history distorted to conform to your preconceived notions.

This ready agreement and confirmation of every implied symptom or detail can be sensed. When it is, you must carefully phrase each question so that it contains no hint or clue as to the answer. Instead of asking, "Is the pain worse in the morning?" you can ask, "When, during any 24 hr, is the pain worse?" You can ask, "Are your bowel movements as they always have been?" rather than, "Are you constipated now?" You may have to challenge answers in a polite fashion with "Are you sure about that?" or "Please describe it for me." If you sound doubtful, the answer may change completely. At best, it will be time-consuming to sort out valid facts, and you may need another informant to obtain a satisfactory history.

The Unreliable   Some patients are unreliable historians. The mentally deficient, the incoherent, or the senile, deteriorated patient, and the person with psychiatric or neurological disease may be incapable of giving accurate or meaningful information. With such a patient it is pointless to go on questioning. You will have to find some other informant if possible.

Most patients make mistakes, but they will make the same one twice or will note that they have corrected themselves. Thus if you get directly conflicting answers to the same question or a closely related one without the patient remarking on it, you had best doubt the reliability of all other answers.

The Deceitful   Akin to such a patient but more difficult to detect is the deceitful patient who often is a *malingerer.* The patient is deliberately lying in whole or in part, usually hoping to gain something by it. People have faked angina pectoris, internal injury, skin diseases, and a variety of other conditions for various reasons.

The faker may select a disease without signs or laboratory findings and then study the symptoms in a medical textbook. Sometimes the present illness is reeled off in classic form without a single question from the examiner. At other times the present illness is described in medical terms with which the patient should be unfamiliar. The patient can then be trapped by asking questions containing medical terms which the patient will not know. At times the present illness contradicts what is brought out in the background information. Largely, though, the examiner gets his first hint from an experienced evaluation of the patient's personality.

The Uncooperative   A few patients are willfully uncooperative either because they have been brought to the examiner against their wishes or because they have something to conceal. Adolescents accompanied by parents are the largest group of obstructionists, but homosexuals, drug abusers, or alcoholics may resent questioning beyond the present illness. The attitude and often its cause can be detected early. Sometimes a sympathetic, oblique, and friendly approach turns the patient to the examiner. Where something such as homosexuality, drug abuse, or alcoholism is being concealed, the patient often becomes cooperative when the problem is brought out into the open. Your calm, matter-of-fact acceptance of the situation can clear the way to other information.

The Talkative There remains the much more common overtalkative patient. The causes are many—loneliness, fear, anxiety about what the examiner will find, frank psychoneurosis, and plain chattiness. You can often uncover the cause during the interview when the patient volunteers it or routine questions reveal it.

While itself a sign, talkativeness is also a problem. You will usually be busy, even if you are not rushed. Most medical histories can be elicited in well under an hour and many need less than 30 min. A talkative patient may continue for 3 or 4 hr unless interrupted. You must decide whether you are getting information you need. If you are not, you will have to interrupt. Spontaneous histories are in many ways the best, but unrelated chatter only clouds the relevant facts.

The Mistaken One last word about medical histories. Patients easily misunderstand, misinterpret, and "misreport" what physicians and other health care personnel tell them. If you have never been misquoted, you will be. Therefore, report in quotation marks what the patient says the doctor said and do not assume without checking that the physician was really wrong.

EXERCISES

1 Elicit and record in the recommended form the complete medical history on one or more patients.
2 Report orally the medical history in brief form from your record. Do not read the entire thing, rather make a consistent, coherent picture of the patient and the problem.

Chapter 5

The Complete Physical Examination

5-1 GENERAL APPEARANCE, SKIN, PULSE, AND TEMPERATURE

The physical examination described in Chapter 2 is thorough but not complete. This chapter will present other observations, maneuvers, and techniques which extend and expand the simpler examination.

You will not need all of these procedures for every patient, but you should know and be able to use them. You will also find that some terms are not specifically explained. Many of these are discussed in Part 3, since they are sometimes difficult to understand otherwise. A medical dictionary helps also, and you should use one freely.

The page number after each heading refers to the related material in Chapter 2. The former descriptions are not repeated here; you are expected to be thoroughly familiar with them.

General Appearance (page 27) The appearance and behavior of a patient can be described in precise, concise terms that have more meaning than those generally used. With experience you can say that the patient appears acutely or chronically ill, although it is difficult to relate all the signs that lead you to the description. An *acute* illness is one of short duration, a *chronic* illness is a long one. A patient who is apparently robust, well-nourished, and generally seems to have been healthy before the present illness is said to be "acutely ill" even though his condition is serious or he is *moribund*. A patient who is drawn, emaciated, debilitated, and has poor muscle tone is said to be "chronically ill" whether moribund or able to lead a nearly normal life.

You can say also that the patient appears slightly ill, moderately ill, seriously ill, or moribund. Again, experience is a better guide than descriptions. In general the more signs of distress, the more seriously ill is the patient up to the point of collapse. Very seriously ill patients often become nearly inert and show few or no signs of distress near the end. They may be so dulled or unconscious that they seem placid and undisturbed. Other signs such as pulse, respiration, color, or blood pressure will indicate the gravity of their condition.

Growth and Habitus   The patient's height and weight are especially important in infancy and childhood, when retarded growth may indicate a chronic illness. Children differ rather widely and still remain within normal limits of height and weight, depending in considerable part on their heredity. Indeed, the rate at which they grow is more important than their size at any one time. Charts have been developed both to show whether a child is within the normal range for any given age and whether he is progressing typically. Deviation at one time and an abnormal growth rate often indicate trouble.

The range of normal height among adults is wide, of course, but at one extreme are dwarfs and at the other are giants. Roughly any man or woman taller than 6 ft 6 in or so is considered to show *gigantism*; any shorter than 4 ft 6 in to show *dwarfism*. There are several causes of dwarfism and therefore several types. One, the *achondroplastic dwarf*, is easy to recognize because the trunk and head are of normal size but the arms and legs are extremely short.

Just as there is a range of normal height, there is variation in skeletal width independent of the amount of fat. This width together with height determines in large part the patient's "build" or *habitus*. At one extreme is the relatively tall and narrow individual whose bones are lightly structured for their length. At the other is the short, squat, relatively wide person whose bones are heavily structured. Between is the person of more usual build. Various descriptive terms have been given to these normal types. The lanky, linear person is called *asthenic* or *ectomorphic*, the squat, broad person *pyknic* or *endomorphic*, and the intermediate one *sthenic* or *mesomorphic*. The adjective is less important than the realization that other normal variations are associated with the build and that patients with one habitus will tend to have certain diseases while those with another habitus will be more likely to have other diseases.

Desirable Weights for Men and Women
(According to height and frame; ages 25 and over)

Height in feet and inches (in shoes)	Weight in pounds (in indoor clothing)		
	Small frame	Medium frame	Large frame
	Men		
5 2	112–120	118–129	126–141
3	115–123	121–133	129–144
4	118–126	124–136	132–148
5	121–129	127–139	135–152
6	124–133	130–143	138–156
7	128–137	134–147	142–161
8	132–141	138–152	147–166
9	136–145	142–156	151–170
10	140–150	146–160	155–174
11	144–154	150–165	159–179
6 0	148–158	154–170	164–184
1	152–162	158–175	168–189
2	156–167	162–180	173–194
3	160–171	167–185	178–199
4	164–175	172–190	182–204
	Women		
4 10	92–98	96–107	104–119
11	94–101	98–110	106–122
5 0	96–104	101–113	109–125
1	99–107	104–116	112–128
2	102–110	107–119	115–131
3	105–113	110–122	118–134
4	108–116	113–126	121–138
5	111–119	116–130	125–142
6	114–123	120–135	129–146
7	118–127	124–139	133–150
8	122–131	128–143	137–154
9	126–135	132–147	141–158
10	130–140	136–151	145–163
11	134–144	140–155	149–168
6 0	138–148	144–159	153–173

Note: Prepared by and reproduced by permission of the Metropolitan Life Insurance Company. Derived primarily from data of the *Build and Blood Pressure Study*, 1959, Society of Actuaries.

Our ideas of "too fat" or "too thin" are culturally determined, but body weight is important medically. Obesity is associated with more illness and a shorter average life than is leanness. The verified "ideal weight" as judged by length of life is determined by sex, height, and body build. It is not primarily determined by age during active adult life. The accompanying table indicates ideal weights for adults.

In recording the general appearance, it is common to describe the patient as "poorly developed" or "well developed." The amount of fat is noted as "emaciated," "thin," "well nourished," "slightly or moderately overweight," "obese," or "very obese." The habitus can be given if important and a phrase added, such as "heavily muscled," if appropriate.

Posture   The patient's posture and gait can also be well described. The posture is, of course, erect when the head, trunk, and legs are in normal alignment. A *kyphotic* posture resembles a slouch but is due to an excessive "bowing" of the upper spine. The patient cannot straighten and the curvature remains when the patient lies down. The *scoliotic* posture, with one shoulder higher than the other, results from an S-shaped curvature of the spine from side to side. *Kyphoscoliotic* posture combines the two.

The *lordotic* posture appears when the lower spine is thrown into an exaggerated forward curve. It is normal in late pregnancy and occurs in a rather weak patient with a heavy, prominent abdomen.

Bedridden patients sometimes assume a characteristic posture in bed. Abdominal pain may prompt a sufferer to lie on his side with knees drawn up. Some patients can breathe reasonably well only when sitting. A person with an injured arm or leg or with painful arthritis often lies so that the extremity will not move.

The posture of an infant, especially when placed on his stomach, is characteristic of his age. The child, like the adult, who is extremely quiet usually is very ill.

Gait   The gait and body movements usually are described together. A *spastic* gait results from tenseness in all the muscles of one or both legs. The affected leg is thrown to the side as it moves forward and often overshoots across the other foot as the foot strikes the ground. This results in a *scissors* gait when both legs are spastic. Often the arm of the same side is also spastic. It remains stiffly bent and does not swing as the patient walks.

In contrast to *spasticity*, *flaccidity* is a loss of the ability of muscles to contract. A completely flaccid leg prevents walking, but a partially flaccid one causes a gait characteristic of the muscles affected. A *flail foot*, which cannot be raised toward the shin, is usually thrown to the side to clear the ground but is placed in proper alignment. If the flaccidity is less complete, the flail gait is replaced by one in which the foot is picked up high and thrown forward in a *steppage* gait.

Festination is the gait characteristic of advanced rigidity in which the muscles do relax but do so too slowly. The result is that the steps are short and the trunk leans forward so that the patient seems to be falling forward and trying to recover his balance.

There are numerous other gaits characteristic of specific conditions, including too tight shoes, dislocated hips, and serious neurological disease. You should describe those for which you have no specific terms.

Movements   The patient may also make uncontrollable movements. The most common of these is *tremor* or trembling. You should describe this as "very fine," which usually can be felt but not seen; "fine," which can be seen, "moderately coarse" or "coarse," in which a hand or foot is moved through several inches. You should also characterize the movement as regular or *rhythmic* or as *irregular* and determine whether it is constant and always present; is evident "at rest" and disappears when the patient makes a purposeful movement of the trembling part; or occurs "on intention" when the tremor begins just before or during movement of the part.

Patients may show irregular, uncontrollable movements of an arm or leg or even of the whole body. These movements can be writhing in character or totally disorganized. They may include the face as a series of grimaces.

There is a somewhat different set of involuntary, repetitive movements which the patient is able to control but which return when the patient's attention is distracted. These *tics* usually involve the face, neck, or shoulders and are in themselves normal motions. One common tic is repeated turning of the head to one side and pulling down one corner of the mouth as the head is returned. It is exactly the motion made normally by a man whose collar is too tight. Another tic is repeated shrugging of one or both shoulders.

You can make all the observations discussed so far in the few moments that the patient takes to walk toward you. They are confirmed and extended during the remainder of the examination.

EXERCISES

1   If patients or subjects are available, see briefly those with gigantism, dwarfism, and the different body types. You should be able to describe the characteristics after a very brief view.
2   If available, watch patients with abnormal postures and gaits. Name those you can recognize and describe those you cannot.
3   Examine briefly patients with various tremors and abnormal movements. Describe what you observe.

Face and Hands   Other parts of the physical examination are readily apparent on quick inspection of a clothed patient and so can be considered in the general appearance. *Pallor, flushing, cyanosis,* and *jaundice* can all be seen in the face, lips, or sclerae. A glance at the hands will show many joint changes in the fingers as well as *clubbing.* The latter is an enlargement of the fingertips beyond the first joint. The nails are broad and rounded, so that each finger does, in fact, look like a small, knobbed club.

Speech   The patient's speech is also easy to observe, both for defects in the act of speaking and for any abnormalities in what is said. You are already acquainted with some speech defects—stammering or stuttering, lisping, hoarseness, and the flat, loud, monotonous speech of the deaf. Another is a peculiar, slow, interrupted rhythm of speech called *scanning*, which in extreme form sounds as though the patient were spelling out each word. Other patients have a tortured, *explosive* speech which often goes with spastic paralysis. Still others cannot form or use words, often saying they forget them or substituting a word that is totally inappropriate. Some patients, while obviously trying, cannot manage to say a single word.

The content of the speech is also revealing. It may be completely responsive and appropriate, but it may also be completely irrelevant and even bizarre. It may be exaggerated and overflorid or confined to monosyllables. It may be so disjointed that, while each word and phrase is distinct, they mean nothing when taken together. In such cases you will gain little by trying to get a history. The quality of speech is the most valuable observation.

Consciousness   Speech, responsiveness, and obvious awareness are usually sufficient to judge the state of consciousness. In testing the level of consciousness, you can try to rouse an inert patient by asking him a question. You can then shake him with increasing force if he does not answer and finally see whether he rouses in response to pain. One common way to cause pain harmlessly is to squeeze very hard the large tendon of Achilles at the back of the heel.

It is well to add a word of caution. Patients apparently completely unconscious or in coma sometimes are aware of what is going on around them. It will always be wise to assume that every patient can understand what you are doing and saying.

EXERCISES

1   If they are available, listen to the speech of patients with some defect either in the mechanics or in the content of speech.
2   If possible, watch the instructor determine the level of consciousness of a patient.

See Section 9-8.

Skin (page 28)   The skin may reflect a general or *systemic* disease as well as disease in a single internal organ. It may be the site of a localized or widespread disease affecting only the skin itself. Thus the eruption of measles is a sign of systemic disease. Jaundice may be due to liver disease. Acne, on the other hand, is a localized disease of the skin alone.

Similarly, changes in the hair and nails may be signs of systemic or local disease. It is therefore important to discover and record abnormalities in the skin, hair, and nails.

Changes in skin color are usually easier to see the lighter the skin. It is difficult to detect erythema or reddening of the skin, especially in macules, when the patient is black. To detect the change when obscured by pigment, strong light is necessary. Macules may be seen only as somewhat darker and very slightly redder areas when compared to the surrounding black skin. Loss of pigment, on the other hand, may be visible only by close inspection in the blond or redhead.

Lesions are said to show *primary* and *secondary* signs. Macules, papules, pustules, and vesicles are usually primary. So are very large vesicles called *bullae* and *urticaria* or hives. This is true because they usually appear first. Scaling, exfoliation, induration, fissuring, exudation, crusting, and excoriations are secondary changes in that they appear later. *Erythema* or general reddening, in contrast, may be primary—as in sunburn—or secondary when produced by rubbing to relieve itching. Similarly, dilated veins near the surface may be primary or secondary.

In describing *discrete* lesions of the skin, you can characterize the number and distribution as single, isolated, clustered, widespread, or generalized. Except for the last, you should give the location and, if generalized, you should say what areas are spared.

It is well to give the size of a lesion, of course, but the shape should be described as well. The outline is regular, irregular, or *confluent* when separate areas "run together." In larger lesions the boundaries may be sharp and abrupt, fading gradually to normal, elevated in relation to the central areas, or *undermined*, as in some ulcers where a ring of loosened skin overlaps the margins.

An area is *gangrenous* when it is dead and disintegrating. This usually is visible as a black or dark brown area, often with a sharp boundary. Sometimes the area is "dead white" with an *erythematous* or reddened border. Smaller areas of dead flesh are usually called *necrotic* and occur most often in the centers of lesions as secondary changes.

As healing occurs, the deeper layers of the skin begin to grow as pinkish, moist *granulation tissue*. Sometimes this overgrows and rises above the skin surface as *exuberant granulation* or "proud flesh." Normally, granulation tissue becomes covered by the outer layers of skin with complete healing or with tough scar tissue.

If scar tissue is very extensive, it may draw up into *contractures* that distort and limit motion. Occasionally scar tissue overgrows and forms raised masses called *keloids*.

Bleeding into the skin can occur as the result of injury—as in bruising—or as a result of disease without injury. When it results from disease, it often affects the mucous membranes as well as the skin.

Tiny areas of bleeding or *petechiae* may be generalized in the skin, conjunctiva, and oral mucous membrane. In the skin they are more commonly seen on the inner aspects of the arms, especially in the *cubital* area or bend of the elbow and in the *inguinal* folds of the groin. They can appear as splinterlike streaks in the nail beds.

Petechiae, especially as they fade, may resemble macules. Macules, however, blanch if you stretch the skin or press on it with a glass slide. Petechiae in which bleeding must have occurred do not blanch.

Larger areas of bleeding into the skin go through the succession of color changes characteristic of a bruise, whether they result from injury or occur spontaneously. You can therefore tell something of the age of an ecchymosis.

The nails sometimes show pitting or ridging as the result of systemic disease or of injury. Some localized diseases cause thickening and whitening of the entire nail. There may also be scaling of the nail surface or loosening of the entire nail.

EXERCISES

1   Examine patients with various lesions due to localized skin diseases. As you do, distinguish between primary and secondary signs. Try to identify more recent and older lesions by the secondary changes.
2   Examine, if available, patients with the skin changes of systemic disease, including the erythema of fever, jaundice, petechiae, and a macular and papular eruption. Again, try to identify primary and secondary changes.

See also Section 9-11.

Pulse and Temperature (page 30)   *Pulse Characteristics*   The blood pressure as measured determines the amplitude and tension of the pulse and hence its character. The amplitude correlates with the pulse pressure; the greater the amplitude palpated, the wider the pulse pressure. A pulse of great amplitude is sometimes called *large*, one of low amplitude *small*.

The tension of the pulse reflects the diastolic pressure; the greater the tension, the higher the diastolic pressure. A pulse with high tension is said to be *hard*, one with low tension *soft*. This is an important quick diagnostic sign, since the low diastolic pressure of shock is accompanied by a rapid, soft pulse.

The surge of pressure in the arteries which produces the pulse can be recorded as a wave. This may be a sharp, brisk wave clearly followed by a pause, or it may rise and fall more gradually with a less clear interval. You can feel these differences. The brisk wave is described as a *quick* or *bounding* pulse, the gradual one as *prolonged*. These do not describe the pulse rate, which is *fast* or *slow*. In general, however, a fast rate tends to be accompanied by a quick pulse in a healthy person.

Rhythm An arrhythmia of the pulse reflects an arrhythmia of the heart. Except for the *normal* or *sinus arrhythmia* accompanying respiration, any arrhythmia should be considered a probable sign of disease. It is important, therefore, to characterize the arrhythmia accurately.

The most common arrhythmia is ordinarily called a *dropped beat*, although usually it is caused by a premature contraction of the heart, a systole coming so soon after the preceding one that the ventricle has too little time in diastole. The ventricle then fills incompletely and pumps out too little blood to make a palpable pulse wave. Your palpating finger will feel a pause in the otherwise regular rhythm. Such pauses may occur infrequently but may come several times a minute. These frequent dropped beats can be a serious sign.

A variation of this is the *bigeminal pulse* or *bigeminy*. Here your finger will feel two beats followed by a pause, then two more beats and another pause. This *coupling* is repeated regularly over and over. A *trigeminal pulse* is, as the name indicates, the regular recurrence of three beats followed by a pause.

Alternating pulse is another descriptive phrase. A large pulse follows a small one in regular rhythm, so that you feel great- and small-amplitude waves alternately.

Parodoxical pulse also shows a swing from large to small pulses, but here a few large, slower pulses occur during expiration, to be followed by small, rapid pulses during inspiration and so on regularly with each breath. The paradoxical pulse occurs during quiet respiration and, while resembling sinus arrhythmia, is much more marked.

There remains the wildest arrhythmia of all, best called *irregular irregularity*. It used to be called "cardiac delirium" because large and small beats follow one another in no predictable pattern and with no consistent rhythm. The rate may be fast or slow and is difficult to count. Further, if one examiner counts the radial or wrist pulse while another simultaneously counts the beat as heard over the precordium, there is usually a *pulse deficit*, with several beats per minute less at the radial pulse than at the apex. For obvious reasons this is called an *A-R deficit* or *apical-radial deficit* and is usually recorded as P–A124, R100 or as P A/R 124/100.

Sometimes you may have to determine the A-R deficit when you have no one to help you. This is best done by placing your stethoscope where you can most readily count the heart sounds—counting only S_1 or S_2, not both. At the same time, put your fingers on the radial pulse. Then ease the pressure on the pulse until you no longer feel it and count the apical rate for 30 sec. Raise the chest piece slightly and press the radial pulse, counting it for 30 sec. Jot down the two rates and repeat the maneuver. You can then give reasonably accurate A-R rates and calculate the deficit.

This irregularly irregular arrhythmia is a sign of *auricular fibrillation* or AF. The rhythm is sometimes reported as AF, but this is an interpretation, not a description of the sign, and you should avoid it.

Comparing Pulses   A useful maneuver is to feel both radial pulses simultaneously. Anything which blocks the free flow of blood through the artery to one arm will reduce the tension and the amplitude on the affected as compared to the normal side. Obviously you should palpate both pulses if the one you feel first is small and soft.

Arterial Wall   The changes so far described all relate to the pressure waves traveling within the artery. You can also palpate the wall of the artery to detect *atherosclerotic* changes or "hardening of the arteries." To do so, lightly palpate up and down the artery as far as you can follow it. The wall normally is smooth and reasonably straight. A very atherosclerotic vessel may feel *beaded*, with irregular differences in diameter. It may also be twisted or *tortuous*. You can accentuate the beading and with practice can gauge the stiffness of the wall by emptying the blood from it.

To empty the arterial segment, place your two middle fingers side by side on the arterial wall and compress it as much as you can. If you now move these fingers apart, still compressing the artery, you will empty it. You can then palpate with an index finger between the two middle fingers.

A very hard arterial wall may actually crackle as you compress it. You feel this as a tiny gritty sensation. It does not cause bleeding, however. You can examine the walls of the carotid and temporal arteries by palpation but it may prove more difficult to do, and the carotid should not be completely compressed for more than a few seconds.

EXERCISES

1   Examine the pulse of patients with hypertension and heart disease, describing and characterizing the character, rate, and rhythm of the beats.
2   Examine the pulse of a patient with auricular fibrillation and count the radial pulse until you can get consistent results. What would you expect to hear between the systolic and diastolic levels as you take the blood pressure? Try it, lowering the pressure slowly in the cuff and listening carefully. With another student, determine the A-R rates.

3 Palpate the arterial wall of a patient with severe atherosclerosis, examining the radial and temporal arteries. Compare the signs with the normal arterial wall of a student or of another patient.

Temperature The body temperature is reasonably constant in healthy people and is little influenced by age. It is, however, considerably influenced by physical activity, extremely hot or cold environments, and by disease. Ideally, the temperature would be measured inside the abdomen or chest. Practically, it is measured, of course, under the tongue, in the rectum, or in the axilla. Since these differ, you must remember that the normal oral temperature is 98.6°F (37.0°C) for a person at rest. The rectal temperature is 0.7°F higher, or 99.3°F (37.4°C); the axillary is 1°F lower, or 97.6°F (36.3°C).

These figures are not so precise as they seem. Normally the body temperature is lower during sleep and rises during the active hours. The difference can be as much as 2°F (1°C) by oral measurement and usually is about half that. Obviously an oral temperature of 99°F (37.2°C) does not mean fever; any oral temperature over 100°F (37.8°C) in a quiet patient usually does. Young children develop fever more readily and their temperature goes higher. A temperature of 104°F (40°C) to 105°F (40.6°C) in a child is roughly equivalent to 101°F (38.4°C) to 102°F (38.9°C) in an adult.

A malingerer can fake a fever by rubbing the thermometer on the bedclothes, and patients can knowingly or unwittingly conceal a fever by slipping the bulb from under the tongue and then inspiring over it. If the measurement is critical and suspicious, you will have to watch the entire procedure yourself.

5-2 HEAD, NECK, AND BACK

Skull and Scalp (page 33) Deformities and defects of the skull are usually visible and palpable. These may include an abnormally large cranium or an abnormally small one with an essentially normal face. The cranium may also be enlarged and bulging just above the forehead and on top. It may have a depressed area, usually as the result of an injury. Any part of the cranium may have a bony knob or a tumor. Rarely, you may feel an area of softened or weakened bone.

Hair The hair, of course, differs in color and texture with race. Women usually have finer hair than men, but repeated use of cosmetic preparations may coarsen, roughen, and dry it. Baldness also differs with the sex. *Male baldness* includes a retreating hairline at the forehead and a patch of baldness on the back of the crown. You should note such a distribution if you find it in a woman.

A general loss of hair—thinning—occurs in elderly men and women. It is noteworthy in younger patients and may occur rather acutely during a severe illness. It can precede total baldness, which usually is temporary if due to illness.

There is another type of *alopecia totalis*, or total baldness, in which the beard, eyebrows, eyelashes, and even the body hair may be absent. In *alopecia areata* the hair drops out completely in patches even in the beard. The result is often described as "motheaten."

Extremely fine or very coarse hair may be normal, but it may also indicate disease. Dandruff is a local condition with scaling of the scalp. It usually is associated only with oiliness; but if it occurs as scaling on erythematous areas or elevated, flat lesions called *plaques*, it may be a sign of a generalized skin disease.

The scalp often has tumors that are really *cysts* called *wens*. They are not dangerous or signs of disease.

Face   Deformities and defects of the face are usually more obvious than those of the skull. They may result from inherited defects, injury, or disease.

One side of the face may show flaccid paralysis. If this is slight, you can see it best by asking the patient to smile. The paralyzed side does not respond well and there is little or no deepening of the normal fold from the nose to the corner of the mouth.

There are other changes that reflect more systemic disease. The wasting of severe, chronic disease is evident in the face and in the extreme form, *cachexia*, produces the sunken temples and cheeks, sharp nose, and drooping eyelids of many terminal patients. An accumulation of *edema*, on the other hand, plumps out the face but may be difficult to detect. Usually an early change is puffiness of the eyelids and "bags" under the eyes.

This puffiness around the eyes can extend to the cheeks and eyebrow regions. If it is accompanied by coarse, dry, cool, skin and pallor, with a dull, lackluster expression and sparse, dry, coarse hair, it is a sign of *myxedema*. The reverse condition in most respects is seen in *thyrotoxicosis*, where the face is usually somewhat flushed with warm, moist, fine skin, fine hair, and an overly alert, eager expression.

Erythema or reddening of the cheeks extending up and across to meet at the bridge of the nose forms a *butterfly lesion*. This may be incomplete or may extend up onto the forehead. It should not be confused with a tannish pigmentation of the cheeks and forehead, the *mask of pregnancy*, which can also appear in women taking contraceptive hormones. Both lesions usually occur in younger women.

The face may be fat and round out of proportion to the body, with a flushed appearance and acne. This is the *moon face* caused by corticoid hormones.

In children as well as adults, the facial expression or rather the lack of it and the dull, lackluster eyes may give you a strong hint of mental deficiency. Similar changes occur acutely in very ill people or those in shock.

EXERCISES

1   If possible, examine patients with defects or diseases of the skull, scalp, and hair. Describe what you find.
2   Examine the faces of patients with the changes of chronic, severe disease; with mental deficiency; and with various lesions. Try to identify the outstanding characteristics of each.

See also Section 8-1.

Ears (page 34)   *Hearing Tests*   Detailed tests of hearing require rather elaborate equipment, but you can discover a great deal with a *tuning fork*. The usual one used is called 128 C because of the frequency at which it vibrates. To set it vibrating, you tap one of the free arms or tines gently and briskly on your palm or knuckle. It must always be held by the stem; it will stop vibrating if you touch the arm.

During the test, cover one of the patient's ears with your free hand, tap the fork gently, and hold it about 3 in from the uncovered ear. Ask the patient to tell you the moment he can no longer hear the humming ring. Then swing the fork immediately up to 3 in from your own ear. If you know that your hearing is normal and you can still hear the fork, the patient probably is somewhat deaf in that ear. Then repeat the test in the other ear.

You have tested the hearing by *air conduction* and if it is normal, nothing more is needed. Sound waves can reach the sound sensors in the inner ear by *bone conduction* almost as well as by air. In one kind of deafness, the ear is defective in such a way that it fails to carry the sound waves to the inner ear. This is called *conduction deafness*. In the other type, the sensors of the inner ear or the nerves running from them to the brain are defective, and this is *sensorineural* or *neural deafness*. In this type any sound waves reaching the inner ear either by air or by bone conduction fail to be perceived. You can distinguish between these two types of deafness with the tuning fork.

One test begins as before, but the moment that the patient fails to hear the note, you pull the external ear forward and press the end of the tuning fork's stem firmly against the bone just behind that ear. You ask whether the patient now hears the note, and if he does, he probably has conduction deafness.

This test, comparing the patient's air conduction (AC) with his own bone conduction (BC), is the *Rinne* (pronounced Rinn-ay) test. It is usually recorded as "Rinne AC > BC" when, as is normal, air conduction is more sensitive than bone conduction. In conduction deafness it would be "Rinne BC > AC."

To be more certain of the deafness, you can compare the patient's bone conduction to your own by alternating pressing the stem behind his ear and your own. A patient whose ear has a conduction defect may hear the hum better than you do because he hears less distracting noise from the surroundings. When the patient has sensorineural deafness, you should hear the hum longer than he does. This is the *Schwabach* test.

A third test, the *Weber* or *lateralization* test, is performed by pressing the stem of the vibrating fork in the center of the forehead about 2 in above the bridge of the nose. The room must be very quiet. You ask the patient to show you in which ear the sound is loudest. If hearing is normal or reduced equally in both ears, the sound will seem to be in the middle of the head. If there is conduction deafness in one ear, the sound will be louder in that ear. If there is sensorineural loss, the sound will be louder—or *lateralized*—in the normal ear. This is often recorded as "Weber =" when there is no lateralization and as "Weber → L" or "Weber → R" when there is lateralization to the left or to the right ear, respectively.

Young children and even infants can be tested for deafness, but not so thoroughly as adults. You can snap your fingers near an infant's ear and the baby will blink if it hears. Even so soft a sound as snapping or clicking a fingernail may elicit the response. An older child will turn his head to see what made the sound. A totally deaf youngster will not blink even at a loud handclap; a baby who hears may cry; and an older child may turn his head in response to the motion of your hand or the sensation of the breeze you create. It is best, therefore, to clap behind him.

External Ear   Detailed examination of the ear itself begins with a quick inspection of the outer ear and the area behind it for any lesions of the skin. Palpation may disclose small nodules called *tophi* along the edge of the ear. These may look whitish through the skin. The bony process just behind the ear is the mastoid, and the skin over it may be reddened in a severe ear infection. If it looks normal, tapping it lightly with the fingertip may elicit pain if the mastoid cells it contains are diseased.

Removing Cerumen   If the speculum discloses cerumen in the canal, you can wash it out safely. To do so, force water from an ear syringe into the canal with increasing pressure. This water should be at about body temperature. The patient may become very dizzy if hot or cool water is used. If you catch the irrigating water in a small pan, you can see the wax plug or pieces of it come out. A clean canal will then let you examine the tympanic membrane.

Tympanic Membrane   The tympanic membrane has a tiny bone attached to its center and visible through it as the whitish ridge running upward and slightly toward the forehead (see Figure 5-1). An imaginary line can be drawn along this ridge and continued to the lower margin of the membrane. If another line is now drawn at right angles to the first through the central bony attachment, the tympanic membrane is divided into four *quadrants: anterior-superior, anterior-inferior, posterior-inferior*, and *posterior-superior.* You can help identify these by remembering the position of the patient's face and by noting a shiny "cone of light" running from the membrane's center outward in the anterior-inferior quadrant. If it were a real light, it would shine at the patient's feet and light his way like a flashlight.

The quadrants are used to locate any defects in the membrane. These may be open holes or *perforations* through which pus or blood may be coming. You may see white scars of old perforations. Such lesions are often near the margin of the tympanic membrane.

There are other generalized changes. The entire membrane may be reddened or *infected.* It may visibly bulge outward toward you, and you may be able to see fluid with bubbles or white pus behind it. It may be *retracted* as though sucked inward. In both bulging and retraction, the cone of light is broken up and distorted.

The entire tympanic membrane may be destroyed, so that you look directly into *middle ear chamber.* Here you may see granulation tissue like

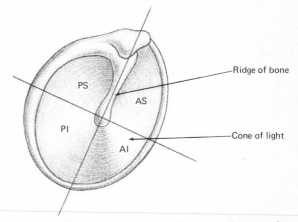

Figure 5-1 Right tympanic membrane. PS, posterior-superior quadrant; AS, anterior-superior quadrant; PI, posterior-inferior quadrant; AI, anterior-inferior quadrant.

that in healing skin. There is often pus and sometimes a little bleeding, scabbing, or crusting.

EXERCISES

1   Try the various tuning-fork tests for hearing on a normal subject and on yourself. Close one ear with a fingertip and try the Weber, Schwabach, and Rinne tests on that ear.
2   If possible, test in the same way the hearing of a patient with partial deafness. Determine the type of deafness.
3   Examine with the otoscope patients with scarred, perforated, and destroyed tympanic membranes. Locate the lesions you see by quadrant.

See also Section 9-1.

Eyes (page 35)   *Vision*   Reasonably accurate testing of distant visual acuity can be carried out with an inexpensive cardboard *Snellen chart*, the familiar random arrangement of letters of decreasing size. After this is mounted on a wall and well illuminated, the patient must be placed exactly 20 ft in front of it. He covers first one eye and then the other while you point to individual letters or entire rows. You begin with the row marked 20/20 and ask him to call off the letters. If he does so, you move your finger to the next smaller letters. If he cannot, you ask him to read the next larger size. You continue in this way until you find the smallest letters that he can read with only one error in the row.

The 20/20 beside the row of letters means that at 20 ft the patient reads what most normal eyes read at 20 ft. If the patient can read only the row marked 20/100, with its larger letters, he reads only what the normal eye can read at 100 ft. He has, therefore, less than normal vision. When he reads this without glasses using his left eye and reads the 20/50 row with his right eye, you record this as "Vision, uncorrected L 20/100, R 20/50."

You should retest the vision with the patient's glasses on if he wears them. If your patient with glasses reads 20/25 with each eye, you add "corrected L 20/25, R 20/25." In this instance the glasses do not give him vision that is quite as good as normal.

Eyelids   The eyelid itself contains small *glands* which can become plugged to form *cysts* and may become infected. With or without infection, these cysts occur on the lids just inside the edge. They often cause a bulge which can be seen when the eyelids are closed. A reddened infection at the base of an eyelash is more easily seen and is a *hordeolum* or *sty*.

Higher on the outer surface of the upper lid are sometimes yellowish, rather stiff plaques called *xanthomas*. A similar *xanthoma* may occur elsewhere on the skin.

Ptosis is a condition in which an upper eyelid cannot be retracted and so droops. In other conditions, including facial *paralysis*, the patient may be unable to close the lids completely over one or both eyes.

With or without ptosis, it may be necessary to open the lids so that you can see the conjunctiva and eyeball. This occurs often when an injured or diseased eye shows *photophobia*, pain on exposure to light. You should never press on the eyeball in opening the lids, especially when the eyeball may be abnormal. The correct way to open the lids is by placing your thumb on the bony rim just below the eye and your forefinger against the bone above the eyeball. By pressing firmly while you move your thumb and forefinger apart, you can force the lids open without any pressure on the eyeball.

Eyeball A severe infection or injury of the eyeball is usually evident as soon as you see behind the lid. The eye easily becomes fiery red in acute conditions and there may be edema which bulges the conjunctiva of the lids or of the sclera. Pus forms readily and may streak over the cornea.

Less severe injury, such as a speck of dust embedded in the outer part of the cornea, may not redden the eyeball, but it causes copious tearing and photophobia. Infections within the eye itself often produce a circle or *corona* of redness around the cornea.

You may find a *pinguecula*—a small, raised, yellowish spot—on the sclera to one side or the other of the cornea. You may also see tiny brownish or black areas on the sclerae. Neither pinguecula nor pigment spots are important except as they may alarm the patient or the beginning examiner.

Eye Muscles Weakness or paralysis of one or more muscles moving the eyeball may be evident when the patient looks straight ahead. If one eye swings inward, in which case the patient is commonly called "cross-eyed," the patient has an *internal strabismus* or internal squint. The opposite, with one eye turned outward, is an *external strabismus* or squint. If the patient sees double in either condition, it is recent; if he never sees double, it is chronic or one eye is blind.

Abnormal spontaneous eye movements are as important as obvious strabismus or weakness elicited by testing the eye movements. Completely blind patients often have random "searching" eye motions. Other blind patients may roll their eyeballs upward until the cornea is almost concealed by the retracted upper lid.

Nystagmus is a much finer movement, regular and rhythmic and usually back and forth. It may be rapid or be slow enough for you to see that it has two components—a slower "drift" in one direction and a fast "jerk" back to the original position. When you can distinguish these, you describe the direction of the nystagmus by its quick component. "Right nystagmus" means that the quick "jerk" is to the patient's right (your left).

You may see nystagmus when the patient looks straight ahead, but his eyes may be steady in that direction. You can then demonstrate it by having him turn his eyes to follow your finger to one side or the other. If you then see nystagmus in both eyes when he looks to the left but not to the right, your complete description of the side-to-side movements would be "Right horizontal nystagmus on left lateral gaze."

Many normal people show a few swinging movements when they look as far as they can in either direction. You must learn to distinguish these normal *nystagmoid jerks* from true nystagmus, which is an important sign.

EXERCISES

1 Test the vision of a subject using the Snellen chart. Accurately record the results.
2 If possible, examine patients with abnormalities of the eyelids, conjunctiva, and sclerae. Compare the color of the sclera in the normal eyes of white and blacks. Look carefully for pigmented areas and pingueculae.
3 Try to elicit nystagmoid jerks on extreme lateral gaze in several subjects. Then spin one normal subject around, as children spin themselves around, until he is dizzy. Have him look straight ahead while you watch his eyes carefully. Can you characterize the movements? As he feels less dizzy, try the results of lateral gaze. What symptom would suggest an immediate test for nystagmus?

Cornea, Anterior Chamber, and Iris   Detailed examination of the eyeball itself begins with the cornea. It is seen best in a darkened room and with the beam of a flashlight directed from the side. It should appear as a clear, smooth, completely transparent dome. You can inspect it quickly for *opacities,* which look milky or gray; for ulcers, which are pits usually with gray rims and which are very painful; for foreign bodies, which are usually seen as black specks; and for irregularities.

The anterior chamber behind the cornea should be filled with completely clear fluid which you cannot see. Blood or pus, usually settling to the lower part of the chamber, is easily visible.

The iris separates the small anterior from the larger posterior chamber, and these two compartments communicate through the pupil. You are interested primarily in the edge of iris at the pupil. This should be almost perfectly round. Any departure from this shape is a sign, as is any hole in the iris.

Lens and Posterior Chamber   Behind the iris lies the *lens,* normally completely clear and so invisible to you. Equally clear and invisible is the jellylike substance that fills most of the *posterior chamber*, but the wall of that chamber is visible. This wall is composed of an inner coat, the *retina,* in which you can see blood vessels; a black *choroid* layer backing it; and the tough white *sclera* as the outer layer. In order to see the retina and its blood vessels, you will have to use an ophthalmoscope.

Ophthalmoscopy The ophthalmoscope consists essentially of a small light bulb with a focusing lens, a prism to direct its beam forward, a shield to keep stray light out of your own eye, and a hole in the shield through which you look. A dimming switch lets you adjust the intensity of the light and a series of lenses allows you to correct for nearsightedness or farsightedness in the patient's eye (see Figure 5-2).

These lenses are mounted on a disc and, by turning the disc with your finger, you can bring one after the other in front of the hole through which you look. Some ophthalmoscopes have colored filters that can be moved into the beam of light, but these are rarely necessary. The power for most instruments is supplied by flashlight batteries in the handle.

The beam of light from the ophthalmoscope must be correctly focused. Directions for doing this accompany a new instrument, but you should get help from someone already acquainted with the model when you have to adjust it.

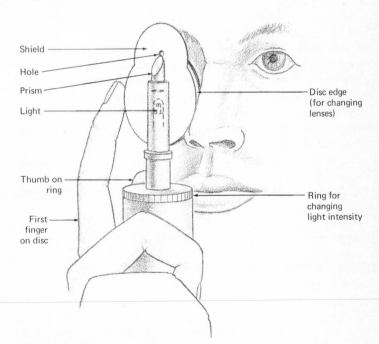

Figure 5-2 Ophthalmoscope in use.

To examine the patient's right eye, hold the ophthalmoscope in your right hand in front of your right eye. Keep your index finger on the disc so that you can change the lens, and anchor the hole directly in front of your eye. During the examination, move your entire head, keeping the "scope" fixed in relation to your own eye.

You usually start with the 0 lens in place. This really is plain glass. The increasing red numbers marked "+" mean that the focus moves closer, the white numbers marked "−" that it recedes from you. To test your positioning of the instrument and your ability to use the lenses and their effects, you can start with the 0 lens in a darkened place. Holding the instrument before your right eye, look through the hole at the spot of light shining on your left hand. Move that hand backward and forward until you find the closest point where it is sharply in focus and then backward to satisfy yourself that it remains in focus.

You can now change to the 1+ red lens and repeat the hand focusing. Going up the red numerical series, you will find that you must move your hand nearer each time and are magnifying it. Returning the lenses to the 0 position, you can run through the − white series and note the reducing action. Always keep the hole firmly in front of your eye. You can then execute the same maneuver with your left hand and eye.

You must have the patient's cooperation to examine the interior of the eye—the *fundus*—satisfactorily. It is best to have him seated comfortably, his head at about the same level as yours, with the room almost totally dark. You can do a satisfactory examination with the patient lying on his back while you bend over from the head of the table, and with experience you can work under even less ideal conditions.

You begin by indicating a spot on the wall directly in front of the patient and asking him to stare constantly at it, even if your head gets in the way momentarily. You can explain that you really want him to keep his eyes steady.

With the light on and the 0 lens in place, look through the hole of the ophthalmoscope and locate the eye. It is usual to start a foot or so away, and many examiners put the free hand on the patient's shoulder to help orient themselves.

For the right eye, stand just to the patient's right and aim the light through the pupil at a point behind the patient's nose. Move your head toward his along the path of the light. If you lose sight of the pupil, move back and start again. The pupil looks increasingly red rather than black, and by the time your forehead touches the patient's, you should see more or less clearly some branching blood vessels that are actually in the patient's retina. If they are fuzzy, try the 1+ red, then the 1− white lens. Continue up the series that makes the image sharper until it is in good focus.

Anatomy of the Fundus   In order to examine the fundus properly, you must know something of its anatomy (see Figure 5-3). Extremely small sensory cells in the retina are the sense organs of sight and send long fibrous processes to a central point. Here they come together to form the *optic nerve* going to the brain. This central point is the *nerve head* or *optic disc,* a white or grayish, round area easily seen in the red retinal field.

Normally it is flat with a slightly elevated, ringlike margin, but it may be *concave* or "cupped," especially in nearsighted people. It may, on the other hand, bulge into the eye, which is a sign of disease. The disc, because it is easy to see, is the principal landmark of the fundus, and its width or diameter is used as the measure in describing distances on the retina.

The small *arteries* which nourish the retina enter the fundus through the middle of the optic disc, and the *veins* which return the blood from the retina exit at the same point. Both divide as they lie farther from the disc, much as a river branches if you proceed upstream from its mouth or as branches arise from a tree trunk. Usually an artery and a vein run near one another and are seen together.

Their branching forms an easy guide to the optic disc. You will almost certainly see a vessel and easily locate a point where it branches. Follow the resulting larger vessel as you would follow a river downstream and you will come to the disc.

One other retinal point must be identified. It is the most light-sensitive part of the eye and the part that is responsible for the detailed, fine, *central vision*. This *macula* lies a little less than two disc diameters from the edge of the disc, away from the nose. It is hard to see in blond people, where it is a tiny yellow dot surrounded by a blushing reddish area. The yellow is more easily seen against the darker red retina of a

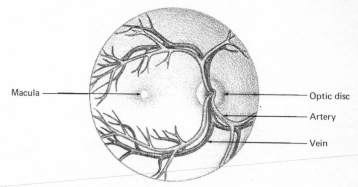

Macula ——————

Optic disc

Artery

Vein

Figure 5-3 Anatomy of fundus of right eye as seen through ophthalmoscope.

brunette or black. You can see the macula easily by asking the patient to look at your light. It will, however, be uncomfortable for him, will make the pupil contract, and—like any bright light looked at directly—will cause temporary blindness. For that reason it is best to examine it last.

Retinal Blood Vessels   The arteries of the retina are smaller than the accompanying veins, usually with an average ratio $A/V = 2/3$. This varies from point to point on the retina, but if *on the average* the arteries are less than two-thirds the width of the veins or if they are much more so, it is a significant sign. The artery is narrower than the vein, but down it runs a strip of light or highlighting—the *light reflex*—which is wider than that of the vein. In some diseases this light reflex becomes even wider than normal.

The normal artery has invisible walls and the bright red column of blood in it has smooth, regular sides. The vessel gradually narrows as the distance from the disc increases. If the arterial walls are *irregular,* the edges of the blood column will be roughened or show indentations. When the walls can be seen as whitish or gray lines on either side of the red column, it is called *sheathing,* and like the irregularities is abnormal (see Figure 5-4).

The veins are wider and darker red than the accompanying arteries. Generally their appearance is less important except when they greatly exceed their normal size. It is most important to examine them where they cross arteries.

The *arteriovenous (AV) crossing* normally shows the vein passing

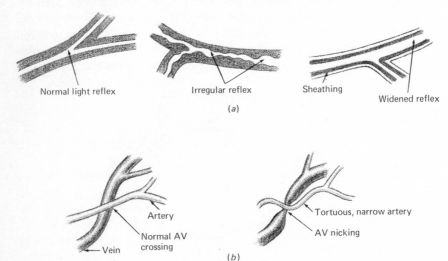

Figure 5-4 (*a*) Normal and abnormal retinal arteries (*b*) Normal and abnormal arteriovenous crossing.

unchanged under the artery. It is as though the artery lay loosely across the vein. In *atherosclerosis* or hardening of the arteries, you can see the vein apparently narrow as it passes under the artery and then widen as it leaves the artery. This is *AV nicking.* Occasionally the vein disappears at the crossing as though it could not pass, and the upstream side may be dilated as if the artery were pressing down on it to reduce the flow.

Retina Between the vessels the retina will normally vary in color from a light pink in blonds and redheads to a dusky brown in dark-skinned blacks. Disease can cause lesions visible against this background. *Hemorrhages* may be small and tend to streak toward the optic discs, the so-called *flame hemorrhages.* Tiny, distinct, round red dots are more apt to be *microaneurisms,* minute little blood-filled sacs on very small vessels.

White areas, usually irregular, occur in the diseased retina and may take various shapes, often as discrete small patches called *hard exudates* or more fuzzy, larger, more grayish *soft exudates.* Some are star-shaped, some are streaky or linear. Often they are associated with hemorrhages and almost always easy to see.

Black pigmented areas, sometimes small and occasionally rimmed with white, can be seen in some diseases. The small areas are usually well out from the disc.

Examination of the Fundus In order to detect any disease, the examination of the fundus must be systematic; since the examination is somewhat uncomfortable for the patient, you should organize it so that you waste no time. Ordinarily the sequence runs something as follows. You will see blood vessels and, as you follow them to the disc, you note their size, light reflex, contours, and the AV crossings. You can also form an impression of that part of the retina. At the disc, you note its color and whether it is flat, deeply cupped, or bulging, the latter being called *papilledema.* You follow quickly another pair of vessels, examining them and the retina, repeating this in each of the four quadrants of the eye. Swing your light and vision quickly around the fundus as far from the disc as you can see it. Then ask the patient to look at your light while you examine briefly the macular area for changes like those in the retina.

Any changes can be located by considering the fundus as a clock face. A hemorrhage is then said to be "at 6 o'clock" if it is directly below the disc and "out two disc diameters" if it is that far below the margin of the disc.

Since small children will not cooperate, the ophthalmoscopic examination is largely a catch-as-catch-can procedure. You should be well acquainted with the fundus before you attempt to see anything but the macula.

Lesions of Lens and Chambers   All the preceding assumes that you can see the retina and its components. This is not true, for example, if the lens contains a *cataract,* which you will see as a white or gray opacity in the pupil when you bring the ophthalmoscope up to it. If the cataract is not dense, you may see a grayish-pink reflex instead of the usual red one. If the cataract is small, you may be able to see part of the retina around it.

Bleeding into the posterior chamber gives a red reflex, but everything remains a reddish haze when you look for the retina. A patient who wears very strong glasses may have to keep them on during the examination. Otherwise you may be unable to focus on the retina.

Some patients have pupils that are very small or that contract vigorously when your light shines into the fundus. You will not be able to see well under these circumstances and it is therefore common to dilate the pupils with eyedrops to facilitate the examination. This carries a risk for some patients, and you should not attempt it unless you have been taught how to test beforehand for the danger.

EXERCISES

1   Handle the ophthalmoscope, position it correctly, and practice keeping it firmly in place. Test the light beam's focus. It should form a small, sharp-edged circle of light about 2 in from the hole and directly in front of it. Get help in adjusting the instrument if necessary.
2   Try using the various lenses by looking at your fingernail until you are at ease in changing them with the disc. Remember to hold the ophthalmoscope firmly before your eye as you do this.
3   In a darkened room, examine both eyes of a student-subject. Locate arteries and veins, optic disc, and macula, if possible, on the first trial. After a rest, repeat the examination, this time concentrating on the blood vessels. Determine the AV ratio, the regularity of the arterial walls, and the width of the light reflex on arteries and veins. Observe the AV crossings, the general course of the vessels, and the ways the vessels relate to one another. After another rest, concentrate on the optic disc and the retina near it and as far out as you can see it in all directions. Finally, look at the macula briefly but carefully.
4   Examine the fundus of another two or more student-subjects, preferably individuals having different skin colorings. Can you relate retinal tints with skin hues? Does the macular region appear different in different-colored retinas?
5   If feasible, examine ophthalmoscopically the eyes of patients with different vascular changes, retinal lesions, and cataracts. In each instance concentrate on and be ready to describe the abnormalities.

See also Sections 8-1 and 9-1.

Nose (page 37)   You need at least a nasal speculum to examine thoroughly the anterior part of the nasal chamber. This speculum is a scissorslike instrument with two rounded blades at right angles to the shafts. It is made so that the blades spread apart when the handles are pressed together. These blades are inserted into the nostrils, and then gently spread apart as far as possible without hurting the patient.

The most convenient light is that from a head mirror or a light mounted on a headband, since these leave both hands free. A flashlight is a reasonable substitute.

The position of the patient and of his head is important. He should sit bolt upright with his head thrown back. You should be able to guide his head into various positions by means of your fingers even while you hold the speculum in one hand and the flashlight in the other.

Nasal Cavity   You can examine the septum by tilting the patient's head away from you. You should look for *septal deviations* that are great enough to cause obstruction, for sharp angles or *spurs,* and for *perforations* or holes. You may see an area of distinct small blood vessels forming a network. Such an area frequently bleeds in *epistaxis* or nosebleed. Note any *ulceration* or *crusting* on the septum as well.

If the nasal chamber is large and roomy, you may see the anterior ends of the inferior turbinate and the middle turbinate above it. They curve out into the cavity from its lateral wall and may appear pale, swollen, and glistening—*boggy* turbinates—due to edema, or they may be swollen and dusky red. Look for any strands of shiny *mucus* or creamy pus streaming over them.

Nasal polyps appear as pale or white, shiny balls which can move about. Each is attached by a stalk or *pedicle* which you may be able to see, since it often arises from the inferior turbinate.

Children notoriously put things up their noses. You can usually see a bean, pea, or other foreign object with the speculum or even without it.

All the above changes cause obstruction. *Atrophic rhinitis* does the reverse. In it the mucous membrane withers away to leave a shiny gray surface that is often covered with hard crusts. There is a characteristic objectionable odor, but the patient may have no sense of smell.

Nasal Sinuses   Hollow cavities, the *nasal sinuses,* lined by mucous membranes lie in the facial bones (see Figure 5-5). They connect with the nasal cavity by several openings. One group high up in the roof of the nose—the *ethmoid* sinuses—can be examined only with special instruments or x-rays. You can inspect, palpate, and percuss the two larger sets.

The *frontal sinuses* lie above the inner ends of the eyebrows and between them. They may be large or small and frequently are unequal. When infected or simply blocked off by the nasal mucous membranes which are swollen around their openings, they fill with fluid or pus and are tender. You palpate for tenderness by pressing firmly over them above the inner ends of the eyebrow and by pressing upward, just to either side

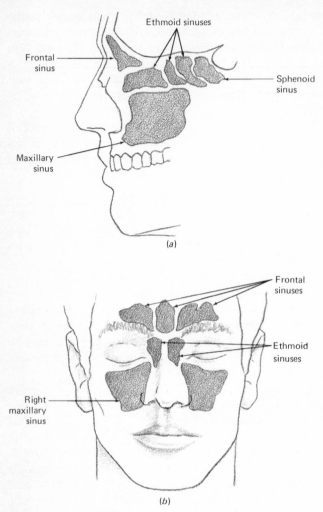

Figure 5-5 (a) & (b) Nasal sinuses, lateral and frontal views.

of the nose, against the bony ridge that forms the upper rim of the eye socket or *orbit*. You can percuss for tenderness by tapping the forehead just above the eyebrows.

There is a *maxillary sinus* in each maxilla on either side of the nose. It can be palpated and percussed for tenderness at that point.

To visualize the sinuses, you need a small pen flashlight and a really dark room. The frontal sinuses can be seen as a series of connected chambers if they contain air. You press the flashlight bulb upward and inward just behind the bony upper rim of the orbit. You will have to put your hand over the patient's orbit to shade the light itself from your eyes.

You must illuminate both sides, and if you see no translucent chambers, the frontal sinuses are probably filled with fluid or pus.

You can visualize the maxillary sinuses by placing the light inside the patient's mouth and having him close his lips around it. You may have to shade the lower part of his face, but you normally see two bright areas, one under either eye. If one of these areas is dark, the maxillary sinus is probably full. A patient wearing upper dentures must remove the false teeth before you carry out this maneuver.

EXERCISES

1 Using a nasal speculum and flashlight, examine the anterior part of each nasal chamber of several subjects. Insert and spread the leaves of the speculum carefully after first inspecting the nostril area. Identify the various parts. How much space for airflow is there beneath the lower turbinate and, if you can see it, between the middle and lower turbinates? Between them and the septum? Can you identify individual small blood vessels on the septum? Pay particular attention to the color and apparent thickness of the mucous membranes.

2 Palpate and percuss the frontal and maxillary sinuses of a normal subject. Compare the sensitivity to that higher up on the forehead. (*Note:* You are only trying to elicit pain; the "feel" and percussion notes mean nothing.)

3 Transilluminate the frontal and maxillary sinuses of several normal subjects. Note the variation in apparent size and the amount of light transmitted.

4 If possible, examine the noses of patients with acute and chronic changes due to disease, including one with allergic rhinitis and one with visible polyps.

5 Transilluminate the sinuses of a patient with fluid in one or more sinuses. Compare the result to that obtained in normal subjects.

See also Sections 8-1 and 9-2.

Mouth and Pharynx (page 38) *Lips* Lesions on the outer surface of the lips are usually obvious, and inspection should center on the outer angles and inner surfaces. To see the former, ask the patient to open his mouth rather wide. To inspect the latter, ask him almost to close his mouth so that you can sweep a tongue depressor along inside the lower and then the upper lip while you inspect the mucous membrane. You may see small yellowish glands in clusters on this inner surface. You may also find whitish, soft, elevated areas with scraped or broken mucous membrane if the patient has bitten his inner lip.

The deformity of *harelip* is seen mainly in infants, since it is commonly repaired surgically while the child is young. The deformity is a cleft running upward from the lip's edge to or toward the nostril. There may be one on each side. Surgical repair leaves a narrow scar running from lip to nostril.

Buccal Mucous Membrane The inner surface of the cheek, the *buccal membrane,* like the inner surface of the lip, may show small, normal glands. There is also an elevated ridge, sometimes whitish, along each buccal surface opposite the line where the upper and lower back teeth come together. This also is normal.

The opening of *Stensen's duct* is harder to find. This duct leads saliva from the *parotid gland* lying outside the mouth and just above the angle of the jaw. The opening is on the buccal membrane opposite the upper first or second *molar* or large grinding tooth. It may appear as the forward end of the elevated ridge. You can identify the opening by pressing on the parotid gland above the angle of the jaw so that saliva flows into the mouth.

The parotid glands are the ones which obviously swell in *mumps,* and their openings become surrounded by reddened, swollen mucous membrane. *Measles* also appears early on the buccal membrane near the opening of Stensen's ducts. Here, small bluish-white spots with red margins are the characteristic *Koplik's spots.* Reddened macules scattered over the buccal membrane occur in *German measles.*

The buccal membrane of infants and some chronically ill adults may show large or small white patches that look like milk curds. They do not, however, brush away easily, and if scraped off, they leave a fiery red base. This is a sign of *thrush,* an infection.

Vesicles appearing on the buccal mucosa usually are those of *herpes* and break down to form shallow whitish ulcers. It is more common to see torn, whitish mucous membrane where the patient has bitten his cheek.

Gums You can turn your attention immediately from the buccal membrane to the buccal surface of the gums opposite it. The margin where the gum joins the teeth and the little points of gum between the teeth should be examined closely. The gums may be *retracted,* shrinking back from the teeth, or *hypertrophied,* overgrowing with thick points between the teeth. It is more difficult to see an abnormal bluish-gray line that appears just below the gums' edge; this is the "lead line" of lead poisoning.

An *infected* tooth often shows a swollen, red, tender area of gum at its root. In *pyorrhea,* pus appears at the gum margin and the teeth may be loosened. Painless *tumors* can also appear on the gums as hard, nontender swellings.

Teeth A complete examination of the teeth is not a routine part of the "physical," but health is both reflected in and influenced by the teeth. Normally the infant and young child cuts twenty teeth, beginning with the first when he is about 6 months old. These *milk teeth* are replaced over several years by the *permanent teeth*, beginning when the child is about 6 years old. The adult usually has thirty-two teeth, eight on each side of each jaw. These consist of two *incisors* in front, with a pointed *canine* or "eye" tooth behind them. There follow two rather small *premolars* and two or three larger *molars*. The back or third molar appears late if at all and is the *wisdom tooth*.

Normally the teeth form a smooth arch in each jaw; any deviation from this is a *displacement*. Failure of the upper and lower teeth to come together properly in biting is *malocclusion*. In proper occlusion the molars and premolars meet, but the lower canines and incisors slide just inside their upper counterparts.

Some teeth fail to erupt, but more are pulled or *extracted* because they decay or become loose. Dentists commonly replace a few missing teeth with artificial ones on a bridge or other *partial denture*. If all the teeth of the upper or lower jaw are extracted, the replacement is a full or *complete denture*.

Your examination should, of course, disclose the absence of teeth as well as their replacement with dentures. You can also detect displaced teeth and malocclusion. Broken teeth are usually obvious, but you can also detect badly decayed teeth. The surface may have broken away to leave a jagged edge with a dark, rough, unroofed cavity. In an earlier stage, you may find a dark pit or hole in one or another surface of the tooth or along the gum margin. If the cavity has been filled, you can see the *gold,* silvery *amalgam,* or white *porcelain* filling.

Palate   You can examine the inner or lingual surface of the gums by displacing the tongue with the depressor, and then continue the examination upward to the hard and soft palates. The hard palate may show macules or ulcers. It is also a place in which you can detect jaundice. One rather common irregularity is a bony knob which is technically a tumor but causes no difficulty.

Cleft palate is easy to detect, but it usually is seen only in infants, since it is repaired early, as is harelip. Indeed, the two often occur together. The hard palate shows a midline slit, often rather wide, up into the nasal cavity. You should note whether this cleft involves the hard palate, the soft palate, and the uvula.

Floor of the Mouth   To examine the floor of the mouth you ask the patient to put the tip of his tongue on his hard palate; if he cannot, you must move it upward. The frenulum rarely is so short that the patient cannot move the tip of the tongue freely and is *tongue-tied.* If he can protrude his tongue between his teeth and can pronounce "n," "t," "d," and "l," a short frenulum has no clinical significance. It is also important to look for ulcers and tumors beneath the tongue.

Back of the Mouth   Since the tongue is kept inside the mouth during the examination of the pharynx, you may find it easier to depress it immediately after examining the floor of the mouth. The tonsils normally are so small in the adult that the folds of the fauces almost hide them. They are relatively larger in children. In *acute tonsillitis* they enlarge, sometimes almost meeting in the midline. They are usually bright red when enlarged and often show white pits filled with pus. Some smaller, normally pink tonsils show similar *crypts,* which are generally accepted as signs of *chronic tonsillitis.* Enlarged tonsils may be covered with a dirty-looking, ragged, gray membrane in some infections. Or they may show the white patches of thrush, which can extend onto the fauces.

The uvula may be swollen, almost translucent, or red in tonsillitis or pharyngitis. You have the patient say "ah" for two reasons: to detect *paralysis* of the soft palate and to expose the pharynx for inspection. If half the palate is paralyzed, the uvula swings upward and off toward the normal side.

Pharynx   In *pharyngitis,* the posterior wall is reddened, swollen, and may have pus on it. In some infections there is a dirty gray membrane on the surface, and the white spots of thrush may also occur there.

You will more often see strands of mucus or pus coming from above and lying on a relatively normal posterior pharyngeal surface. This is a *postnasal drip* and is common in sinus infections.

Young children sometimes have a severe infection called *posterior pharyngeal abscess,* a collection of pus behind the mucous membrane. It causes a swelling forward of part or all of the posterior wall.

Tongue   The tongue should protrude in the midline when you ask the patient to stick it out. It will deviate to the right or left if it is partially paralyzed.

If you also ask the patient to open his mouth wide, you may be able to see the entire upper surface of the tongue. You will find a normal V-shaped row of large papillae at the extreme base of the tongue. You should note whether the tongue is normally moist or unusually dry, whether it is thick and swollen, and whether it is of normal color. A bright red tongue is a sign of trouble. Examine the surface to see whether it has the normal velvety appearance; has a rough, coated appearance; or is smooth and shiny. A patch of black or an irregular mottling usually means no trouble. Smooth, raised, white *plaques* are signs, as are tumors and ulcers of the tongue. You should also look for scars—teeth marks—which indicate that the patient has bitten his tongue badly.

Breath   You will probably have noted the odor of the patient's breath before this point. In some conditions it is a sign. The odor of alcohol may make the diagnosis, but it may be incidental. An odor like that of urine occurs in some patients with severe kidney disease, and a fruity odor in severe diabetics. Extremely bad odors may be signs of disease in the lungs, throat, nose, or mouth. Patients with severe liver disease have an odor sometimes described as like that of a mouse's nest or of fresh meat. *Diphtheria* produces an odor described as "mouselike."

EXERCISES

1 Carefully inspect the lips and buccal membranes of normal subjects. Can you identify the small glands? Stensen's ducts? Can you press saliva from the latter?
2 Examine the teeth and gums of a normal subject. Can you identify each tooth? Are any filled? Is there an unfilled decay cavity? Are any teeth displaced? Is occlusion normal?
3 Examine, if available, the mouths of patients with obvious dental and gum defects. Describe what you see.
4 Examine the mouth and pharynx of any available patients with oral or pharyngeal lesions. Can you describe the signs?
5 If possible, try to examine the mouth and pharynx of a child aged 2 or 3. The child may find this unpleasant even if he is well. Usually another person will have to hold him on the lap, using one hand to restrain the arms crossed over the child's chest and the other hand to steady the child's head. The tongue depressor should be the smaller pediatric size, and you should use it gently to displace the lips and cheeks. If the child is not crying, you may then be able to sneak up onto the tongue and depress it. If you cannot, you will have to glimpse the fauces, tonsils, and pharynx as he cries. Do not try to force the tongue down or you will cause the child to gag.

See also Sections 8-1 and 9-2.

Neck (page 41) The posterior region of the neck consists principally of the muscles which hold the head erect and the vertebrae which support the skull. These are examined by determining the range of motion and by palpating for *spasm* and tenderness in the muscles.

At the front of the neck under the jaw are muscles of the tongue attaching to the U-shaped *hyoid* bone about at jaw level when the head is held normally. This bone can be palpated when the head is thrown back, is quite movable, and should be handled gently (see Figure 5-6).

Below the hyoid and also in the midline is the irregularly shaped, firm larynx, which extends almost to the *sternal notch* when the head is in the usual position. With the patient's head thrown back, you can feel the trachea just below it and embraced near the notch by the lower ends of the *sternomastoid muscle.* You can trace this cordlike muscle up to the

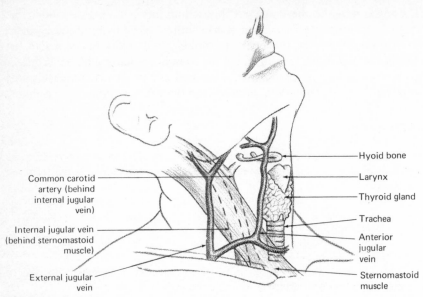

Hyoid bone

Larynx

Thyroid gland

Trachea

Anterior jugular vein

Sternomastoid muscle

Common carotid artery (behind internal jugular vein)

Internal jugular vein (behind sternomastoid muscle)

External jugular vein

Figure 5-6 Anterior region of neck.

mastoid bone. These are the principal *landmarks* of the *anterior cervical* or *neck region.*

The pulsating *carotid artery* running upward along each side of the trachea and larynx is accompanied by the large *internal jugular vein,* which you cannot identify. You can see the *external jugular vein,* however, just under the skin on each side of the neck. Behind the larynx and trachea the *esophagus* runs downward into the chest, but you cannot feel it.

Thyroid Gland   The *thyroid gland* has a *lobe* on either side of the lower part of the larynx and upper portion of the trachea. Each lobe lies beneath the sternomastoid muscle, which covers most of its lateral surface. The two lobes are joined by a thin *isthmus* of gland passing in front of the trachea.

The normal gland is firm but not hard, with a smooth surface. Each lobe is about 2 in long and almost as wide, but only about $1/2$ to 1 in thick. It is firmly bound to the larynx and moves with it in swallowing.

The thyroid gland can become very large as a *goiter,* but more commonly it enlarges enough to give a visible fullness on one or both sides of the lower neck. Even less obvious enlargement can be detected by palpation, but the normal gland varies in size and is larger in some parts of the country than in others. Perhaps more importantly, palpation reveals the presence of discrete *nodules* as firm, rounded masses of various sizes.

Some examiners palpate the thyroid from the front, some from the back, and some from both positions. In either position the patient should be sitting with the chin dropped slightly to relax tension on the larynx. It may be necessary to raise the chin upward if the patient has a short, fat neck. The patient's head should be tilted slightly to the side you are going to examine so as to relax the muscles on that side.

To examine the right lobe from behind the patient, tilt his head to the right and gently but firmly push the larynx to the right with the first two fingers of your left hand. You can then slip your right thumb behind and under the sternomastoid muscle and place the first two fingers of your right hand just below the most prominent part of the larynx. As your fingers sweep laterally and inward toward your thumb with gentle pressure, you will feel the thyroid as a firm pad of tissue. You can outline its upper, median, and lower margins by shifting your fingers. You may be able to feel the lateral margin with your thumb. Ask the patient to swallow, and—as the larynx moves upward—you can feel the thyroid go with it. If he cannot swallow easily, have the patient hold water in his mouth while you place your fingers and then have him swallow it. You then tilt the head to the left and reverse the procedure to examine the left lobe.

You can then palpate the isthmus by sweeping a finger up and down the lower part of the larynx and the upper part of the trachea to feel a little pad of tissue running across between the two lobes. The size and position of the isthmus vary a good deal and you may not feel it distinctly. It may, however, contain a small nodule; therefore you should palpate the region.

To examine the thyroid from the front, the maneuver changes only in the way the hands are placed to examine the lobes. You displace the larynx toward the examining hand with the opposite thumb. The first two fingers of the examining hand slip behind the sternomastoid muscle, and the thumb of that hand palpates the more exposed surface of the lobe.

You should follow a definite routine in palpation: first one lobe, then the other, followed by the isthmus. The size and consistency of the gland are noted, whether it is tender, how it moves with swallowing, and whether it is attached to any surrounding structures. The same order is followed with any nodule that is found.

Auscultation is used when there is any enlargement. You place the chest piece over the gland, have the patient hold his breath, and listen for a *bruit*. This is a soft blowing or humming sound heard during systole or as a to-and-fro swish during both systole and diastole.

Cervical Lymph Nodes   The lymph nodes of the neck lie chiefly near the sternomastoid muscle as the *lymphatic chain* runs down from the head into the thorax. Just in front of the upper part of the muscle and so just under and behind the angle of the jaw are the *superior nodes*, which enlarge and become tender during infections of the tonsil and pharynx. Along the back edge of the muscle lies the *anterior superficial chain,* and farther back still is the *posterior chain,* which really ends at the edge of the heavy shoulder muscles. The *anterior deep nodes* run down beneath the sternomastoid muscle. There is still another group lying just above and behind the *clavicle* (see Figure 8-11).

When any of these nodes except the deep ones become enlarged, they can be felt or seen. You should palpate any detectable node, noting its location, size, consistency, tenderness, movability, and whether it is fused with adjacent nodes.

EXERCISES

1 Examine the thyroid glands of normal subjects from the front and from behind. Pay particular attention to size and consistency. Also pay attention to any complaints from the subject. Since the area is fairly sensitive, you should learn a gentle but thorough technique.
2 Palpate in normal subjects the areas in which are located the superior cervical nodes, the anterior superficial chain, the posterior chain, and the supraclavicular nodes. You probably will feel no nodes, but you should become acquainted with the normal findings.
3 If available, examine patients with enlarged thyroids and thyroid nodes. Listen carefully for bruits.
4 Examine patients with enlarged cervical lymph nodes. Describe carefully and completely what you feel.

See also Sections 8-1, 9-7, and 9-10.

Back (page 42) *Lower Back* The regions of the back most apt to cause difficulty are the *lumbar* and *sacral* areas. A complaint of low back pain may be the only evidence of trouble, but there are sometimes clear signs accompanying it. These usually arise from *splinting,* the normal defense against pain on motion. The pain is avoided by contracting the muscles that prevent the painful movement, thus holding rigid the joints affected. With low back pain you may be able to feel the hard contraction of the muscles along the spinous processes of lumbar and lower thoracic vertebrae. This, of course, limits the motion of the lumbar spine and may flatten the lower back, with loss of the normal forward *lordotic* curve. If one side is more involved in the contraction, the entire back may be held tilted to one side.

You may sometimes be able to elicit pain by pressing or tapping one spinous process. Similarly, pressure over the *sacroiliac joint* may show it to be tender. This joint, where the large sacrum below the last lumbar vertebra joins the pelvis, is just inside a bony ridge running downward on either side between the hips.

A further test—*straight leg raising*—is carried out with the patient lying on his back. You raise one leg passively, keeping the knee straight. If the patient complains of pain, ask him its location and whether it spreads to other areas. Also note how far up the leg can be raised before there is pain, and express this as degrees (with the leg flat on the table as 0° and straight up as 90°). If you can raise the leg to 90° without pain, briskly bend the foot downward at the ankle. If this produces no pain, the test is negative. Then repeat straight leg raising with the opposite leg.

The lower back is the location of several midline signs of *congenital* or inborn *defects*. The posterior part of the vertebra, including the spinous process, may be split down the midline, a condition called *spina bifida*. There is often a dimple or tuft of hair over this spot, a little above or below it. You may feel the process as broader than the adjacent ones or may even identify the split halves. This defect usually occurs in the lumbar spine or sacrum.

The same area is a common one for the more serious *meningocele*, a fluid-filled sac bulging outward through a vertebral defect. Such a lesion can occur anywhere along the spine; it is found only in infants, since it usually is fatal unless repaired.

Young adults can show a *pilonidal cyst* which has a midline opening, usually between the small *coccyx* or tail bone and the *anus*. The opening may resemble a dimple and sometimes has hair protruding from a small hole in the skin. If infected, as such a cyst usually is when first noted, it may be thought to be a boil or small abscess. The cyst itself extends up under the skin over the coccyx and lower part of the sacrum. When it is infected, this area may become swollen and tender, with reddened skin over it.

Upper Back The most common defect of the upper spine in children and young people is *scoliosis*, the lateral curvature of the spine. There is not only an S-shaped displacement but the vertebrae are partially rotated so that the ribs are more prominent on one side than on the other when seen from behind.

In elderly people, *kyphosis* is more common. The backward curvature of the thoracic spine is exaggerated. An exaggerated lumbar curve is *lordosis* and is, of course, normal in late pregnancy. Children also have a normal lordosis, as do fat people with pendulous abdomens. In others it is a sign of difficulty.

EXERCISES

1 Examine carefully the lower back of a normal subject, identifying the spinous processes of the five lumbar vertebrae, the sacrum, the coccyx, and the sacroiliac joint.

2   Perform straight leg raising on both legs of a normal subject. Note the angle to which you can raise the leg and where discomfort comes when you reach the extreme position.
3   Examine the lower back, including straight leg raising, of a patient with a herniated lumbar disc if such a patient is available.
4   If feasible, inspect the backs of patients with scoliosis and kyphosis, with pilonidal cyst, or with other back defects.

5-3 THORAX

Thoracic Wall and Respiration (page 43)   The thoracic wall shows changes due to disease and provides landmarks to locate signs within the chest. It is customary to include with the chest wall the *shoulder girdle,* consisting of the clavicles attached to the sternum in front and to the scapulae at the shoulders, as well as the scapulae themselves and the muscles which move the shoulders.

Sternum   The *sternum* itself has three parts: an upper *manubrium,* to which attach the clavicles and first ribs; the longer *body,* to which the second to tenth ribs attach; and the small lowermost *xiphoid process* (see Figure 5-7). You can palpate each of these. The broad manubrium begins at the sternal notch and joins the body at a rather prominent *angle.* The xiphoid, at the lower end of the body, is narrow and movable. In infants, it sometimes angles upward when the abdomen protrudes during the

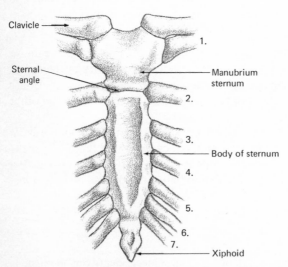

Figure 5-7   Sternum and attachments. Costal (rib) cartilages numbered 1 through 7. Cartilages 8 through 10 attach to 7.

exertions of crying. Frightened parents may think this is a dangerous abnormality, but it has no significance.

The lower end of the sternal body may, however, be depressed inward or protrude outward in an abnormal fashion. These deformities, although slight, should be noted.

Ribs Each of the twelve bony *ribs* ends anteriorly in a firm but elastic *costal cartilage*. This strip joins the first seven ribs to the sternum. The costal cartilages of ribs eight through ten turn upward to join the cartilage of the seventh rib and so attach to the sternum indirectly. The cartilages of ribs eleven and twelve are short and do not attach to the sternum, so that these are commonly called *floating ribs* (see Figure 5-8).

The costal cartilages become progressively stiffer with age. At almost any age they may become painful or may be injured where they join the sternum. The symptoms may be confused with the pain of more serious disease, but firm pressure on each cartilage at the sternal edge will produce pain in the area affected by these minor conditions. Redness and swelling may accompany the tenderness and help locate the trouble.

The ribs themselves are bowlike bones of graduated lengths, the shortest of the true ribs being the first. They attach by movable joints to the twelve thoracic vertebrae and curve downward as well as forward. The posterior end of each rib then is considerably higher at the back than it is in the axillary line or at its front end. You must remember this in using the ribs as landmarks and in identifying ribs on a chest x-ray. Once this is clear and you can see it on a lateral x-ray of the chest, the films will help orient you on the thorax (see Figure 8-12).

You can follow the costal cartilage and bony ribs most of the way from the sternum laterally and posteriorly for ribs eight through ten. The higher ribs get lost in the back muscles and under the scapula. The posterior ends of all the ribs are buried under the strap muscles of the back; hence you will need other landmarks on the posterior surface of the chest.

Thoracic Vertebrae The spinous processes of the thoracic vertebrae provide these marks. To locate each of these, first palpate the highest, prominent process at the base of the neck. This is the seventh cervical vertebral spine. The one next below it belongs to the first thoracic vertebra. You can then count each process below it to the twelfth. If you continue counting downward, the next are the five *lumbar spines*.

Use of Landmarks To locate accurately the level of anything on the posterior chest wall, the number of the spinous process is used. A sign on the level of the sixth thoracic spinous process is said to be at T 6.

On the lateral chest wall, you use the number of the rib or of the *intercostal space* which has the number of the rib just above it. Thus you can refer to "the level of sixth rib in the midaxillary line" or say "in ICS 5 in the MAL."

Anteriorly the ribs and intercostal spaces are used as marks of levels below the angle of the sternum. Above that you can say "on the level of the manubrium" or "of the sternal notch." More commonly the areas are simply called *supraclavicular* or *subclavicular.*

On the back also, the general area below the lower pole of the scapula is *subscapular.* The area between L 9 or L 10 and the diaphragm is usually called the *base of the lung.*

The vertical reference lines, of course, cross these more or less horizontal ones. On the back, there are the *midline* and the *right* and *left scapular lines,* the latter drawn up and down through the lower pole of each scapula. On each side are the posterior, mid-, and anterior axillary lines. On the front are the two *midclavicular* lines and the *midsternal* line or *midline.* The right and left *sternal margins* are also used.

You can locate quite specifically on the chest wall anything you find by using these vertical and horizontal reference lines. You can say, for instance, that there is "a fracture of the fifth rib just anterior to the right AAL" and so locate it within an inch or so.

Rib Defects   Ribs frequently are fractured. You can usually palpate a point of tenderness even in a break which is not complete. You may feel the jagged ends grinding together when the patient breathes, but it is important to distinguish between this and a friction rub. The two often feel somewhat different but the distinction can be made most easily by *springing* the rib. To do this, you position the patient on his back, and then you place your hand on the sternum, usually over the lower part. If you now push down lightly and release the sternum quickly, the patient will feel a jab of pain at a fracture site. He will not feel the pain at a friction rub unless you push down hard. This maneuver will not work for fractures of the eleventh and twelfth ribs and sometimes not for the tenth, but they lie below the level of the diaphragm for the most part and so are not where friction rubs occur.

A fracture may itself produce a friction rub, especially if a bony piece tears the pleura lining the chest wall. You will then find pain on springing the rib. Auscultation may let you discover the characteristic squeaky rub even though you hear the bones gritting together at the same time.

Inspection and palpation will show irregularities and asymmetries of single ribs. They almost never have any significance except when there is a distinct bony nodule or tumor. This usually is not tender. Even without changes in the rib, there may be areas of tenderness in the intercostal spaces when patients complain of localized pain on deep breathing.

Children may show a series of bony knobs along the costochondral junctions, where the ribs join their cartilages. This is the *rachitic rosary* due to *rickets*. These children also have the lower part of the rib cage flared outward and this flaring persists in adulthood.

Increased Chest Size   A general *overdistention* of the chest is more common. It is due to *obstructive pulmonary disease* and is *acute* during an asthmatic attack, subsiding when the respiratory distress passes. In older persons it may be persistent and indicate *chronic* obstructive pulmonary disease.

The early stages of overdistention are hard to detect because chest shape differs with habitus. Pyknic people have deep, wide chests; asthenic ones have shallow, narrow chests. Then too, muscular development, breast size, and the amount of fat confuse the evaluation. It is important to judge only the condition of the bony thorax.

In overdistention, there is an increase in the *anteroposterior* (AP) *diameter* of the chest. The ribs are permanently raised, as in inspiration, and so have raised the body of the sternum. They have swung laterally as well, widening the chest but less obviously. The movements of the ribs and sternum are restricted and the bony thorax may not move at all during attempts at forced respiration.

This, of course, hampers breathing, and the patient is breathless on exertion or even at rest. He uses the neck and shoulder muscles just to achieve shallow respiration and may be cyanotic.

An overdistended chest forces the shoulder girdle upward, raises the shoulders, and apparently shortens the neck. Again, the same configuration can be normal in a pyknic person.

Chest Asymmetry   One shoulder is almost always a little higher than the other in normal people. In scoliosis the curvature and rotation of the spine exaggerates this. The changes also distort the architecture of the chest wall, so that one side appears overdistended.

Paralysis of one side of the chest or unilateral splinting to relieve pain may collapse the wall on one side. This exaggerates the appearance of the slight overdistention on the normal side. This active side will, however, be moving through a greater range than normal, as it essentially is doing the work for two.

Respiratory Patterns   You probably have noted the pattern of breathing during your general observations, but it is well to check it while inspecting the chest. The rate may be slower than normal, called *bradypnea,* or more rapid, called *tachypnea.* The respiration may be shallow or deep. *Hyperventilation* implies simultaneously rapid and deep breathing.

The rhythm of respiration normally is regular unless interrupted by speech, coughing, sighing, or voluntary action. In *periodic respiration,* also called *Cheyne-Stokes breathing,* the patient alternately stops breathing and then gradually builds up to hyperventilation. This is followed by a subsidence into *apnea,* the term for no breathing. The entire cycle may last as little as half a minute or extend over a minute or more. It is a serious sign. So is the totally chaotic breathing called *ataxic.* In ataxic respiration, there is no rhythm and breaths differ in depth as well as rate.

Patients may grunt, wheeze, or snore with each breath. Children especially may show a *crowing* respiration, which is well described by the name. *Stertorous* respiration is marked by rattling or gurgling in severely ill patients, especially in unconscious ones. It is the "death rattle" and often does indicate imminent death.

EXERCISES

1 Examine chest x-rays (PA and left lateral) of normal chests. Systematically locate the vertebral column, the sternum with its parts, all twelve pairs of ribs, the clavicles, and the scapulae. Locate the lungs, heart, and diaphragm.
2 If possible, compare normal chest x-rays of pyknic, sthenic, and asthenic adults, and of elderly, adult, and child subjects.
3 Compare the chest x-rays of normal persons and those with chronic obstructive pulmonary disease.
4 Palpate the ribs as far laterally and posteriorly as possible in a normal subject, beginning with the second rib and proceeding in order downward. It will help to mark the line of each rib with a ballpoint pen or wax pencil. Note especially the level of each rib in the MCL, AAL, MAL, PAL, and scapular line. Percuss the diaphragm and record its position in each of the above lines.
5 Similarly locate and mark the spinous processes of each thoracic and lumbar vertebra. What is the level of the *scapular* process? Of the lower scapular pole?

See also Section 8-2.

Lungs and Pleura (page 53) *Voice Sounds* Vibrations of the vocal cords can be heard as well as felt through the chest wall. These *voice sounds* provide information on auscultation that supplements what you get from listening to breath sounds alone. But to get the maximal information you must try to have the patient produce a consistent sound; this is done by asking the patient to say "eee" over and over. He should always use the same level of loudness, and this need not be more than the normal speaking level. Your examination proceeds in the same order that you used for palpation, percussion, and auscultation for breath sounds.

Normally the voice sounds differ from place to place on the chest. In areas where you hear vesicular breath sounds, the voice sounds are muffled and distant. Where you hear bronchovesicular breathing, voice sounds are louder and more distant. In areas of bronchial breathing, the voice sounds seem almost in the chest piece itself but sound somewhat "brassy." The "eee" sounds much more like "ay." This is called *bronchophony* when it occurs in any abnormal area.

Voice sounds usually parallel breath sounds. When one type of sound changes in character or intensity, so does the other. You may, however, use voice sounds to confirm a change in the breath sounds.

Pleural Cavity   Each lung lies within a *pleural cavity* and normally occupies it completely (see Figure 5-8). The thin lining—the pleura—of this cavity forms the innermost layer of the chest wall and then turns inward near the midline. Here the right and left pleura form the median "walls" of the pleural cavities and the lateral walls of the *mediastinum*. The mediastinum occupies the central area of the chest from top to bottom and from the vertebrae to the sternum. Through it run the esophagus, the aorta, and the great vessels. In its upper part it holds the trachea and largest bronchi, in its lower part the heart. There are other structures within it as well, but only the trachea and bronchi are air-filled.

The lung in a sense begins where the large bronchus, pulmonary artery, and vein enter it from the mediastinum. At this *hilum* the pleura turns out over the surface of the lung to form its outer coating. The pleura follows the lung surface where it dips inward toward the hilum at the separation of the lobes. It thus lines the pleural cavity inside and out just as the rubber lines the cavity of a balloon when you push in the wall with your finger. The difference is that the pleural cavity normally contains no air and has no opening to admit any.

Air can get into the pleural cavity, however, and there it is a sign of injury or disease. A hole through the chest wall or one in the lung admits air, partially collapsing the lung. Such a *pneumothorax* can result from disease which forms a pathway for air from the bronchus to the pleural cavity (see Figure 5-9). This is a *bronchopleural fistula.* A smaller patch of disease may admit a small amount of air without forming a true fistula.

Both injury and disease more often produce liquid in the pleural cavity. The name given to the condition depends upon the nature of the fluid. *Hemothorax* means blood in the pleural cavity, *empyema* means pus, *pleural effusion* means that a more or less clear fluid is present. When air accompanies the fluid, the result is *hemopneumothorax, pyopneumothorax,* or *hydropneumothorax,* respectively.

Pneumothorax   Air alone in the pleural space produces signs by four mechanisms. It interposes a barrier to the vibrations of fremitus so that they cannot be heard or felt normally. It can itself vibrate and so produce

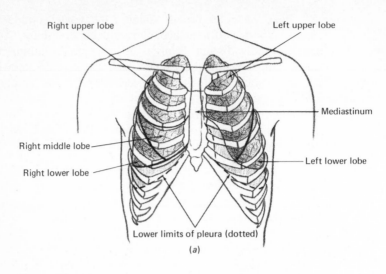

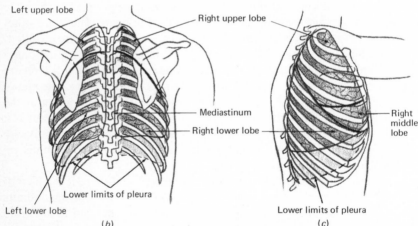

Figure 5-8 Pleural cavity with lung lobes. (*a*) Anterior, (*b*) posterior, and, (*c*) lateral projections.

tympany on percussion. If present in large enough amounts to collapse the lung, it interferes with movement and so reduces the breath sounds and abnormal noises. If the pneumothorax is under considerable pressure, it pushes outward, displacing the cavity walls, especially the thin-walled mediastinum and its contents.

The signs of pneumothorax on inspection depend upon the presence of air under pressure. Small amounts produce no visible changes. Large amounts tend to immobilize the affected side, and the normal side then overbreathes; respiration is rapid and labored. It may be possible to see the PMI displaced to the left of the MCL with right-sided pneumothorax,

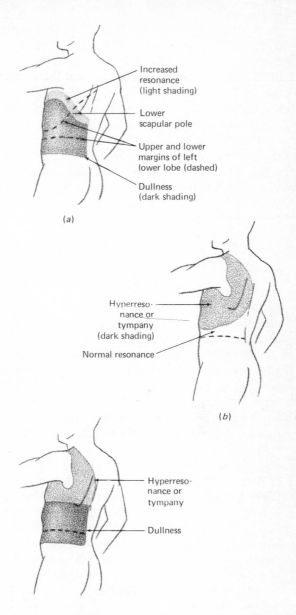

Increased
resonance
(light shading)

Lower
scapular pole

Upper and lower
margins of left
lower lobe (dashed)

Dullness
(dark shading)

(a)

Hyperreso-
nance or
tympany
(dark shading)

Normal resonance

(b)

Hyperreso-
nance or
tympany

Dullness

Figure 5-9 Percussion signs in hydrothorax (a), pneumothorax
(b), hydropneumothorax (c).

and it may be obliterated in left pneumothorax as the mediastinum and
heart are displaced to the right.

Palpation is more informative. Vocal fremitus is reduced where the air is located. Unaffected parts of the lungs often show increased vocal fremitus. This sign may be absent if there is very little air but quite marked if there is more. When the mediastinum is displaced, the position of the PMI on palpation changes and the trachea shifts. You can detect this shift by feeling the trachea behind the sternal notch. It should lie in the midline, and movement to right or left indicates upper mediastinal displacement without revealing the cause.

Percussion is the most revealing maneuver. The affected part of the chest is *hyperresonant* or even tympanitic. If the lung is only partially collapsed, there is an area of relative dullness just below the pleural air. With large amounts of air, the diaphragm is lower and moves little or not at all on the affected side. Cardiac dullness is displaced toward the unaffected side as the mediastinum shifts.

Auscultation shows reduced or absent breath sounds and voice sounds over the involved area. The heart sounds also shift as the heart is displaced.

Fluid in the Pleural Cavity   Air being light moves into the uppermost part of the chest if it is free to do so. Fluid, on the other hand, settles to the lower part of the space available to it. For these reasons it is usually advisable to examine the patient sitting upright when either is suspected.

Fluid alone in the chest produces signs chiefly by masking the vibrations from the air-filled lung. It collapses the lung and so alters the production of sound within it, but it rarely causes mediastinal displacement.

Inspection may show some overbreathing of the normal side with restricted motion of the affected side when there is fluid on one side only. Palpation reveals reduced vocal fremitus, and percussion alone will discriminate fluid from pneumothorax. Fluid in the chest causes dullness or flatness, depending on the amount. The boundary of dullness may be fairly distinct, and there is often a narrow band of hyperresonance above it. Even with the patient sitting upright, the upper boundary of dullness is not level if fluid alone is present. The line of dullness then usually is higher in the midaxillary line than in the scapular or midclavicular lines. Auscultation shows reduced breath and vocal sounds where the fluid is present. There may be bronchovesicular breathing just above the fluid.

When both air and fluid are present in the pleural cavity, the line between them is distinct as a shift from hyperresonance to dullness. This line is horizontal. Another sign is a distinct splash, heard best by holding your ear against the patient's chest and rocking him to and fro.

Pleuritis   A pleural effusion often is preceded by a friction rub, which disappears as the fluid forces the pleural surfaces apart. After the fluid subsides, especially in empyema or hemothorax, the space may be filled with scar tissue. This persistent *fibrous pleuritis* produces the same signs as does fluid in the cavity.

The two conditions can be distinguished if the area of dullness is sufficiently great. To do this, mark the level of dullness in the midclavicular line after the patient has been sitting upright for 5 min or so. Then percuss above and below the mark again after the patient has lain on his back for 5 min. If the previously dull area has become resonant, it means that the fluid has flowed to the back of the pleural space. This cannot occur, of course, with scarring, so that *shifting dullness* is a sign of fluid.

Fluid in the Lungs   Fluid can accumulate within the lung, specifically in the alveoli. The signs it produces depend upon the amount of liquid and the location of the accumulation within the lung. Obviously the closer to the lung surface, the more obvious the changes will be at the chest wall, and small abnormal areas near the hilum cannot be detected.

Small amounts of fluid in the alveoli and small bronchioles do not prevent the air from moving in and out. The liquid does, however, produce sounds which are called *rales,* pronounced "ralls."

Rales are classified as *fine, medium,* or *coarse;* as *soft* or *loud;* as *inspiratory, expiratory,* or both; and as *postptussive* if they appear only after a cough. Their *distribution* in the chest is important, and they can be *constant, occasional,* or in *showers.*

Fine rales are almost always high-pitched, usually are soft, and commonly are heard at or near the end of inspiration. You can mimic the sound by rolling a strand of hair between your thumb and finger near your ear. In the patient you can make them more audible by having him take a short, quick breath in and then exhale slowly. You should not, of course, attempt to characterize the breath sounds while the patient is breathing in this fashion.

Medium rales are often somewhat fewer, each sound seems to last longer, and they are usually somewhat louder than fine rales. They sound a little like the breaking bubbles you hear when you hold the neck of a bottle containing soda water to your ear after opening it. They tend to occur earlier in inspiration than fine rales.

Coarse rales can be described as bubbling or gurgling, are usually loud and discrete sounds, and come early in inspiration. They may be accompanied by squeaks or whistles and can continue into expiration.

Rhonchi are even louder and coarser than coarse rales. *Sonorous* rhonchi are low-pitched and somewhat like snoring or rattling. They are frequently palpable. Conscious patients often cough when sonorous rhonchi appear, and the sounds then change drastically or disappear. *Sibilant* rhonchi are high-pitched and often musical. They may be squeaking or whistling. They are, in common terms, wheezes. You can mimic them by forcing the last bit of air from your own lungs, and they are more often expiratory than inspiratory, although they may appear in both phases.

Having the patient cough is a useful maneuver in auscultating for rales. You may hear fine and medium rales only after a cough, but this is best done in an artificial way. You ask the patient to exhale, cough gently, and immediately inhale. You listen to the inspiration following the cough. Exhaling before a cough is the reverse of the natural action, and you will have to demonstrate what you want.

A cough may accentuate or abolish rales and rhonchi. When they disappear after a cough, it is important to listen for their return after the next few respirations.

Pulmonary Edema   Fluid may enter the alveoli as *edema*, often in small amounts. Edema forms first in the lowest part of the lungs—the bases—if the patient is upright and along the back or lower side if he is lying. Palpation and percussion may yield no signs. On auscultation, you will hear scattered, fine rales, usually at both bases, and they will generally disappear after a cough only to reappear after a few breaths. This reappearance is important because fine rales sometimes appear in the lung bases of normal obese or elderly subjects who have remained seated or lying in the same position for some time. A cough or a few deep breaths will make these rales disappear, and they will not return until many minutes later.

More edema in the lungs changes the signs dramatically. The lowest area becomes dull to percussion, the breath sounds become bronchovesicular, medium and coarse rales appear, and fine rales are heard mostly at the upper border of the area. With still more edema, the lowest part becomes almost flat, without rales or breath sounds at that level.

Pulmonary edema may develop very slowly, but it can also progress rapidly and fatally. The patient with even moderate edema will struggle to sit upright and in more advanced stages will have respiratory distress and cyanosis.

Pneumonia   The *consolidation* of pneumonia is caused by pus rather than edema in the alveoli and bronchioles. There is often, however, some edema around the area of consolidation. If the area is small or deep in the lung, you may find no signs on palpation and only a small area of diminished resonance or none at all. Fine rales and sometimes medium rales may be present, but you may have to listen for postptussive rales.

Large areas of pneumonia increase vocal fremitus, cause dullness on percussion, and produce bronchial breathing with bronchophony. Small areas of consolidation or edema can produce bronchophony even before you can hear breath sound changes. There are usually numerous fine, moist, and often coarse rales. If the consolidation is just below the pleura, a friction rub may appear.

Atelectasis   *Atelectasis* like consolidation or edema can make the lung "solid," but this occurs as a result of the air leaving the alveoli rather than because of fluid entering them. The alveoli then *collapse* and, because no air enters, can produce no sound. An atelectatic area of sufficient size will show no vocal fremitus and will be dull on percussion. There will be no breath sounds or rales in most instances.

This is particularly true when the atelectasis results from the *obstruction* of a bronchus. Air absorbs rapidly from the alveoli when none can enter, and if the bronchus is a large one, an entire lobe may collapse. As it shrinks, it pulls the mediastinum toward it, with displacement of the trachea, the heart, or both toward the affected side. The remaining lung on that side will also tend to overexpand somewhat, but the respiratory movement of that side may be restricted. When an entire lung is atelectatic, the affected side is collapsed and the mediastinal shift is marked.

Compressive atelectasis involves no obstruction. It occurs whenever there is pneumothorax or pleural effusion and when anything such as a very large heart or a paralyzed half of the diaphragm encroaches on the pleural cavity. Usually the signs of the air, fluid, or solid organ over-shadow those of atelectasis.

One kind of compression atelectasis is quite common and harmless. The small area of the lung at the extreme base may be squeezed against the chest wall by the diaphragm when it is not moving actively. This is what causes the transient fine rales that you hear at the bases in obese and elderly patients.

Another type of atelectasis is seen in newborns. It is caused by failure of a part of the lung to expand when breathing begins.

A related but serious condition occurs when a branch of the *pulmonary artery* becomes blocked. There is often a friction rub and the alveoli collapse to produce a type of atelectasis.

Overdistention   The opposite of this collapsed lung is the *overdisten-ded* one in *obstructive pulmonary disease.* Air enters the alveoli but is partially blocked from leaving them, so that they balloon out. Besides the fixed thoracic wall and increased diameter, the changes reduce vocal fremitus. The chest becomes hyperresonant and percussion shows the diaphragm to be low with almost no excursions. You hear diminished breath sounds and their bronchovesicular character is obscured even where you normally hear it. When you can hear breath sounds, the expiratory phase is prolonged and there are often sibilant rhonchi.

Bronchial asthma is acute obstructive pulmonary disease and the changes are usually less marked. The one exception is the prolonged expiration with sibilant rhonchi. These are usually generalized but may be patchy when the attack is beginning or ending. Chronic obstructive pulmonary disease is also called *emphysema* and generally has less marked sibilant rhonchi.

EXERCISES

1 Examine the chest of one or more normal subjects for voice sounds. Listen especially just below the middle of the right clavicle. Associate the quality and intensity of vocal sounds with those of breath sounds in the same area by listening first to one and then the other there.
2 If available, examine the chests of patients with chronic and acute obstructive pulmonary disease, atelectasis, pleural effusion, and pneumothorax.
3 If possible, examine the chest in cases of pneumonia and bronchitis.
4 In the above examination, determine the location of the signs using the landmarks of the chest wall and describe the findings in the medical terms for signs, not diagnoses.

See Sections 8-2 and 9-3.

Heart (page 63) *Pericardium* The heart, like each lung, lies in a smooth-walled cavity, this one saclike and lined with *pericardium*. Like the pleura, the pericardium turns at the great blood vessels to form the outer covering of the heart, so that there is a *pericardial space*. The heart itself lies free in the pericardial space except where it is attached to the great vessels (see Figure 5-10).

The *great veins, pulmonary veins, aorta,* and *pulmonary arteries* enter and leave the heart in a rather tight group almost directly behind the sternum. Their endings lie between the level of the third rib where it joins the sternum and the diaphragm. They are in the middle of the mediastinum as seen from front to back. Most of the heart then lies in front of and to the left of these attachments.

The Heart The large left ventricle occupies most of the back, left side, and part of the front of the heart. Its pointed end to the left is the apex. The smaller right ventricle is chiefly on the right at the front. The right atrium lies above and behind the right ventricle. The left atrium is behind and slightly above the left ventricle.

This is further complicated because the pulmonary artery swings to the left as it leaves the right ventricle and the aorta swings to the right as it leaves the left ventricle. This explains why the pulmonic valve sounds are loudest to the right of the sternum, the aortic sounds to the left. The mitral sounds are more logically to the left of the tricuspid sounds.

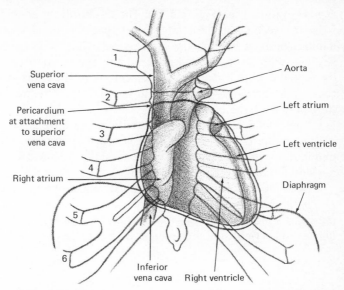

Figure 5-10   Heart, great vessels, and borders of pericardium, from in front.

The anatomical relationship is important because it allows you to understand the meaning of changes in the heart's size and shape. You can, of course, determine these to some degree by percussion.

If you were to cut across the heart, especially the ventricles, you would find—from the outside inward—the *pericardium,* the *myocardium* or muscular wall, and the *endocardium* or smooth lining. Muscle requires blood to function and the myocardium is supplied by a special pair of arteries—the *coronary arteries*—which run on the heart's pericardial surface. The thin valves within the heart contain neither muscle nor blood vessels of any size, but around each valve is a tough *fibrous ring* which keeps the opening its proper size.

Disease can change the pericardium, the myocardium, the endocardium, the coronary arteries, and the valves. If extensive enough, the changes interfere with function and produce signs.

Pericardial Changes   If roughened, the pericardium rubs audibly and at times palpably. Pericardial rubs often are quite transient, being audible for only minutes or hours. They are most often the result of damage due to interruption of the blood supply in the coronary arteries.

Fluid can accumulate in the pericardial sac from several causes. Usually it is watery, but it may be bloody. It is undetectable if scanty, but in larger amounts it makes the PMI disappear both to inspection and palpation. Percussion shows that cardiac dullness is increased in size with typical outlines (see Figure 5-11). The left border is almost a straight line from the second or third intercostal space at the sternal margin to the diaphragm at or beyond the midclavicular line. The right border is also straight, with its lower end at the diaphragm several centimeters to the right of the sternal margin. On auscultation, the heart sounds are much reduced in intensity—especially in the mitral and pulmonic areas, where they may be inaudible.

Since fluid changes position with posture, it is possible to detect *shifting dullness* in a large enough *pericardial effusion.* This is easiest to find in the second interspace, where the dullness is wider when the patient lies down than when he sits upright.

Scarring may follow an acute episode and produce *chronic constrictive pericarditis.* As the name implies, the scarred pericardium restricts the heart's movements. Normally, the PMI shifts as a person turns from his left to his right side. In a patient with constrictive pericarditis, the PMI

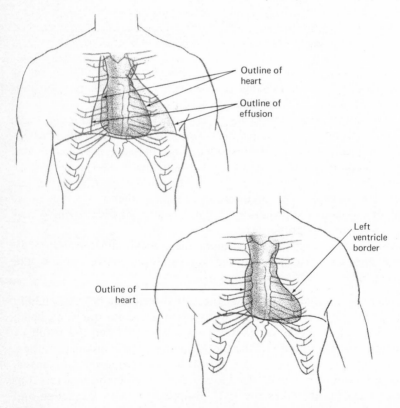

Figure 5-11 Pericardial effusion (above) and left ventricular enlargement (below).

does not shift. Some patients will show a retraction of the interspace instead of an outward push during systole. There may follow a heave in diastole, so you will have to time the palpable movements by simultaneously listening to the heart sounds. There is often a short, loud, extra heart sound—called S_3—after S_2. The size of the heart is usually normal, as is the shape.

Cardiac Enlargement A large area of precordial dullness usually is due to an enlarged heart. The increased size may result from *dilatation* and excessive stretching of the myocardial walls. The stretching reflects muscular weakness and past a certain point interferes with the heart's ability to contract in systole. This is what occurs in the more common forms of *heart failure* or *decompensation.* The heart, specifically one or both ventricles, becomes too weak to pump enough blood to sustain the body's needs and, being weak, dilates.

A special type of stretching occurs if one area of myocardium is weakened. The weakened area balloons out locally as a *ventricular aneurysm.*

Dilatation can involve any of the four chambers of the heart. If it affects the right atrium, it may disorganize the heart's rhythm to produce *auricular fibrillation,* although there are more common causes. The normal rhythm can also be upset by ventricular dilatation.

Ventricular hypertrophy increases the heart's size by quite a different mechanism. It is the myocardium's response to a continued heavy work load, such as moving the blood against increased resistance. It occurs, for example, in *chronic hypertension* or continuing high blood pressure.

You can detect an enlarged heart by seeing or feeling the PMI farther to the left than normal. Unless the mediastinum is shifted to the left, a PMI lateral to the MCL suggests an enlarged heart. A very forceful beat further suggests ventricular hypertrophy as a cause; a weak but often enlarged area of the PMI hints at ventricular dilatation. The ventricle may, in fact, become hypertrophied and then dilate; enlargement usually appears as dilatation under those circumstances.

Percussion confirms cardiac enlargement (see Figure 5-11). Further, it can give evidence of which heart chambers are involved. If only the left ventricle enlarges, you will find a *"boot-shaped heart."* The right border percusses as normal, as does the width in left ICS 3; that is, the left border of dullness is 2 to 4 cm from the midsternal line. The width in ICS 4 may be about at the upper limits of normal, 7 cm from the midline or a little more. In ICS 5 and ICS 6, however, the left border of dullness is well beyond the usual 8 to 10 cm and is often 12 to 16 cm.

If the right ventricle is also involved, the left border is nearer a straight line, with some widening in ICS 3 and ICS 4. The right border may be widened in ICS 4 or ICS 5 to 3 or 4 cm.

Direct Percussion   Percussion must be carefully done to make these determinations. It is best to percuss softly in a quiet place. Sometimes *direct percussion* is even more sensitive to the border of dullness. In this maneuver the middle finger of one hand is used and held extended. You hold your palm near the chest surface and snap the middle finger downward, bending only the joint where the finger joins the hand. The fleshy end of your middle finger should strike lightly parallel to the ribs in the intercostal space. You let your finger remain where it hits rather than bounding it up again. In this way you can feel as well as hear the vibrations of resonance.

Heart Sounds in Myocardial Disease   Myocardial changes are also reflected in the heart sounds. More accurately, changes that affect the heart sounds accompany changes in the myocardium. In left ventricular hypertrophy, S_2 in the aortic area (also called A_2) is louder than in the pulmonic area (P_2) and recorded as $A_2 > P_2$. In right ventricular hypertrophy, the reverse is true, noted as $P_2 > A_2$.

Ventricular hypertrophy also produces the fourth heart sound gallop. The fourth sound (S_4) can be heard normally, but only in young children. Then and in the gallop, it immediately precedes S_1; that is, it occurs very late in diastole. It sounds something like "pul-lubb dup." In left ventricular hypertrophy you hear it in the aortic area, in right ventricular hypertrophy in the pulmonic area. In both it is a short, soft, low-pitched, dull sound, and you can hear it better with the bell than with the diaphragm. The sound can be louder and more distinct between the apex and the sternum in ICS 4 or ICS 5.

Hypertrophy is also associated with an *early systolic click.* This is brief and high-pitched, as the name suggests, and follows just after S_1. It again is in the aortic or pulmonic area as the left or right ventricle is hypertrophied.

Both S_4 and a systolic click occur in other conditions as well. Indeed, all the signs found in a patient must be taken into consideration in deciding what heart lesion he has.

Dilatation of the ventricles also alters the heart sounds. S_1 becomes softer than S_2 even in the mitral area, and S_2 may be louder than normal. In more severe dilatation, both heart sounds are decreased in intensity and are somewhat slurred; they have been described as "mushy."

Dilatation is also accompanied by an S_3 or an S_3 gallop. The *third heart sound* follows S_2 after a brief pause and so is early in diastole. It has been said to sound like "lubb dup-puh." It is a low-frequency sound best heard with the bell of the chest piece and is usually loudest at the apex in left ventricular dilatation and nearer the sternal border in right ventricular dilatation.

A *gallop rhythm* results when either S_3 or S_4 is almost as intense as S_1 and S_2. The cycle of "sound-sound pause sound pause sound-sound pause . . ." has the rhythm of the hooves of a galloping horse. You may have trouble distinguishing between an S_3 gallop and an S_4 gallop, particularly if the heart is beating rapidly. Both, however, are serious signs in most instances.

Arrhythmias The various arrhythmias are also associated with disorders of the myocardium. Most arise in the atrium but some in the ventricles. The most common are *premature beats* arising in the ventricles and are serious if frequent, especially after a coronary occlusion.

Coronary Occlusion Occlusion or block of a coronary artery branch with death of part of the myocardium may produce no signs, lead to heart failure with dilatation, or produce arrhythmias which can be fatal. The rate is usually rapid, premature beats are common, and there may be a gallop. The most characteristic sign is a pericardial friction rub which usually lasts only a few hours.

Murmurs and Thrills Within the heart chamber, changes that produce sounds usually are in the valves. In addition there can be holes in the *septum,* the sheet of myocardium and endocardium that separates the right from the left atrium and the right from the left ventricle.

These sounds are *murmurs* and sometimes they can be felt as *thrills,* rapid vibrations best felt with the edge of the hand or the base of the palm. It is common to describe the feel of one kind of thrill as being like that of a purring cat. It may also resemble the tingling, rapid vibration you feel in a rubber tube if you reduce the stream of water by pinching it.

The latter illustration serves also to explain how murmurs and thrills arise. A fluid—water or blood—flowing smoothly and uninterruptedly through a pipe or heart chamber with a smooth lining does not vibrate and will not set its container in motion. A narrowed section of the container, however, makes the moving stream swirl and eddy. This turbulence is a vibration and shakes the walls of the container. In general, the vibration will be stronger downstream from the partial obstruction and will be carried along by the moving fluid.

A thin membrane partially obstructing flow is itself set in vibration by the fluid eddies and adds its component to the turbulence. Even an abrupt widening in a segment of the container wall produces eddies as the fluid swirls within it.

A second stream of fluid joining the first and especially meeting it head-on causes eddies and so vibration. Finally, if the fluid moves faster and faster, it will reach a point where the container no longer carries it smoothly, and eddies form at the walls in a turbulent flow with vibration.

It is vibrations set up by these mechanisms that are the audible murmurs and palpable thrills in the heart and blood vessels. The frequency or rapidity of the vibrations determines the pitch, their strength controls the loudness, their point of origin determines the location.

Valvular Lesions   Valvular changes are the most common cause of murmurs and thrills. Any of the four heart valves can be at fault and each can be involved in two ways. The opening through which the blood passes can be too narrow, either because the ring around the valve is too tight or because the leaves of the valves are distorted and cannot swing back out of the way. Such abnormal narrowing is *stenosis.*

A valve may also fail to close completely, so that blood flows back through it when it should not and meets an oncoming stream of blood. This can occur when the valvular ring dilates or when the leaves are distorted so that they cannot close. This is *insufficiency* (see Figure 9-2).

Stenosis and insufficiency can occur in the same valve simultaneously, as, for example, when the leaves stick to one another where they join near the ring. This reduces the degree to which they can open and, by shortening the free edges, prevents them from closing completely.

It is possible then to have aortic stenosis, aortic insufficiency, aortic stenosis and insufficiency, mitral stenosis, mitral insufficiency, mitral stenosis and insufficiency, pulmonic stenosis, etc. One valve may have stenosis and another insufficiency or stenosis in any combination.

Other Causes of Murmurs   All these are *organic valvular changes* with anatomical lesions. There are, however, *functional murmurs* in which there are no local lesions. Murmurs can appear when the heart is pumping blood so rapidly that even normal valve openings produce eddies. Functional murmurs are common under certain circumstances and must often be considered normal findings. Certainly they are not always signs of heart disease.

Murmurs also are produced by a hole or defect in the septum which separates the left from the right side of the heart. Pressures are higher in the left cardiac chambers, and the resulting flow of blood through the defect produces a murmur.

Similarly, the higher pressure in the aorta forces blood into the pulmonary artery when these remain connected after birth. This occurs in *patent ductus arteriosus,* in which the connection that is normal before birth persists into infancy, childhood, or even adult life.

Air moving in the lung with each heartbeat can cause an audible sound, the *cardiopulmonary murmur.* It is a normal finding and indicates no disease.

Aids to Hearing Murmurs   Murmurs can be difficult to hear either because they are of low intensity, because the left lung is overdistended, because there is fluid in the pericardium, or because the chest wall is thick or fat. You can use certain maneuvers to accentuate them.

Exercise increases the intensity of most murmurs. This can be shown by having the patient sit up and lie back from three to five times; younger patients and those in better physical condition may require even more exercise.

Murmurs high in the precordium—aortic and pulmonic areas—or at the *base of the heart* near the sternum in ICS 3 through ICS 5 are usually best heard if you have the patient sit up—or finish exercising in a sitting position—and bend forward. It also helps if he exhales as fully as he can and holds his breath while you listen.

Murmurs at the apex near the PMI are accentuated by having the patient lie on his left side while you support him with your left arm. Again you can hear better if he exhales and holds his breath.

Murmurs that are high-pitched are more audible with the diaphragm of the chest piece. Low-pitched murmurs are best heard with the bell. To use it properly, you must hold the bell lightly against the skin, anchoring it so that it does not rub but not pushing hard enough to stretch the skin beneath it. You really create a poor diaphragm if you stretch the skin.

Description and Geography of Murmurs   To characterize a murmur completely, you must determine its *location* and *transmission;* its *timing, duration,* and *course;* its *pitch* and *quality;* and its *intensity* or loudness. You can determine only location and transmission without having listened to murmurs themselves.

The *location* of a murmur is the point at which it is loudest and most distinct. This may be a small area or one several centimeters in diameter. If you can hear the murmur only in a small area, it is *sharply localized.* When it is loud and distinct over a larger area, it is *diffuse* and *centered* at the loudest point.

The exact location is usually in one of four valve areas. It may be at the apex, just inside it, or at the *base of the heart* near the left sternal margin. You can be much more specific by measuring the distance in centimeters from the midsternal line in a definite intercostal space.

Transmission is simply the spread of the murmur's sound outside its location. Usually the sound will become fainter the farther you move from the point of maximum intensity. If it does not fade out or if it fades and then becomes louder again, say as you move from the aortic to the mitral area, you should suspect a murmur in each area.

Some murmurs are transmitted into the axilla, some to the inter-scapular area, and some into the carotid artery low in the neck. Obviously only loud murmurs will be so widely transmitted. Soft ones will not usually be heard outside the precordium.

Chronology of Murmurs   The *timing, duration,* and *course* of a murmur are the most difficult characteristics to master, but they are among the most important. You can successfully determine them only if you can identify heart sounds and listen differentially to the various parts of the cardiac cycle.

The first distinction to make is whether the murmur is *systolic, diastolic,* or *continuous.* This is relatively easy if the heart rate is slow and the heart sounds are distinct. Murmurs can, however, cover up heart sounds. If you have trouble telling S_1 from S_2, the first maneuver is to feel the carotid pulse and identify systole by the surge of arterial blood. If a heart sound is obscured, you can sneak up on it by moving your stethoscope far enough away to pick up both S_1 and S_2 distinctly. You then inch it back to the point where the murmur is loud enough to be timed.

Once you decide in which *phase* you hear the murmur, you must determine its specific *timing* and *duration.* Some murmurs last throughout systole, beginning with or masking S_1 and continuing into S_2. Such a murmur is called *holosystolic.* Similarly, a murmur can continue through diastole from S_2 to S_1, and this is *holodiastolic.*

Holosystolic murmurs usually and holodiastolic murmurs often sound louder at the start than at the end. This diminishing intensity is called *decrescendo.*

It takes careful listening to distinguish between a truly holosystolic murmur and a *midsystolic* one. The difference is that there is a clearly distinguishable S_1 before the murmur and a very slight pause before a distinct S_2. A late *systolic* murmur, of course, begins after a clear pause following S_1 and continues to S_2, which it may obscure. This murmur may start at low intensity and increase in loudness. Such increasing intensity is called *crescendo.*

Diastolic murmurs can also occur at different times. A *middiastolic* murmur has a pause after S_2 and before S_1. It may increase in intensity and then die away. This is a *crescendo-decrescendo* murmur. An *early diastolic* murmur may begin almost as soon as S_2 stops, and it ceases about halfway to S_1. The *late diastolic* murmur is usually called *presystolic.* It usually is crescendo and often obscures S_1.

A *continuous* murmur extends without interruption throughout the entire cardiac cycle. It may be slightly crescendo-decrescendo, but there is no murmur-free period as there is with combined systolic and diastolic murmurs.

Such careful characterization as this is difficult when there is only one murmur in an area. It is even harder when there are two, as may occur when the same valve has both stenosis and insufficiency. Aside from differentially listening to the phases and simultaneously timing with the carotid pulse, another maneuver helps. One murmur frequently is better transmitted in one direction than in the other. By listening in various directions, you may find the systolic or the diastolic component relatively clearer. In doing this, however, you must remember that another source may contribute still another murmur, so it is well to stay near the area of maximal intensity.

Sound Properties of Murmurs The *pitch* of a murmur is easy to characterize after you have heard a variety of them. The high-pitched murmur sounds somewhat like air escaping from a small pressure hose or valve. A low-pitched murmur more nearly resembles the sound of air escaping from a partly filled balloon with a rigid neck. A *median-pitched* murmur is between these sounds.

The pitch assumes more meaning when you consider the *quality* or timbre of the murmur. The words so graphically describe the sounds that you should have little trouble distinguishing them. A *puff* is a very brief, low-pitched sound. A *blowing* murmur may be median- or high-pitched but it is smooth in quality and not musical. A *harsh* murmur is higher-pitched, more rasping, and not so smooth. A *rasping* murmur is rougher still. A *rumbling* murmur is low-pitched and even less uniform, while a *musical* murmur sounds a clearer note like that of a whistle or pitch pipe.

A continuous murmur may have a *machinery* quality, humming or even whining. Occasionally a murmur can be accurately described as *crowing* in quality.

The *intensity* or *loudness* of a murmur is judged at the point where it is best heard. It is often reported as *very soft, soft, moderately loud, loud,* or *very loud.* Other clinicians grade the intensity, but some use a system of I to IV, others of I to VI. In each, the highest number is the loudest. If you use such a grading system, you should always indicate the scale. Thus a very soft murmur is reported as Grade I/VI, read as "Grade one of six." A very loud murmur on another scale would be Grade IV/IV.

To characterize a murmur completely, you will have to describe it under each of the separate categories. For example, a complete description of one murmur would be "Moderately loud, harsh, high-pitched, holosystolic decrescendo murmur in the aortic area, transmitted toward but not to the apex and into the carotid artery."

Thrills Palpable thrills accompany murmurs and are characterized in much the same way by *location, timing* and *duration, quality* and *intensity.* Even the same maneuvers of exercise, position, and respiration are used to accentuate them.

Usually the location of the thrill is the same as that of the murmur that it accompanies. Ordinarily, though, the thrill is more sharply localized and less often transmitted.

Timing a thrill at the apex usually is a matter of determining where it comes on the palpable heartbeat. In other areas and even at the apex it is easier and often necessary to listen simultaneously and time the thrill by the heart sounds. Ordinarily it is accurate enough to describe the thrill as short or long, systolic or diastolic. At the apex, however, you should try to distinguish a presystolic thrill from a systolic, midsystolic, or early diastolic one.

The quality of a thrill is usually described as *fine, coarse,* or *rough.* The terms give a fairly clear picture of the differences, and you should have no difficulty identifying each.

The intensity can be described as *barely palpable, palpable,* and *easily palpable.* You should not be misled by the loudness of the murmur which the thrill accompanies. Usually the two characteristics prove roughly parallel; the loudest murmurs are those with easily palpable thrills. But the loudest may have no thrill, and a barely audible murmur may be accompanied by a distinct thrill.

Vascular Lesions   Lesions in blood vessels as well as those in the heart can produce murmurs and thrills. Patent ductus arteriosus is one example, but others are more common. An *aneurysm* or dilated sac on a large artery such as the aorta may cause a pulsation on the chest wall, a murmur, and a thrill. A connection directly from a fairly large artery to a vein can produce a humming murmur. Such an *arteriovenous fistula* can occur in many parts of the body, often after injury.

Examination of Children   Infants and young children have relatively thin chests with large, loud hearts. They also can cry loudly enough to make auscultation difficult. You will find it easier to inspect, palpate, and percuss the chest and abdomen before you examine the head or use your stethoscope. You can then auscultate the heart and lungs or abdomen. This you should be able to do calmly and quickly so that the child does not become alarmed or restive. The rapid normal heart rate will make it more difficult to time murmurs, but they generally are easier to hear than in adults.

EXERCISES

1   If available, examine a patient who has pericardial effusion and one who has left ventricular hypertrophy. Examine only the anterior chest and compare the findings by inspection, palpation, percussion, and auscultation.

2   Examine a patient with cardiac dilatation. Can you distinguish this from either or both of the above? Does the patient have a gallop rhythm?

3   If possible, auscultate and palpate for thrill the precordium of a patient with only aortic stenosis. Characterize the murmur as to location, transmission, timing, duration, and course. Your instructor may have to help you decide on its pitch, quality, and intensity.

4 Listen to and characterize completely as many murmurs as cases and time will permit. You need an instructor who will check your findings, but report them to him fully before he gives his own. Above all, do not kid yourself that you can discriminate between various characteristics unless you really can.

5 Phonograph or tape recordings of murmurs may be available. Listen to them, but remember that each will sound a little different through your stethoscope. The records or tapes usually identify the murmur by the valvular lesion that produces it. You should concentrate on what you hear rather than on this interpretive label.

6 You may be able to produce an innocent functional murmur in one or more of your fellow students. Have him do sit-ups or jog briefly in place, then ask him to bend far forward and hold his breath in expiration while you listen at the mitral and pulmonic areas. If this fails, repeat the exercise, having him lie on his back and exhale while you listen at the pulmonic area. Do not expect anything very dramatic and notice what happens to the murmur when he inhales. Characterize the murmur you hear.

See also Sections 8-2 and 9-3.

5-4 ABDOMEN, HERNIAS, AND MALE GENITALS

Abdomen (page 66) *Abdominal Landmarks* On the anterior abdominal wall as on the chest, landmarks are used to locate signs more precisely than by quadrant. The lower costal margin and the xiphoid process of the sternum are used in the upper abdomen. Below, the pelvis and its palpable *ligaments* serve. The large bone on each side of the pelvis is the *ilium,* and it is fused in front to the *pubic bone,* which partially surrounds the genitals. You can feel both the *crest* of the ilium—the hipbone—and the pubic bone. You can also feel the tough *inguinal ligament,* which stretches from the front part of the iliac crest to the pubic bone. These serve as landmarks of the lower abdomen. The *midline* and *umbilicus* are also reference points, as is each lateral edge of the large *rectus abdominis* muscle, stretching from the ribs down to the pubis (see Figure 5-12).

It is common to refer to the *epigastric* region, which covers the upper end of the rectus abdominis from the xiphoid about halfway down to the umbilicus. The area around the umbilicus is called the *umbilical* region, and that just above the pubic bone is the *suprapubic* region. The *inguinal* region lies along that ligament, and the lateral area between ribs and iliac crest is the *lumbar* region or flank.

The anterior end of the iliac crest where the inguinal ligament begins is the *iliac spine,* although it is really a very blunt knob. If you draw an imaginary line from the right iliac spine to the umbilicus and move along it about a third of the way toward the umbilicus, you are at *McBurney's*

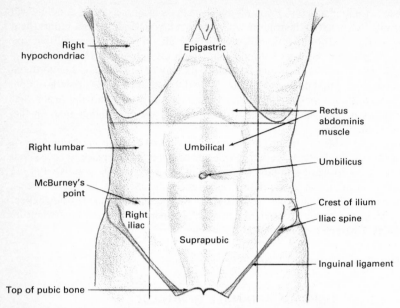

Figure 5-12   Anterior abdominal wall with landmarks and names of regions.

point. This overlies the appendix and is usually the point of greatest tenderness in *appendicitis.*

Abdominal Hernias   The supporting muscles of the abdominal wall are not everywhere equally strong. Pressure rises inside the abdomen with many activities, and the abdominal wall may stretch outward at some weaker point. When this becomes permanent, it is a *hernia.*

The naturally weak points are the umbilicus and the inguinal regions. Any scar where the abdominal muscles were cut may also form a hernia. The hernia will protrude when a cough, straining at stool, or lifting increases pressure inside the abdomen. The hernia, if small, may subside completely when the pressure is lowered. You use this in examining for hernia. During inspection of the abdomen, a cough will usually cause an *umbilical hernia* to protrude as a soft, rounded mass. It will also make a hernia bulge in a scar or recent *incision* if it is weak.

The umbilical hernia usually subsides when a reclining patient relaxes. If it does not, you can usually push the contents gently back inside the abdominal cavity. It is *reducible.* A hernia that you cannot reduce by firm pressure is *incarcerated;* if it is also tender, it may be *strangulated.* You can understand how this can happen when you palpate the rather tough ring that surrounds a reducible umbilical hernia.

Inspection will also show a condition similar to a hernia and seen most often in older women who have borne many children or in younger women soon after childbirth. This is a spreading apart of the two sides of the rectus abdominis muscle. The weakened wall forms a broad midline bulge when the patient raises her head or starts to sit up.

Abdominal Muscles   The entire abdominal musculature may be weak in older patients, those who have been chronically ill or malnourished, very obese people, and those who have some neurological diseases. The abdomen, especially the lower part, becomes protuberant when they stand but less prominent when they lie down. The relaxed abdominal wall can be distinguished more easily when it is not also fat; but when the patient stands, a fat wall bulges more below the epigastrium if the muscular support is poor.

Palpation of the abdominal wall lets you judge further the strength and tone of the abdominal muscles. A relaxed wall feels flabby. In contrast, severe disease with pain in the abdomen may produce muscular *spasm* of the abdominal wall. You can visualize the palpation, since it is commonly described as a *boardlike abdomen* when all the muscles are spastic. No amount of distraction can induce the patient to relax it.

Abdominal Distention   Enlargement of the abdomen, as distinct from changes in its wall, is best seen with the patient flat on his back. You can see whether there is a symmetrical, uniform enlargement, whether it is asymmetrical and more pronounced in one part or another, or whether it is localized.

You may also see exaggerated wavelike movements of the intestine if the distended abdominal wall is thin. This is especially true in young children and it may mean, regardless of age, that something is obstructing the large or small intestine.

Palpation will confirm and extend the findings of inspection in distention of the abdomen, but it is less likely to do so in distention of the intestine within it. Generalized swelling that is slightly asymmetrical sometimes is a large *tumor* or a *cyst* filled with liquid.

Ascites   Fluid within the abdominal cavity is usually watery, like the fluid in edema, and is called *ascites*. It can cause distention and must be distinguished from fat within the abdomen, tumors, or cysts. Even a distended intestine can look like ascites. Since ascites often accompanies other edema and/or pleural effusion, either of these should prompt you to search for it even when the abdomen is not distended.

Detection of ascites depends upon the fact that the small intestine contains gas and so floats on water. It is able to move rather freely within the abdomen and is of course resonant or hyperresonant on percussion. Ascitic fluid also moves freely in most cases and gives a dull note. You can roll the patient to one side and then the other or sit him up to percuss for *shifting dullness*.

Another maneuver, more apt to disclose small amounts of fluid, uses the elbow-knee position with the patient on elbows and knees. You then percuss the hanging anterior abdominal wall. If the umbilical area has become dull, it usually means fluid. Whether there is little or much ascites can be estimated by determining the borders of the dullness.

In addition to shifting dullness, you can use another maneuver to discriminate between fluid, fat, and a solid mass. Another person must assist you by pressing the edge of his hand firmly in the midline just above the umbilicus while the patient lies on his back. Place the palm of one hand on the flank below the upper border of dullness, then slap or percuss sharply with the fingers of the other hand on the opposite flank. You will feel a sharp tap or slap against your stationary hand if fluid is present. This is the *fluid wave.* A fat abdomen often gives a very similar result unless you have someone's hand in the midline to block the wave along rather than within the abdominal wall.

Abdominal Tenderness   Many diseases cause tenderness as well as pain in the abdomen. A swollen or distended organ may be tender, as may tumors or other masses. This both limits and informs the examiner. You must first determine whether there is truly *diffuse* tenderness, whether there is a *point of maximal tenderness,* or whether it is truly *localized.* You must gauge the intensity of the tenderness and whether you can produce local pain by pressing at some point on the abdomen away from the painful or tender area.

It is also important to test for *rebound tenderness.* To do this, press gradually but deeply on the abdomen, well away from the tender, painful area. Then snap your hand away so that the abdominal wall rebounds to its original shape. This may cause a sharp jab of pain in the already painful or tender area, *not* where you pressed. You must always ask the patient where he felt the jab—unless, of course, he volunteers the information.

It is a good idea to ask the patient exactly where he has pain as you start to palpate the abdomen, even when he has told you during his history. This may guide you in deciding where to begin your palpation, but *referred pain* is frequent. In this, the pain is felt rather far removed from its source. For example, pain from the kidney may be most intense in the inguinal region. You must be prepared, then, to discover localized tenderness in some region other than the painful one.

Abdominal Organs and Masses   A visible, localized swelling is often associated with a palpable organ or mass. You must, of course, determine the *location* of any palpable mass as accurately as possible in all three dimensions. This is fairly easy in terms of its position in the vertical and horizontal dimensions but is more difficult in relation to anterior or posterior. You will have to palpate deep to feel a posterior tumor or to try to feel part way around an anterior one. You must do this gently but firmly or you may do damage as well as hurt the patient.

In the process you will doubtless determine whether the tumor or organ is *movable* and in what directions. Some are completely *fixed,* some move easily in certain directions, and some are freely movable. You may also detect whether it moves with *respiration* or the *heartbeat.* You can best check movement with respiration while the patient breathes deeply and slowly.

If you find movement with the pulse rather than respiration, you should try to determine whether an artery—usually the abdominal aorta—is displacing the mass with each beat or whether the mass is *pulsatile,* expanding with each beat. You can determine its pulsatile character best by feeling the mass between your two hands. Your hands will move apart with each beat if the mass is pulsatile and move simultaneously back and forth if it is being *displaced.*

The size of an organ or mass can only be guessed, especially if the patient is fat. It should, however, always be estimated in terms of the three dimensions. If the abdominal wall is fat, you can subtract from the apparent size the thickness of the fat that, according to your estimate, lies between your fingers and the object.

A fat wall also obscures the *shape* and *consistency* of the mass or organ. It is important, where possible, to determine whether the mass is a smooth sphere, has an irregular or scalloped edge, or is grossly irregular or lumpy. It may be compressible, soft, firm, or hard.

This assumes that what you feel is not too painful or tender to prevent palpation. You should, of course, report whether an organ or mass is *nontender, slightly tender, tender,* or *exquisitely tender.* In judging this and in deciding how vigorously to examine the abdomen, you must consider how the patient reacts to pain.

A truly stoic patient will tell you that you are hurting him only if you ask him. He may wince or grimace and not utter a sound. A tense, apprehensive, or emotional patient probably has already announced that the blood-pressure cuff was painful or that it hurt when you tapped his skull. Such a patient winces and grimaces at the mildest discomfiture but will tolerate the usual amount of prodding while discussing grandchildren, taxes, the cost of food, or the insolence of a cab driver. Only when you palpate a truly tender area will he cry out, grimace, or wince.

Liver and Gallbladder The liver edge is usually more easily palpable when it is abnormal than when it is normal. When you feel it, you must determine whether it is soft, firm, or hard; whether it is blunt or sharp; regular or irregular. The terms are descriptive, but only experience can let you discriminate between them. Having felt the edge, you should trace it down into the right lumbar area and as far to the left as possible. It usually is fairly easy to feel whether the liver surface between the edge and the lower rib margin is smooth, nodular like a cobblestone pavement, or contains one or more nodules.

The gallbladder lies on the deep surface of the liver, normally just peeping below the lower margin at a point a little inside the right MCL. Normally it is not palpable or tender. When diseased, it may enlarge so that you feel it as a smooth round body extending from the liver edge. More often, it is tender and you will not be able to palpate it carefully.

The gallbladder may be exquisitely tender even when the liver is not enlarged or palpable. If you have the patient breathe deeply as you palpate for the liver margin, he will check his inspiration abruptly as the tender gallbladder touches your finger.

Another maneuver can detect a slightly tender gallbladder. Have the patient exhale, then hook your fingers under the costal margin where the gallbladder will descend. The idea is to get your fingers deep and high under the ribs. When the patient inhales deeply, he will check his inspiration if the gallbladder is tender.

The liver is less often tender than the gallbladder. Unless it is enlarged, it cannot be palpated, so tenderness is determined by *fist percussion.* To do this, thump the ribs about midway between the diaphragm and the lower costal margin. Use the edge of your fist next the little finger and strike just hard enough to jolt the liver against the ribs.

Liver in Heart Disease   The liver may enlarge in heart disease, and two maneuvers are carried out on the liver to determine the condition of the heart. The first involves placing the fingers of your right hand, held palm up, as far as possible under the edge of the enlarged liver. You then put your left hand on the liver surface above the fingers in order to determine whether it is *pulsatile.* It does no good simply to press down on the surface, since each pulse of the aorta may *displace* an enlarged liver upward.

The second maneuver—producing an *hepatojugular reflux*—is somewhat more complex. The patient is placed on his back and the height of his head is adjusted until the column of blood visible in the large neck veins extends one-third or halfway up their course. It is a good idea to mark the level with a ballpoint pen. You instruct the patient to breathe normally and watch that he does so, since the maneuver will fail if he does not. You then press slowly and gently in the right upper quadrant with one or both hands, gradually increasing the pressure over the course of a minute. If the liver is tender, you can press away from its edge, either lower down or near the umbilicus. The patient should feel little or no discomfort.

Watch the column of blood in the neck as you press. Normally it will not change, will become a little lower, or rise no more than a centimeter. In a positive test, the column of blood will slowly rise well above that amount, usually by two fingerbreadths or more.

Spleen   The spleen, even enlarged, is usually more difficult to feel than the liver. Often it is extremely soft, although it may be hard. It may lie just under the anterior abdominal wall or considerably deeper. It is well to percuss its dullness before you try to feel the organ and then to begin palpating superficially just below the lower margin of dullness.

If the spleen seems only slightly enlarged to percussion and you cannot feel it, you can turn the patient on his right side and have him curl up so that his chin comes close to his knees. Then gently push the tips of your extended right fingers deeper and deeper under his left rib margin as he breathes slowly and deeply. You may have to try several locations before you feel the tip of the spleen tap your finger.

Pregnant Uterus   The uterus rises above the pubic bone as pregnancy progresses and comes to lie just under the anterior abdominal wall (see Figure 5-13). Abdominal palpation will not usually detect the uterus during the first 2 months of pregnancy or even the first 3 months if the woman is fat. After that, you can estimate the approximate month of

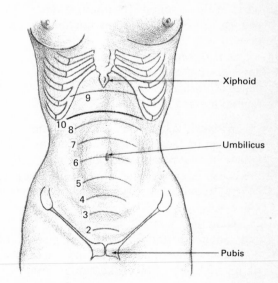

Figure 5-13 Location of upper edge of uterus during pregnancy. Number beside each level indicates lunar month of pregnancy. Month 10 is lower due to lightening.

pregnancy by the height of the uterus. It is, however, only an estimate and often a month or so off the true duration.

The top of the uterus reaches the umbilicus at 5 months and the xiphoid by the start of the ninth month. After that the bottom of the uterus often slips deeper into the pelvis and the uterus tips forward, a process called *lightening*. The top of the uterus then descends until it is only about halfway between the xiphoid and the umbilicus.

The mother will feel fetal movements at about the end of the fourth month. You may not be able to palpate them until several weeks later. You can hear the *fetal heartbeat* at about this time if the baby's position is favorable. You will have to push rather hard with the bell chest piece at several places over the enlarged uterus, starting low in the midline about the pubic bone.

With practice you can palpate the *fetal body* and *head* during the last 3 months of pregnancy. This is important in locating the fetus before delivery. The point of maximal intensity of fetal heart sounds may be of assistance as well. You may be able to establish the presence of twins by detecting two fetal heartbeats.

Bowel and Vascular Sounds   Auscultation for bowel sounds reveals how active the intestine is. True absence of the sounds, especially after "bouncing," indicates little or no movement of the bowel. High-pitched and frequent "rushes" of sounds often accompanied by cramping pain are evidence of an overactive intestine. It is sometimes difficult to tell a short burst of these sounds from normal ones, and you will have to listen long enough to be sure that they continue to recur with only short interruptions.

Aneurysms in the abdomen produce murmurs. You should listen to any pulsatile mass you detect. You may also hear a swishing murmur, called a *bruit,* above an abnormal artery in the abdomen even though you feel no mass.

Kidney   When you can feel the kidney easily, it usually is abnormal at least in its location. It often is impossible to feel even a very enlarged kidney in a fat patient. In really thin patients, you may be able to tell that the organ is enlarged and even to feel a mass connected to it. This, of course, requires experience that you can get only by feeling normal kidneys.

Generally you will learn more by detecting tenderness. If palpation and "bouncing" the CVA cause no pain, you can carry out a more drastic maneuver. The patient sits up and you use fist percussion over the twelfth rib on each side. You strike harder than over the liver but not as hard as you can.

EXERCISES

1 Carry out the maneuver to produce the hepatojugular reflux sign in one or more normal subjects. How much does the blood column rise or fall in the neck veins?

2 If a patient with a reflux is available, repeat or watch a repetition of this test.

3 Test a normal subject for gallbladder tenderness and for hepatic tenderness. Ask the patient to describe what he feels.

4 If feasible, examine the abdomen of several women 3 or more months pregnant. Note the height of the uterus, fetal movements, fetal heart sounds, and—if possible—find the fetal back and head.

5 Carry out the maneuvers to elicit CVA tenderness in one or more normal subjects. Ask for a description of the sensation with each maneuver.

6 If they are available, examine patients with abdominal tenderness, determining its degree, location, and distribution as well as the response to rebound tenderness. Pay attention to the feel of the abdominal muscles. Remember that you are producing pain, and do a thorough·examination without making the patient any more uncomfortable than you must.

7 Examine one or more patients with ascites, using all the maneuvers for this.

8 Examine one or more patients with a tumor of the intestines, stomach, or liver. Auscultate as well as inspect and palpate.

9 Examine one or more patients with an enlarged liver. If possible examine a patient with liver disease and one with heart failure. Test for pulsation as well as determining the other characteristics.

10 If available, examine a patient with a tender gallbladder and one with an enlarged gallbladder.

11 Examine a patient with an enlarged spleen and be prepared to describe it.

12 Examine, if available, a patient with a kidney tumor and one with CVA tenderness.

13 Percuss and palpate a distended urinary bladder. If possible, examine the patient again after his bladder is emptied.

See also Sections 8-3, 9-4, and 9-5.

Male Genitals (page 72) *Penis* The penis consists of three *erectile bodies* running along its length—two side by side on the upper surface and a third along the middle of the underside. The tubelike urethra, running through the lower body of the penis, leads from the urinary bladder to the meatus.

The glans is a terminal enlargement of this lower body and is separated from the other two by a groove or *sulcus*. The *prepuce* is attached just beyond the sulcus and is surgically removed by circumcision.

The prepuce is relatively longer in boys before maturity; this, with a small, undeveloped penis, is a sign of *infantilism* in an adult. Conversely, a premature increase in the size of the penis with the appearance of pubic hair indicates *virilism* in young boys.

The prepuce may be so constricted at the end that it cannot be pulled back over the glans. This is *phimosis*. If the retracted prepuce cannot be pulled down again over the glans, it is *paraphimosis*, usually a more immediately serious condition. You should not try to retract the prepuce if that proves difficult, because you may convert phimosis to paraphimosis. Rather, you should carefully palpate the glans and sulcus through the prepuce, since phimosis may occur with a tumor there. If possible, you should also inspect the meatus through the opening in the prepuce, looking especially for a pussy discharge.

Tumors, ulcers, and nodules or vesicles are most apt to occur on the glans or in the sulcus. You must determine whether they are tender, and you had best wear a glove when you palpate them. You should note whether they are soft, firm, or hard and whether they have a watery or pussy liquid coming from them.

Any of these lesions should lead you to examine the inguinal lymph nodes on both sides. If you find any, you should determine their *location, size, tenderness, hardness, movability,* and whether they are *separate* or *matted* together.

The urethra may be imperfectly formed so that it ends as a groove rather than as a tube. When this occurs, there is no true meatus but rather a slit on the undersurface of the penis. Much more rarely, the urethra may open on the upper side of the penis. You will generally find these conditions in infants or very young boys since they are corrected by surgery during infancy.

The penis and the scrotum, being covered with thin skin which stretches easily, are often involved in *edema*. The fluid collection, unless it is extreme, is soft and yields to the touch.

Scrotum and Contents   Several kinds of masses occur within the scrotum, either connected with the normal contents or independent of them. The mass is often visible, especially if it is on only one side, but in other instances it may be detectable only by palpation.

You should determine the *location* of the mass, its *consistency,* and whether it is *connected* with the testis or epididymis. It may be soft and yielding, firm and rigid, or hard. You may be unable to tell its exact shape if it is very soft, but you may feel a smooth rounded surface, a tangle of cords—often called a *bag of worms*—or a generally irregular surface. You should determine whether the mass moves easily or is firmly anchored. Since a soft, movable mass may be a *hernia,* you should try to reduce it (see "Inguinal Hernias," below).

It is important to determine whether the mass is tender. This is easy if it is away from the epididymis and testis or is very sensitive. If it is in the epididymis or testis, you will have to decide whether it is more tender than these structures usually are. You can do this by comparing the lesion to the normal side if only one side is involved.

One entire testis may be enlarged or may have a distinct nodule on its surface. In contrast, one or both testes may be smaller than normal.

You should examine the scrotal contents both with the patient standing and with him lying down. Some lesions are better felt in one and some in the other position.

When you feel a mass, you should try to *transilluminate* it. You will have to darken the room and then put a small flashlight behind the mass. A solid body like the testis will look dark; one containing a clear fluid—a *hydrocele*—will transilluminate and pass light.

There may be only one testis in the scrotum, and occasionally you may feel none. Unless the man was *castrated,* this is almost always because the testis has not descended. The testes develop in the abdomen of the fetus, but normally they move or *descend* into the scrotum before birth. This descent is through an oblique channel, the *inguinal canal,* which begins near the middle of the inguinal ligament and just above it. The testis moves toward the midline and then downward into the scrotum. It remains attached to the inside of the abdomen by the spermatic cord, and this cord occupies the inguinal canal.

When the testis is not in its normal position, you should feel up along the normal course of the spermatic cord. You may feel the undescended testis high in the scrotum, under the skin near the top of the scrotum, or even within the inguinal canal above the ligament. Usually it is softer and smaller than normal and slips upward toward the abdomen as you palpate it.

EXERCISES

1 Examine, if available, the penis and inguinal lymph nodes of patients with tumors, ulcers, vesicles, and nodules of the penis. Determine whether they are tender and be prepared to describe them.
2 Examine or observe the examination of a patient with a urethral discharge. Describe the appearance of the meatus and of the discharge itself.
3 Examine patients with scrotal masses, including the use of transillumination. Carefully determine the attachments, movability, tenderness, etc.
4 If possible, examine a boy with an undescended testis. Describe the location and characteristics of it if you can feel it.

See also Sections 8-3 and 9-6.

Hernias The abdominal wall contains two weak points in the inguinal region on either side. The first is the inguinal canal, in which the spermatic cord lies above the inguinal ligament. The second is the femoral area below the ligament through which the large blood vessels of the leg leave the abdomen. As you would expect, inguinal hernias occur almost exclusively in men; they are occasionally seen in girls, however, since the muscles are similarly attached in the two sexes.

Inguinal Hernias The oblique inguinal canal has an *internal ring,* where the spermatic cord passes through the inner layer of abdominal muscles and an *external ring,* where it passes through the outer muscular layer. Between the two rings the cord is in the canal walled by the two muscle layers (see Figure 5-14). This arrangement allows *herniation* at

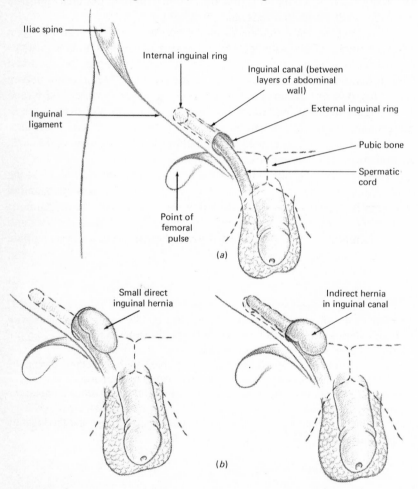

Figure 5-14   Inguinal region of the male (*a*) with direct and indirect inguinal hernias (*b*).

two points. The abdominal contents can enter the canal through the internal ring, pass through it and the external ring, and so enter the scrotum. This is an *indirect hernia.* Or the inner layer of muscle may give way along the canal, so that the hernia passes more or less directly out through the external ring. This is a *direct hernia.*

A large hernia that enters the scrotum distends it and is visible as a swelling. A smaller hernia causes fullness above the inguinal ligament along its lower inner third. You can see these changes best if you sit while the patient stands in front of you. In this position, you can also best palpate for a hernia that is invisible or causes only a swelling above the ligament.

To palpate the right side, have the patient bend his right knee slightly by raising his heel off the floor. Then place your right little finger near the bottom of the scrotum and, pushing the loose scrotal skin ahead of the fingertip, pass it upward along the spermatic cord. Your fingertip normally encounters a taut, sharp-edged ring of tissue that will not admit it. You may find the ring large enough for your fingertip to enter at least part way. At this point, ask the patient to cough. As the patient does so, a small inguinal hernia will tap your fingertip.

As your finger moves upward near the ring, you may feel a soft, yielding mass when the hernia is somewhat larger. Usually you can *reduce* this by pushing gently toward the canal, and your finger will slip through the external ring. Then have the patient cough. If the hernia taps the *tip* of your finger it is an indirect one. A direct hernia strikes the *side* of your finger which is nearest the abdominal cavity.

Use your left little finger and direct the patient to bend his left knee when you examine the left side. You should always examine the opposite side when you find a hernia, since hernias are frequently *bilateral.*

A hernia large enough to enter the scrotum as a visible mass usually is indirect. You had best examine it with the patient lying on his back. Try to reduce it by having him relax and breathe quietly while you push the mass gently upward toward the canal with one or both hands. Often it slips easily back into the abdomen, and then you can insert your finger through the relaxed external ring.

A hernia is *irreducible* or *incarcerated* if you cannot get it to return to the abdominal cavity. The return or reduction is usually a painless process and the contents of the hernia are soft, not tender. If the contents are tense, painful, and tender, the hernia may be *strangulated* and you should not attempt to reduce it.

Femoral Hernia   A femoral hernia of sufficient size can be seen bulging *below* the inguinal ligament over the point where the pulse of the large femoral artery is felt. It is usually a soft, yielding, nontender mass which can be reduced. If it is small, you may not be able to see or feel it distinctly, but you can feel the bulge on coughing.

EXERCISES

1 Examine the inguinal ring on both sides in a normal male, paying particular attention to the sensation at your fingertip when he coughs. Ask him to describe his sensations during the examination. If you hurt him, you did not palpate properly.
2 Examine the femoral triangles of a normal subject. You can identify the triangle by feeling the pulse there. Include the cough while you palpate.
3 If they are available, examine patients with inguinal and femoral hernias. Try to reduce each one under guidance of the instructor. Determine, if possible, whether the inguinal hernias are direct or indirect.

5-5 RECTUM AND FEMALE GENITALS

Rectum (pages 73 and 77) *Anus and Rectal Canal* In attempting to palpate the rectum, you may find that your fingertip does not enter the anus even if you exert gentle pressure for several seconds. This may indicate either a spasm of the anal *sphincter* or a *stricture.* Spasm accompanies pain if the patient has a fissure or a painful hemorrhoid. Stricture is a permanent narrowing due to tough, fibrous scar tissue formed in the ring. Usually continued gentle pressure eventually allows your finger to slip through an anus with spasm but not through one with stricture.

The anus may be so relaxed that your finger enters with no resistance at all, and this will certainly be true if there is prolapse of the rectum. You will note that normally the anal sphincter remains tight about your finger. This indicates normal *sphincter tone.*

In infants and young children, the rectal examination is carried out much as in the adult except that it is easier to have the child on his back with his legs spread apart. You can usually palpate with your little finger and cause less discomfort to the child.

The anal canal just beyond the external anus runs somewhat toward the front of the body and then turns sharply as it becomes the rectum to run toward the back and upward along the inner curving surface of the sacrum. The rectum actually extends upward beyond the reach of your finger before it joins the large intestine coming from above. It lies in the midline, and any displacement from this position is abnormal.

Your finger may encounter a hard or soft mass of *feces* as it leaves the anal canal or passes higher in the rectum. You can displace this rather easily, and it presents a problem only because you may mistake it for a tumor or it may mask one. You should note whether the feces are *soft*, *hard* or *very hard*. If necessary, you may have to repeat the rectal examination after the patient defecates.

Prostate   In the male, you should palpate the prostate, carefully noting its size, shape, consistency, and tenderness. The shape is usually symmetrical, with the two lobes about the same size. Any irregularity in shape and any nodule on the surface should be carefully felt (see Figure 2-15).

The normal consistency is about that of the tip of your nose. An abnormal gland may be much softer and "boggy." It may be generally more tense and then usually is tender. It may also be stony hard either generally, over one lobe, or as a raised nodule. A hard mass may extend from the lower, lateral, or upper surface, and you should trace this as far as you can.

Vasa and Seminal Vesicles   The vas, arriving through the spermatic cord, on either side loops across the pelvic wall to pass behind the bladder and down into the prostate near the midline. A *seminal vesicle* lies on either side of the vas just above the prostate and extends upward and laterally for an inch or so. The urinary bladder lies just in front of the vasa and seminal vesicles. These latter with the prostate are the principal internal sexual organs of the male (see Figure 2-15).

Usually you cannot feel the vasa and the seminal vesicles and, if you can, you feel them only indistinctly above the prostate. You may, however, find them tender. In young boys you usually cannot distinguish the small, immature prostate, seminal vesicles, or vasa. Your finger then is feeling the posterior wall of the bladder.

Tumors   If your finger encounters any mass aside from feces in the rectum of either a man or a woman, you should palpate it carefully. One site is on the anterior and lateral walls just about as far up as your finger will reach. Here you may feel tumor nodules or a shelflike layer that is actually outside the rectum. Tumors in the tissues around the rectum can occur elsewhere too, and if you feel carefully you may feel the smooth rectal wall covering them.

A tumor in the rectal wall itself is usually irregular with an irregular surface. It may be hard, firm, soft, or so weak that it breaks as you feel it. It may or may not be movable.

In contrast, you may feel a tumor that moves very freely within the rectum and a thinner stalk or *pedicle* occasionally can be felt attaching it to the wall. You should note all these characteristics as well as the location and size of the mass.

When you do a complete examination in a woman, examine the

rectum after you complete the pelvic. The rectal examination then confirms your evaluation of the internal sexual organs and otherwise is carried out as in a man.

EXERCISES

1 If patients are available, examine persons with external hemorrhoids, anal strictures, and poor anal tone.
2 Examine patients with enlarged prostates and prostatic tumors. Pay particular attention to the consistency of the organ. Can you feel above the prostate?
3 If feasible, do rectal examinations on patients with extrinsic, annular, mural, and pedunculated tumors of the rectum. Be prepared to describe each completely.

See also Sections 8-3 and 9-6.

Female Genitals (page 75) *Internal Genitals* The principal internal sexual organs of the woman can be considered as beginning at the introitus. Extending upward and backward from this outlet is the *vagina,* lying in front of the rectum and behind the urethra. The latter runs as a small tube in the midline from the meatus to the urinary bladder, which also lies in front of the vagina (see Figure 2-18).

At its upper end, the vagina contains the neck or cervix of the uterus. This protrudes into the anterior vaginal wall, and the vagina continues on beyond it a little way as a blind sac, the *vaginal vault,* forming a groove around the cervix. The vagina itself is a soft, distensible tube flattened from front to back. It is lined by smooth, pink mucous membrane thrown into rather heavy folds. Its lower end is surrounded by the muscles which support the floor of the pelvis.

The cervix, in contrast, is round and firm, smooth, and usually somewhat paler than the vaginal wall. In its center, the *os* or mouth is a transverse slit, and from it the *cervical canal* extends upward into the uterus.

The cervix is really the lower end of the uterus and expands into the *body* or *uterine fundus* above the cervix. This body is like a rounded triangle and at each upper corner joins a *fallopian tube.* The uterus has a thick, muscular wall surrounding a cavity or *lumen* lined by *endometrium* (see Figure 2-18).

The uterine lumen extends outward into the fallopian tubes, each of which curves around toward the rectum just inside the pelvic bone. They end on either side opposite the upper end of the vagina and a little above it.

The end of each fallopian tube is rather like a ragged funnel opening into the abdominal cavity. The ragged end almost surrounds the *ovary*, where the eggs form on either side. Each ovary is ovoid and about $1^{1}/_{2}$ in long, rather firm, and easily movable.

Pelvic Examination Most of these organs can be palpated under favorable circumstances; the vagina and cervix can be inspected as well. A *vaginal speculum* is required for a complete inspection. This instrument consists of two arched or hollowed metal or plastic blades, one longer than the other. These blades can be brought together for insertion into the vagina and then spread apart by means of a scissorslike arrangement. Light is provided by a flashlight or light fixture so mounted that it can throw a beam between the blades of the speculum.

The pelvic examination is easier for both you and the patient if she empties her bladder and preferably her rectum as well before you begin. This can be done routinely before you start the physical examination, and a urine specimen can be obtained at the same time. A pelvic examination is not done while a patient is menstruating unless there is a specific reason to avoid delay. The rectal examination is usually deferred as well.

You usually will need assistance during the examination. A male examiner should have a woman assist him both to reduce the patient's anxiety and to avoid subsequent claims of misconduct on the examiner's part. The assistant helps position the patient in the stirrups and drapes her for the examination while the examiner is out of the room.

Examination of External Genitals The pelvic examination begins with inspection and palpation of the external genitals or sex organs. The appearance varies with age and in elderly women the labia majora and minora may be shrunken, smooth, and glistening. They may show white *plaques* slightly raised above the surface. These often itch, and you may find *excoriations* due to scratching.

The plaques are quite distinct from ulcers, tissue masses, nodules, or papules. While lesions may appear anywhere on the vulva, you should look for them especially on the inner surfaces of the labia minora from the *glans clitoris* at their front end to the vaginal outlet. In this same area, the meatus may show evidence of a discharge or irritation. Older women sometimes have a *caruncle* at the meatus. This is a bright red mucosal prolapse of the urethra. It sometimes is very tender.

The urethra can be "stripped" if there is reason to suspect a discharge. To do this, put a gloved finger into the vagina about half the finger's length, bend it slightly so that its tip touches the anterior vaginal wall in the midline, and slowly withdraw it while exerting gentle pressure. This forces any discharge out the meatus.

Inspection of the introitus will disclose whether there is a *hymen* partially closing the outlet. Usually you will not palpate or inspect the vagina if the hymen has only a small opening. It is, however, rather delicate and, if a pelvic examination is truly necessary, slight force will rupture it.

The introitus normally has a smooth symmetrical shape, rather oblong front to back. If it is distorted, you should palpate the edges. The irregularity may be due to a firm scar, an ulcer just inside the opening, or a swelling deep at the base of one of the labia minora. If such a swelling is found, you should note its location and size, whether it is firm and whether it is tender.

When you ask the patient to bear down to test for prolapse, you will normally see only a slight bulging of the entire vulvar area. You may find, however, that the introitus gapes open either with or without straining. If this is true, you should determine by palpation whether the anterior vaginal wall appears as the bladder pushes downward from the front or the posterior wall when the rectum is forced forward.

These prolapses are due to weakened or torn muscles supporting the floor of the pelvis. You can test this support further by inserting two gloved fingers just inside the introitus and asking the patient to tighten her muscles. Normally you will feel them contract, but not if they are weakened. You can then spread your fingers within the introitus and pull them downward toward the anus. If the muscles are normal, you will not be able to displace them more than a finger's breadth. If the support is weak, you can depress the whole introitus easily.

Examination of Internal Genitals   At this point in the examination you can follow either of two procedures. Some clinicians prefer to begin with inspection of the vagina because this allows collection of *cell specimens* (for *Papanicolaou tests*) before lubricating jelly is introduced into the vagina. Inexperienced examiners usually find it easier to palpate before introducing the speculum. The latter order is followed here.

You can do the pelvic examination with a plastic or rubber glove on your right hand, your left hand, or both. You will need lubricating jelly on the tips of the first and middle fingers of the gloved hand. Usually very little suffices. You stand facing the vulva and ask the patient to relax and drop her knees apart. You can place your ungloved hand on her lower abdomen beneath the drapes and judge her relaxation by the feel of the muscles there. It is useless to begin the palpation until the patient is really relaxed. To maintain the relaxation, you should tell her each step of the examination.

You next spread the jelly in a thin film over your fingers and then around the introitus. Keep the first and middle fingers straight, your thumb stretched up as far as it will go, and your ring and little fingers curled into your palm. Your thumb should be kept straight up in the air and your wrist in a rigid, straight line throughout the examination. Usually, you can insert the two fingers through the introitus without difficulty. If only the index finger will enter, the examination will be incomplete and another technique must be used.

As your fingers advance, raise your elbow slightly so that your fingers follow the posterior vaginal wall as it slopes backward. Then lower your elbow *and hand* so that you displace the introitus and vagina toward the rectum. You can ask the patient whether she feels any pain as you proceed, and if she does, to describe its location and character.

Examination of the Cervix   The cervix is usually easy to locate by palpation. In the nonpregnant adult woman, it has about the consistency of the tip of your nose. It is smooth and rounded, an inch or so in diameter, and easily movable in all directions. Usually the rounded lower end is directed backward toward the rectum, but it may point downward or even somewhat forward. This simply reflects the fact that the entire uterus moves freely and may lie in various positions within the pelvis. The cervix should, however, lie in the midline.

You should note whether the cervix is harder or softer than normal and whether it is irregular in shape or surface. You may be able to palpate the depression of the os at the extreme tip, but this is not abnormal. It is worth noting whether your fingertip will enter the cervical canal through the os, since it normally cannot. You should also determine whether the cervix is larger or smaller than expected and what its exact position is. Restriction of movability is important, and so is any pain produced by movement.

You now feel inward beyond the cervix into the vault in the midline. Note whether there is any tenderness or mass there. You may feel feces in the rectum at this point, but your later rectal examination will confirm this.

Examination of the Fundus   Returning your fingertips to the cervix, palpate along it upward from the tip and then go on to the *bimanual* part of the pelvic examination. Begin by placing your ungloved hand palm down with the fingertips a little below the umbilicus. By bending your wrist, forcing your fingers into the abdomen, and pulling your hand toward you slowly, you force the uterine fundus down against your palpating fingers.

Usually the fundus lies anterior to the cervix, more or less atop the bladder. It may lie posteriorly and be felt through the vaginal vault. By spreading your fingers slightly, you can determine the *size, shape,* and *regularity* of the surface. You can best judge this after feeling normal uteri. It is not difficult, however, to detect enlargement or smooth irregularities of the surface. It is equally easy to detect any loss of movability, since the uterus is usually easily and painlessly displaced whatever its position.

Examination of the Adnexa   It is much more difficult to feel the fallopian tube and ovary—the *uterine adnexa.* Indeed, you cannot feel the normal tube distinctly. If your right hand is gloved, you feel the patient's right ovary by pressing deep just to the right of the cervix and directing your fingers a little upward toward the abdominal wall. Your ungloved

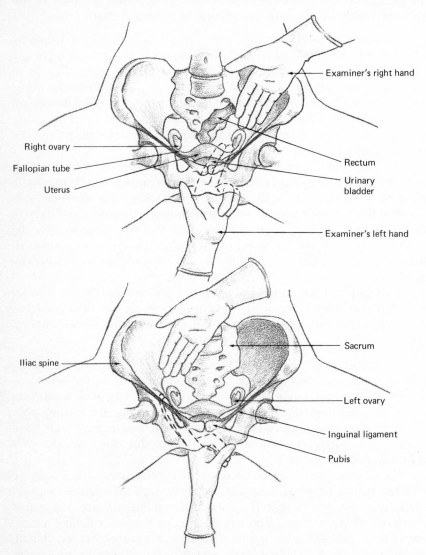

Figure 5-15   Pelvic examination, palpation of adnexae.

hand presses deeply about midway up the inguinal ligament or slightly below that point. You may have to direct this pressure a little toward the midline. The normal ovary is somewhat firm and smoothly oval. Its size is about $1^1/_4$ by $1^1/_2$ in, and it is slightly tender.

To feel the left ovary, your gloved right fingers pass to the patient's left of the cervix; by bending your fingers backward at the base, you move them toward the patient's left side and angle them upward toward the abdominal wall. Your hand on the abdomen, placed as it was on the opposite side, presses downward toward the gloved fingertips. You may have to move the latter a little toward the midline to feel the ovary as it is pushed downward.

You should note the apparent *size* of the ovary, its *consistency,* and the *regularity* or irregularity of its surface. Any true tenderness of the ovary or any area in its vicinity is significant, as is any mass. You should feel an enlarged fallopian tube between the ovary and the body of the uterus, but it may feel much like an enlargement or tumor of the ovary in that direction.

Speculum Examination Palpation allows you to select the proper size speculum to use for inspection of the vagina. Women who have borne children often will take the largest, women who have not may require the medium size, and elderly women or children can tolerate the smallest. It is usually wise to use the largest size that you can introduce without pain or discomfort.

Holding the speculum, blades together, in the ungloved hand, put a little lubricating jelly along each blade. The gloved hand then separates the labia as for inspection of the vulva. Turn the speculum sidewise, the blades firmly together and the sides of the blades pointing almost up and down, then pass the blades into the part of the introitus nearest the rectum and keep the pressure on the posterior vaginal wall.

When the blades are well within the vagina, turn the speculum handle down. This puts the longer blade on the posterior wall so that it can pass into the vaginal vault. Now press the lever that spreads the blades to open them while the assistant directs a light into the vagina. You can usually see the cervix at the tip as the blades spread apart. It is identifiable by the os even when its color matches that of the vagina. If you do not see the cervix, you can withdraw the speculum a little way and it may almost pop into view. You should close or almost close the blades before you advance them again.

Note the color of the cervix as a whole and examine the os. It usually is a transverse slit and may have small whitish scars, especially at the outer ends if the woman has borne children. It is not uncommon to see a red area extending from the os onto the surface of the cervix. Note carefully whether the margin of this *erosion* is regular or irregular.

Occasionally you may see a stalked *polyp* extending through the os as a dark-red, smooth mass. Note especially whether the surface of the cervix is smooth, irregular, or raw, and whether there is any pus or discharge from the os.

Slowly withdraw the speculum with the blades fairly widely opened until the tips are near the introitus, then close them *almost* completely before removing it. You may catch and tug on the vaginal lining if you close the blades tightly.

As you withdraw the speculum, examine the vagina. The walls are usually pink and thrown into folds except in young girls and postmenopausal women. In them, the mucous membrane is folded little if at all and is thinner. The walls are usually glistening, but you should note any *secretion* which may be thin and watery, thick and curdy, or frankly pus.

Rectovaginal and Rectal Examinations   The rectovaginal examination is used for palpation when the vagina will admit only one finger. To carry it out, the gloved and lubricated middle finger is inserted into the rectum and the first finger into the vagina. The ungloved hand is used on the abdomen and palpation is carried out just as in the bimanual examination already described.

You must use the rectal examination alone when the vagina should not be entered. It is conducted bimanually but is much less precise than the usual pelvic examination.

A routine rectal examination follows the pelvic examination in any event. Aside from the internal sex organs, it is carried out as in a man, palpating for the same lesions.

EXERCISES

1   Examine a set of vaginal specula. Note the ways in which the blades can be moved and examine the small nuts or other locking devices which hold them in position. Holding the blades loosely in the fist of one hand, practice opening, closing, locking, and unlocking the blades with the other. Learn to hold the unlocked blades closed, partially open and fully open with your thumb. When you can manipulate the speculum well with one hand, switch hands and learn to do it with the other.

2   If patients are available, inspect the vulva of older women with senile changes and urethral caruncles. Examine vulvar ulcers, nodules, and cysts in younger women.

3   If feasible, do a bimanual pelvic examination in a woman with normal organs. Begin by testing the support of the pelvic floor and continue through palpation of the ovaries. You should do this under the guidance of a tutor who has already examined the patient. Do not fool yourself that you can feel and identify some organ when you cannot. If your fingers are shorter than those of the tutor or if you do not press them as deeply, you may be unable to locate the adnexa.

4 Inspect the vagina and cervix of a normal woman using a vaginal speculum. Be certain that you clearly see the os of the cervix, noting the shape and position. Note also the color and character of the cervix and vagina.
5 If possible, examine women who have relaxed pelvic floors, cervical erosions, vaginal discharges, tumors of the fundus, and abnormal ovaries.

Papanicolaou Test The Papanicolaou test (commonly known as the Pap test) for cancer is made by examining cells you obtain from the cervix and the vagina. Lubricating jelly can make examination of the cells less accurate, and for that reason it may be best to use the speculum before palpating with lubricated fingers. You can use warm water to lubricate the speculum, but if this does not allow its easy introduction into the vagina, you may have to use jelly. If you do, it should be a very small amount smeared only on the outside of the blades.

Cells from the vagina are obtained either with a swab or a suction device from the vaginal vault. Very little material is needed to smear on glass slides held by the assistant. It should be enough to make a distinct smeary blur, however.

You obtain cells from the os and lower cervical canal by putting a tightly wound swab at the os and advancing it a little way as you twirl it gently. The material is again smeared on glass slides by rolling the swab along them.

Cells can also be scraped from the surface of the os and the cervix near it. For this you use a special wooden *spatula* with an irregular tip, one side of which is longer than the other. Place the shorter part in the os and rotate the whole spatula while the tip is firmly pressed against the cervix. One complete rotation is enough, and you then smear the spatula tip on the glass slide.

After the specimens are obtained, the inspection of the cervix and vagina is completed. Palpation then follows.

See also Sections 8-3 and 9-6.

5-6 EXTREMITIES (see page 78)

Upper Extremities *Hand* Lesions of the hand include some that involve the nails, such as *clubbing* of the fingertips and red or brown *splinter hemorrhages* under the nail, both associated with disease in other parts of the body. Others are truly local diseases and may deform only a single nail or the area immediately around it. You should glance at each nail in turn.

The most common deformity of the fingers is stiffness, limited motion, and bony enlargement of the small joints. The enlargement may not be uniform, so that the bones join at an odd angle. Even without very gross distortion, you may be able to feel hard lumps just below the joint next the fingertip, especially on the little finger. These are *Heberden's nodes.*

A joint may *fuse* so that it cannot be moved actively or passively. If this has occurred, you should determine which joint is involved and note the resulting position.

Some joints are painful on active motion but less so on passive movement. Some are tender but not painful, or the reverse may be true. You should, therefore, test both types of motion in a painful joint and determine the tolerated range for both types. Palpate for tenderness and for bony changes at any joint that seems normal.

Individual joints may swell, redden, or both. In contrast, all or most of the finger and hand joints may be involved. These changes are usually easy to detect, but if they are slight, you can compare one hand with the other to discern small differences.

One or more fingers may be largely immobilized by changes in the muscles which normally move them or by *contractions* in the *tendons* and related tissues attached to them. In these lesions you can see or feel the tense, contracted tissues.

This will be true in *spastic paralysis,* where the muscles remain tensed. In *flaccid paralysis,* the muscles are relaxed and the parts they move are limp and powerless, with slack tendons.

Muscles can waste away or *atrophy* as well as be paralyzed. This is not always easy to detect in the hand. You can best see and feel atrophy at the base of the thumb, where the plumpness disappears on both sides of the bone. In the hand itself, wasting is more obvious on the back, where hollows appear between the bones.

You should pay close attention to any change in the color of the fingers, which may blanch or become fiery red at the tips. The palms may also become bright red, especially over the two thicker areas on either side of the palm.

Wrist and Forearm   As you test the motion of the wrist, you may find a swelling on its outer surface. You should notice whether it is hard bone or a firm but fluid-filled sac. The latter is called a *ganglion* and may cause the patient little problem. There may, however, also be tender swellings in this region.

The forearms are quickly examined, mainly for evidence of muscular atrophy. Even in relatively fat people, a good impression of muscle tone or tenseness can be gained by palpating the forearm.

Elbow, Upper Arm, and Shoulder   The elbow can be quickly tested for its full range of *flexion* and *extension* and for the *rotation* of the hand. If there has been pain localized there, it is well to have the patient fully extend his arm while you place one hand on the back of his. He may feel pain on the outer side of the elbow when you resist his attempts to bend his hand backward against yours.

The upper arm gives you further evidence of muscular development and tone. Also, the shoulder joint rather commonly has restricted motion. This is sometimes due to lesions in the tissues near it rather than in the joint itself. In the rather common *bursitis,* the patient has pain when he attempts to put his hand behind his head. You can further examine him by palpation. To do so, feel the extreme tip of the bone at the top of the shoulder joint, drop your fingers $1/2$ to 1 in below this tip, and press gently inward. Hard pressure will always hurt here, but bursitis is much more tender.

Blood Vessels Arteries of the upper extremity are examined in conjunction with taking the pulse. You can examine the veins during your consideration of the heart or of the arms. Blood in the veins is not under great pressure to return to the heart. When pressure rises within the right atrium, the increased pressure is transmitted to the veins. You can see superficial veins on the back of the hand even in an obese person, hence you can use them as a gauge of *venous pressure.*

The patient lies on his back and you straighten his arm, raising it at about 45° with the palm down. You may notice that the hand veins have collapsed. If they have not, stroke them lightly from the knuckles to the wrist. Now lower the arm slowly, watching the veins, and stop when they plump out with blood. Now measure the height of the hand above the sternal angle. Normally the veins fill only when the hand is within 1 cm ($1/2$ in) of the angle's level. It may be necessary to lower the hand even below that level. You can check your estimate by slowly raising the hand to its previous level, stroking the veins lightly if necessary, and watching for the level at which they empty.

Lower Extremities *Feet* The toes are subject to a variety of lesions including the common *corn.* This is a hard, tender area appearing where there has been continued pressure on a toe. Its hallmark is a *horny core,* and it is pressure on this core that causes pain.

Toes are often deformed as people grow older. One deformity, "hammertoe," causes considerable discomfort when the toes "cock up" or bend upward at the first joint and then flex sharply downward so that the tips, rather than the balls of the toes, touch the floor.

Toenails cause trouble by rubbing the skin of the next toe if too long and, if cut too close, by growing out under the skin at the edges rather than on top of it. Such an *ingrown toenail* can be very tender and painful.

Toes are also subject to *gangrene,* in which they die and discolor with or without ulceration. Often there is a rather sharp reddened margin marking off the gangrenous area.

A common lesion in older people occurs at the base of the great toe. A bony swelling or *bunion* angles the great toe against or under the adjacent toe.

The foot itself is subject to deformity. It may be twisted inward so that the person walks on the side of his foot, the so-called *clubfoot*. Or it may flex and turn outward. These deformities are now seen mostly in infants because they are corrected early in life.

Edema   Edema is more common at the ankle and top of the foot than anywhere else. It may, however, extend upward until it involves the entire body and its exact extent should be noted. It may involve one or both legs and may be unequal in the two legs. Pitting edema is usually graded by pressing where it is more marked. A very small indentation is + (read "one plus") and extensive edema in which you can leave a deep imprint is ++++ (read "four plus"). Intermediate grades are ++ and +++.

Unilateral or unequal edema should lead you to have the patient stand while you look carefully for distended *varicose veins* over the upper and lower legs. You palpate along any suspicious vein for firm, hard, or tender areas.

Recent or *intermittent edema* pits on pressure. *Chronic edema* tends to become hard and woody. You often find the thin, distended skin shiny, and it may be discolored. The color should be carefully noted. The thin skin heals with difficulty if injured, and you may find an ulcer or thin scars in the edematous area.

Lower Leg and Knee   The calf shows atrophy clearly. You can also easily distinguish the increased muscular tone of spastic paralysis from the diminished tone of flaccid paralysis.

Knees that have been injured in the past may be *unstable* even though they move normally. You can test this by a series of maneuvers. In the first, you bend the knee about 15° and then force the lower leg outward. In the second, you repeat this with the leg fully extended at the knee. In the third, you fully extend the leg and force the lower leg inward toward the midline. Finally, you bend the knee 90° and try to pull the lower leg forward and push it backward so that it slips at the joint. Normally you cannot move the lower leg independently of the upper in any of these maneuvers. In an unstable knee, at least one maneuver shows abnormal movability.

In adolescents you may find a tender swelling below the *patella* or kneecap without the joint being involved. Swelling of the knee joint is often an accumulation of fluid that distends the *joint capsule* and the saclike *bursae* around it. This collection may feel like fluid, but it may be quite tense. Even under these circumstances, you can usually bob the patella up and down by pushing on it sharply while the leg is extended and relaxed.

Upper Legs and Hip   The thighs show muscular atrophy, spasticity, and flaccidity quite clearly. The hip, except for its movements, is more difficult to examine because the joint is buried so deep under the muscles. The gait often provides the best evidence of deformities. With infants who do not walk, one maneuver should be added to test the range of motion.

To test for *piston motion*, place the infant on his back and roll his leg outward. With one hand, hold his body steady. Your other hand grasps his bent thigh and you gently pull your hands apart. Normally his leg will move $1/2$ in or so, but if it shifts rather easily downward for over an inch and you feel the head of the femur move along over the pelvis, the test is positive.

Arteries   The arteries of the leg are more difficult to examine than are those of the arm. You start by feeling the *femoral artery* pulsating just below the inguinal ligament. You then feel for the *popliteal pulse* behind the knee. The artery lies deep between the two tendons on either side, but its precise location varies. To palpate it, have the patient lie on his back and bend up his knee to a 45° angle. Then hook your fingers between the tendons and with the tips press firmly upward against the bone. You may have to try several spots there. You must be careful to check your own pulse rate to be sure that you are not feeling your own throbbing fingertip pulsations.

Two arteries are accessible to palpation in the foot or ankle. They too vary in precise location and relative size in normal people. To feel the *dorsalis pedis* pulse, press rather lightly just lateral to the large tendon running to the great toe along the arch of the foot. Occasionally you can find the pulse farther laterally.

The *posterior tibial* pulse is on the inner side of the ankle. To find it, locate the bony knob on the inner surface of the ankle and palpate rather firmly in the groove behind it.

As a final test of the arteries, have the patient swing his feet over the edge of the examining table and sit there for 2 or 3 min. Note the color of his feet and then have him lie down again while you support his legs, held straight, at an angle of 45° above the table surface for 2 or 3 min. He then rests with his feet on the surface for the same length of time. During all this, watch the color of his feet. The color changes little in a normal person, and his feet remain warm. If the arteries are defective, the feet become red or reddish purple when hanging down and blanched when elevated. The feet also cool when they are raised and warm up when they are hanging down; this may be the most evident change in blacks.

Veins The *deep veins* of the legs are the site of serious clots, especially in people who have heart disease, have been confined to bed, have given birth, or have just had surgery. The patient usually complains of pain in his calf, but he may not. Sometimes edema or the bluish discoloration of cyanosis may appear suddenly in the foot, ankle, and lower leg. You can detect small amounts of edema by measuring the diameter at the same point in midcalf of each leg. The large calf is the edematous one.

You can also test for calf tenderness by pressing firmly on the back of the calf so that your fingers move inward toward the bone. If this causes pain, you should then squeeze the calf muscle equally firmly by gripping its sides from behind. Tenderness of the muscle responds more to the latter; an involved vein causes little or no pain when you squeeze the muscle.

Another maneuver is to leave the leg fully extended while you bend the foot firmly upward toward the head. Pain in the calf or the popliteal area is a positive *Homans' sign* and suggests clotting in the deep veins.

A more sensitive test is said to be one using the blood pressure apparatus. You place the cuff around the calf and inflate it slowly. Normally there is discomfort only when the pressure reaches 160 mm of mercury or more. If there is pain below 150 mm of mercury, the vein is probably involved.

There is some danger in doing these tests. You should do no more than you need to satisfy yourself that there is trouble in a deep vein.

Lymph Nodes If you have not already done so, palpate for lymph nodes just above the inguinal ligament and in the region of the femoral pulse. You may find a "shotty," nontender node or two in the femoral area even in normal persons.

EXERCISES

1 Palpate the forearm, arm, calf, and thigh muscles of several volunteers, feeling them when the muscles are relaxed and when they are contracted. You are interested in the volume of each muscle group and in the tone of the muscles.
2 Palpate the elbow of a normal person and test the *dorsiflexion* of the hand with the arm extended. Does this cause pain about the elbow?
3 Palpate the normal shoulder and test for tenderness below the peak of the shoulder.
4 Determine the venous pressure of a normal person using the hand veins.

5 Test a normal knee for instability, paying particular attention to the amount of displacement at the knee with each maneuver.
6 Palpate the femoral, popliteal, dorsalis pedis, and posterior tibial pulses in normal legs. Then determine the effect of position *on the feet.* You can expect some color changes. How great is it and how long does it persist with the legs level? Check the warmth on the back of the foot as well as the color.
7 Perform on normal persons the tests for clots in the deep calf veins. Note especially the pressures you must use to produce pain on palpation and with the cuff. Also question the subject on the sensation produced when you dorsiflex the foot (Homans' sign).
8 If available, examine patients with various changes in the joints of the hands, arms, feet, and legs. Determine the range of active and passive motion in the affected joints as well as inspecting and palpating them.
9 Examine a spastic, a flaccid, and an atrophic extremity. Examine available patients who have lesions of hands, elbows, shoulders, feet, knees, and hips.
10 Determine the venous pressure in a patient in whom it is elevated.
11 Examine and evaluate edema in patients with recent and with chronic ankle swelling.
12 If available, examine an unstable knee. Pay close attention to which maneuver or maneuvers will reveal abnormal movability in that patient.
13 Examine a patient with abnormal arteries in the lower extremities, palpating the pulses and testing the response to changing the elevation of the feet.
14 If possible, watch a trained examiner test a leg with a deep clot.

See also Sections 8-4, 9-9, and 9-10.

5-7 NERVOUS SYSTEM (see page 80)

The *nervous system* generally is considered as consisting of the *brain* and *spinal cord,* together called the *central nervous system* or CNS; the *peripheral nerves,* which lead from the CNS to other parts of the body; and the *autonomic nervous system,* which controls automatic functions, such as blood pressure. The *sense organs*—of sight, hearing, smell, taste, touch, pain, temperature, position, and vibration—are considered part of the nervous system.

The system detects changes, called *stimuli,* and converts them into *sensations* which may or may not be consciously perceived. It interprets the sensations and stores them as memory. If appropriate to the life functions, stimuli may prompt *responses* which are initiated by the nervous system and carried out by various *effectors.* Those effectors which cause movements—the muscles—are called *motor,* a term that sometimes includes glands which secrete but do not cause motion.

The so-called "highest functions" of *intellect* or *cognition—perception, interpretation, memory,* and *judgment*—are carried out in the brain. So are the functions which are called *emotional* or *affective.* Simpler reflex functions occur in the brain, spinal cord, and autonomic nervous system.

Even an experienced examiner needs considerable time for a complete examination of the nervous system. Certain key portions, however, are done as parts of a general examination. Some you have already carried out under "General Appearance," "Head and Neck," and "Extremities." Much of the *mental status evaluation* is included in taking the history, and you need extend this only when you detect some abnormality of speech, behavior, memory, or thought.

Mental Status   The mental status can be considered as including four functional parts: *intellect, affect, disordered thought,* and *insight.* You can evaluate each, and it is well to do it systematically.

Intellect   You probably will find it easiest to evaluate the intellectual functions since you are already familiar with similar tests. You will not be "grading" the patient, only determining whether he has rather gross deficiencies. You will cover the areas of *orientation, memory, information, calculations,* and *judgment.*

Orientation simply means that the patient correctly identifies time, place, and persons. You can tactfully ask the date and year; whether he knows the name and nature of the building he is in, or if not, the city, town, or neighborhood; and whether he recognizes the names or occupations of the persons he has seen in the building. Obviously you must make allowances for small errors, but if they are great, you can ask him as well what his relationship is to you.

Memory is tested in three categories—*immediate recall, recent memory,* and *remote memory.* You can evaluate immediate recall tactfully by asking the patient to repeat the last two or three questions you have asked him. A more direct test is to have him repeat a series of random digits after you have given them to him slowly. You can, for example, begin with seven digits, such as 4-6-2-3-1-6-5. Most persons will correctly recall seven or more. You can test recent memory by requesting the patient to tell you the route he took to see you, how he came into the building and arrived at the examining room, or what he did while waiting to see you. You can check remote memory by asking for a description of some event that occurred several years in the past.

Information or knowledge is to a large extent memory. You will have to take into account the patient's background and education. A person in a rural area, even with little education, can correctly tell you when local crops are planted and harvested. You can ask a better-educated person to name in order the last five Presidents or to name the five largest American cities.

You must also allow for the patient's educational level when evaluating calculations. One standard test is to ask the patient to subtract sevens serially from 100. Thus 100, 93, 86, 79, etc. If this proves too difficult, you can ask him to add or subtract small numbers.

Judgment is somewhat more difficult to test. The questions should be reasonably simple and suited to the patient's background. You can ask, for example, "Which of these three doesn't belong with the other two—right, left, and down? Big, blue, and little? Chicken, sheep, and goat?" A more direct question is, "What is the difference between right and wrong?"

Affect   Affect, mood, or emotional state often is obvious. You must judge whether it is *appropriate* and of *normal degree.* The patient who smiles pleasantly or laughs while discussing the death of his mother or child is showing an inappropriate affect, as is one who cries bitterly when discussing some pleasant subject. Violent aggression toward someone trying to help the patient is an inappropriate affect, as is cheerful or even passive acceptance of serious or threatening news.

It may be necessary to question the patient about his mood, especially if he seems very apprehensive or slightly depressed. You can ask whether he has been sleeping well, has cried often recently, feels blue and "down." From this you can lead into questions about whether he has felt that things are getting too bad for him to cope with, whether he feels that life is just not worth living any longer, and whether he has thought that he might as well kill himself. If he admits to all these, you can without strain ask whether he has tried to kill himself. By tactfully leading up to the question of suicide, you can judge the depth of the depression and its effect on the patient.

Disordered Thought   A patient with severely disordered thoughts will often show them in his actions or volunteer remarks that reveal them. He may obviously be looking at or listening to something you cannot detect or may be answering questions no one else hears. Such bizarre behavior should not prevent your questioning him.

You will have to discover whether the patient is having *hallucinations,* that is, seeing, hearing, smelling, tasting, or feeling things undetectable by others. He may be having *illusions*—identifying one object or sound as another—for example, believing a light bulb is the sun or that a chair is some animal. He may have *delusions*—false beliefs—as when he is convinced that he is all-powerful, that he is the victim of a vicious plot, or that he is controlled by some outside force. Occasionally thoughts and ideas become totally disorganized, disjointed, and inappropriate.

Patients who are nearly normal and are suspicious may deny disordered thoughts if you ask questions directly. You can approach the subject by inquiring whether the patient dreams, whether his dreams ever seem real, and then whether he ever hears or sees anything—rather like dreams—when he is awake. From this you can lead into questions about hearing voices no one else hears or seeing things invisible to others. Similarly you can ask whether he has quarreled frequently or has enemies who are trying to harm him.

Insight   Insight may be present even when the patient has hallucinations, illusions, delusions, depression, or inappropriate affect. He may say that he *thinks* he sees or hears things and recognizes that his ideas are unjustified. He may even ask for help because of the mental disturbance.

When the patient does not volunteer evidence that he has insight into his abnormality, you can ask whether he thinks he is all right, has doubts about the reality of his hallucinations, or really believes his delusions. If he has no insight, it may anger him that you do not share his distortions, and he may demand to know whether you think he is crazy. You can hedge your answer by saying that some of his ideas seem a little peculiar, but try neither to arouse him nor to assure him that he is completely normal unless you are certain that he is.

Consciousness and Language Functions   The condition of the brain determines the *level of consciousness,* examination of which is often included in the mental status. You may, however, determine the level at the first moment of the examination.

A patient may be *hyperalert* and then is usually *hyperactive.* He may be in almost constant motion even though he is weak and ill. He may complain of slight noises and even dim lights. Often he speaks rapidly and may anticipate the end of your question. He is keenly aware of what is going on around him and may be unable to sleep even though he is exhausted.

In contrast, the patient may be quiet and *drowsy* but easily aroused by a question. This is a normal state if he is fatigued, but it can also be an early stage of unconsciousness. The patient may progress to the *obtunded* or *semistuporous* state where he is lethargic, apparently sleeps a great deal, and has obviously slowed mental processes. He is, however, able to rouse himself when disturbed and to answer questions.

In *stupor,* the patient is truly unconscious but does respond to commands or to pain. In *coma,* the unconsciousness is so deep that nothing rouses the patient.

You can usually judge the level of consciousness easily and quickly. You should remember, however, that it is possible to fake the various levels. Some patients remain mentally alert enough to remember what they see and hear even though they cannot respond. You should always assume that what you do and say around an "unconscious" patient may be understood.

The brain is also involved in language, written as well as spoken, perceived as well as used. You have already observed the patient's speech in taking the history, but in some instances you may have to ask him to read and write a few words at your direction. Obviously, blindness, deafness, paralysis, or lesions of the respiratory tract may prevent normal speech function even though the speech centers of the brain are normal.

Cranial Nerves The twelve pairs of peripheral nerves connected to the brain are the *cranial nerves.* In a neurological examination, they are considered as a group even though their functions differ widely. Each pair is tested separately and is usually designated by a Roman numeral as well as a name.

I, the *olfactory nerve,* carries the sense of smell. You can test it by holding each nostril closed in turn and asking the patient to sniff and identify tobacco, soap, or anything else with a distinct odor. The patient should keep his eyes closed and name the substance.

II, the *optic nerve,* is the nerve of vision. You have already tested sight and the pupillary reflex, but there is a further examination that you can do without special equipment. It evaluates the *visual field* by *confrontation.* In confrontation you compare your own *peripheral vision* to that of the patient.

You stand exactly in front of the patient with your eyes on a level with his and about 2 ft from him. He then closes or covers one eye and you do the same for your eye opposite that one. Thus you close your right eye if he closes his left eye.

You hold a small piece of white paper between your thumb and forefinger during the test. The hand you are using must move so that it is always the same distance from his open eye as from yours. You tell him to keep looking at your pupil while you look at his and to tell you as soon as he sees the paper.

You then begin with your hand high above your foreheads and held so that the paper will show. Neither you nor he should be able to see it until you lower your hand. He should tell you that he sees it just as you make it out. You then bring the paper up from below, from the right side, and from the left. In each movement he should see the paper as soon as you do.

The test is then repeated with the opposite eye. If the patient cannot see the paper as far out peripherally as you do, he has a *constricted visual field.*

III, the *oculomotor; IV,* the *trochlear;* and *VI,* the *abducent nerves* are motor and go to the muscles which move the eyeballs. You have already examined them in testing the eye movements. Nerve III is also involved in the *pupillary reflex,* which you have already tested.

V, the *trigeminal nerve,* is sensory as well as motor and supplies the jaw muscles. You test the motor functions by asking the patient to clamp his jaws shut while you feel the tensed muscles just in front of the angles of the jaw. Normally they should be as tense on one side as on the other. When he is asked to open his jaw wide, his chin should stay in the midline. It will deviate toward the paralyzed side if nerve V is damaged.

The sensory part of nerve V supplies almost all of the skin of the face and the mucous membrane of the mouth. Sensory testing in simple form consists of stroking the skin with a wisp of cotton and lightly pricking it with a sharp pin.

The patient keeps his eyes closed while you test his sense of touch by drawing a bit of cotton an inch or so across the skin. You ask whether he feels the touch and move to another area. At intervals you make the stroking motion but do not let the cotton touch. You ask the question as at other times, and if the answer is "yes," you repeat the fake stroking about every other time. If he does not discriminate, you may as well abandon the test.

To test for pain, ask the patient whose eyes are closed to say whether he feels something sharp or dull. Then occasionally turn the pin so that the blunt end touches in order to check the patient's accuracy.

Compare the sensation in corresponding areas of the two sides or as you probe from one area to another on the same side. To make such comparisons, you must be certain to stroke as firmly in one place as another and to touch the skin over about the same distance. In using the pin each prick must have the same force. You then ask the patient in which of the two areas he felt the touch most distinctly and the pinpoint more sharply.

For nerve V, you should test the sense of touch and pain above the eye, above the outer angle of the lip, and below the lower lip. This should be done on both sides. If an area seems *insensitive,* compare the two sides and then try to map out the affected area. An area may be *hypersensitive,* so that even stroking with cotton causes a burning or painful sensation. You should map such an area as well.

VII, the *facial nerve,* is chiefly motor but also is involved in the sense of taste on the front part of the tongue. You often can see the distortion of the face in paralysis of the facial muscles. To test the motor function, ask the patient to wrinkle his forehead, close his eyes tightly, and show you his teeth. The movements simply make any weakness more obvious when the paralysis is slight.

VIII, the *acoustic nerve,* is the nerve of the inner ear. You have already tested for perceptive deafness, which may mean nerve damage. Nystagmus may indicate trouble with another part of the nerve or, more often, with the sense organs of balance which, like those of hearing, are in the inner ear.

IX, the *glossopharyngeal nerve,* and *X,* the *vagus nerve,* are tested together. You touch in turn each side of the pharynx with a tongue blade. The normal response is a contraction of the pharyngeal muscles as the patient gags. Imperfect movement of the soft palate as the patient says "ah" is also a sign of difficulty with these nerves.

XI, the *accessory nerve,* is the motor nerve of the sternomastoid muscle, and any weakness or wasting of it may mean nerve damage. A further test is to have the patient shrug his shoulders while you hold them down. Weakness of one or both sides is another sign.

XII, the *hypoglossal nerve,* supplies the tongue muscles. You can examine for tongue weakness by having the patient stick his tongue far out. If one side is paralyzed, the tongue tip will deviate toward that side.

EXERCISES

1   Perform a mental status examination on one or more normal subjects. In doing so, try to make your questions smooth and as natural as possible. Pay attention to the speed with which a normal person calculates, the promptness with which he supplies information, the accuracy of normal immediate recall, recent and remote memory, and how he answers questions of judgment.
2   If possible, examine the mental status or watch the examination of a patient with organic brain deterioration and one with disordered thought.
3   If available, examine briefly patients with various levels of unconsciousness.
4   Do a neurological examination of the cranial nerves on one or more normal subjects.
5   If possible, examine the cranial nerves of a patient with lesions affecting one or more of them. Be prepared to say which nerve or group of nerves is involved.

Spinal Cord and Peripheral Nerves   Examination of the spinal cord and its peripheral nerves can be thought of as having three parts: *motor functions, sensory functions,* and *complex functions.* The brain really is more or less involved in all three, but less directly than with the examinations already done.

Motor Functions   Motor functions, for practical purposes, involve muscles. Normally the CNS acting through the peripheral nerves maintains the muscles in a state of partial contraction so that they feel firm or, in other words, have *normal tone.* Associated with normal tone is usually normal function, adequate strength, quick contraction, and prompt relaxation.

When the CNS control of a muscle is completely lacking, the result is *flaccid paralysis.* Tone disappears, so that the muscle is flabby and eventually wastes away or atrophies. All strength is gone and the muscle cannot contract; rather, it is permanently relaxed. Muscles that are flaccid may show an odd involuntary movement called *fibrillation*. It is a localized twitching or shivering. Fibrillation occurs in normal people also as a twitching of the eyelid or quivering of a leg, arm, or finger muscle.

When the CNS control is out of balance and excessive, the result is *rigidity* or the more extreme *spastic paralysis*. Tone is increased and the muscle feels unusually firm or hard. It remains contracted, and this interferes with motion. It relaxes either very slowly or not at all.

Your examination has already included observation of the gait for evidence of flaccid or spastic paralysis, palpation for muscle tone, and strength testing. In the neurological examination, such palpation is carried out to determine the tone in all parts of the extremities. Similarly, the strength is more thoroughly determined by having the patient move each joint in all possible directions while you oppose the motion with your hands. Obviously an athlete in training is stronger and has better muscle tone than a sedentary elderly woman. You must use experience to judge what is normal for each patient.

One part of the motor examination is particularly sensitive to flaccidity, rigidity, and spasticity. You ask the patient to relax his arm completely and encourage him until he is as relaxed as he can be. Holding his wrist firmly, bend his arm at the elbow and then pull it straight again rapidly but smoothly. Normally you will feel a slight but definite resistance due to the normal muscle tone. A flaccid arm offers less or no resistance, a spastic one may be very difficult to move and may spring back if you let go. In rigidity, the arm offers increased resistance but moves fairly readily. There may be a peculiar off-and-on quality to the rigidity, as though the tone slips at intervals from increased to normal and back again to increased. This is called *cogwheel rigidity*.

Sensory Functions The sensory functions are varied, but those you will test most often are *touch, pain, position*, and *vibration*. The tests require a cooperative and alert patient. False results can indicate poor testing, stupidity, inattention on the patient's part, or outright faking.

Touch and pain are tested as for cranial nerve V with cotton and pin. Position testing is also carried out while the patient keeps his eyes closed. Ordinarily you will test it in the middle finger and in the great toe of each side. You must be certain to place your thumb and forefinger exactly on the side of the finger or toe, near the tip. Grasp it more firmly than you need to and keep up the pressure throughout the test. Unless you take these precautions, the patient will be able to sense differences in the pressure you make as you move the finger or toe.

To test *position sense* in the finger, support the patient's palm with your free hand. Ask him to relax his hand and arm. Then move his finger up and down until you are sure that it is relaxed. Keeping up your pinching pressure, move his finger down about 45° and tell him that when his finger is more or less in this direction, he should say "Down." Move his finger up about 45° above level and explain that this is "Up," then out horizontally and describe this as "Straight." Then repeat a series of brisk up and down movements ending with the finger horizontal, down about 20° to 30° or up a like amount. The normal person can readily tell you the position.

Test the great toes in the same way, grasping the top of the foot to keep it from moving. If necessary, you can test the wrist, ankle, elbow, and knee the same way. You must, however, always exert pressure on the sides of the part you move.

Vibratory sense is tested with a tuning fork held firmly against bone. Usually this is at the thumb side of the wrist, on either side of the ankle, or on the outside of the elbow or knee. It is well to strike the tuning fork fairly hard and hold it on the patient's chin so that he can feel it "buzz." Then test the wrists and ankles, in each place asking him to tell you whether he feels the buzz and to tell you as soon as it stops. You can then compare it to your own sensation at your wrist. If you suspect that the patient is unreliable, you can strike the tuning fork but leave it in contact with your palm or fingers a brief time so that it does not vibrate. The patient may still report a buzz.

The testing for *touch* and for *pain sensation* can be a general survey, a localized examination, or part of a careful, exhaustive maneuver. In any event, you should test any area which the patient says is numb or has peculiar sensations or where there is paralysis.

The localized examination of such an area begins by careful probing with cotton and pin, checking the sensations in the center of the area. If touch or pain sense is absent, much increased, or much reduced as compared to the corresponding points on the opposite side of the body, you test at frequent intervals outward in all directions. You thus *map* the area of abnormal sensation.

The general survey is useful only if the patient has evidence of neurological disease. It requires too much time to use routinely, since you must carefully test around the neck, down the trunk, and around the genitals, moving cotton or pin only about an inch each time. You then test down the front, back, and both sides of the arms and legs, as well as across the front and back of the hands and feet. Any abnormal area then has to be mapped.

More detailed sensory examination requires even more time and includes *temperature sense,* the ability to *discriminate* between one and two points, and the ability to *recognize objects* by touch. These tests are part of the specialized neurological examination.

Complex Functions   Complex functions include *involuntary movements, coordination* of movements, and *reflexes.* You have already examined for involuntary movements while observing the general appearance.

Coordination produces smooth movements always under the patient's control. *Incoordination* may be evident in the jerkiness of ordinary motions. You often can make it more evident by having the patient alternately slap his thigh with the front and with the back of hand, increasing his speed until he is doing it as rapidly as he can. A similar test of *rapid, alternating movements* has him move his feet up and down as rapidly as possible.

The *finger-to-nose test* of coordination is carried out with the patient's eyes closed. You extend his arms to the sides and ask him to touch his nose alternately with the forefinger of each hand. You can use the *heel-to-knee test* in the same way for each leg. With eyes closed, he must place his heel on the opposite knee.

Obviously muscular weakness, paralysis, or tremor may make these tests of coordination seem positive. The distinction between incoordination and such defects is part of a specialized neurological examination.

Testing the various *reflexes* is probably the most common part of the neurological examination. You must take certain precautions to get a discriminating result, especially if the difference between the two sides is slight. The patient must be relaxed even if you have to distract his attention. He must always be in a symmetrical posture. If sitting, he should look straight ahead or straight up. His arms and legs should be in the same position on each side. Usually his legs will be hanging free below the knees, his hands palms down and first fingers touching in his lap. If lying, his head should be in the midline and he should look straight up. Usually his hands are palms down on his chest with fingers touching and his legs straight.

You must be careful to use the same force with the percussion hammer on the two sides. Similarly you must use the same pressure when you stroke the skin.

Reflexes   Three *arm reflexes* are usually tested—*radial, biceps,* and *triceps.* To test the radial, strike lightly on the *radius,* which you can feel as a bony prominence just above the wrist on the thumb side of the arm. Your free hand should lie lightly on the back of both the patient's hands as you test first one side and then the other. You can then feel the jerk as the forearm bends in response.

You elicit the biceps reflex by placing your free forefinger across the inside surface of the elbow with the arm bent. You can feel the large tendon running down the middle of the space, and you strike your own finger with the hammer just where it lies on the tendon. In response, the forearm bends upward.

The triceps reflex can be best obtained if you place your free hand under the patient's elbow and get him to rest his forearm along yours. You strike the tendon at the back of the arm, just above the elbow and in the midline. The responding jerk straightens his forearm.

Two similar reflexes are tested in the *legs*. You have already elicited the *knee jerk*. You test the *ankle jerk* or *Achilles reflex* by striking the large Achilles tendon at the back of the ankle. You must have the patient relax his leg and foot while you place your free hand under the ball of the foot and raise it to a right angle with the lower leg. The response is a downward jerk of the foot.

To test the ankle jerk in bed, you must bend the patient's knee to a right angle while he lets it lie to the side. You then bend the patient's foot to a right angle and strike the tendon.

Patients sometimes tense up as they see the hammer strike for any of the reflexes. This can *block* the reflex. You can avoid blocking by having the patient look at the ceiling. You may have to reinforce the ankle jerk as you do the knee jerk. You can reinforce the arm reflexes by having the patient clench his fist on the side you are not testing.

The arm and leg reflexes are not equally active from person to person. It is customary to grade each one on a scale of $-$, $\pm$, $+$, $++$, $+++$, $++++$. "Negative" means that no jerk is elicited even with reinforcement. "Plus-minus" means that there is response with reinforcement or a barely detectable response without it. A "four-plus" response is a maximal one and the reflex is said to be *hyperactive*. It is seen chiefly in spastic paralysis of the part. Response rates "one-plus," "two-plus," and "three-plus" are between these and are of increasing strength.

Two reflexes involving stroking are often used. To elicit the *plantar reflex,* grasp the ankle firmly and move the great toe up and down to be sure that it is free and relaxed. Then stroke firmly but not hard upward from the heel toward the little toe and then across the front of the instep toward the great toe. You can use the edge of your thumbnail, the end of a retracted ballpoint pen, or even a sharper instrument, but you should not use enough pressure to scratch the skin.

Normally all five toes bend downward and each remains in contact with its neighbor. The abnormal response, called a *positive Babinski,* is the reverse. The toes spread out and the great toe moves upward. If the abnormal reflex is less pronounced, you may find that the great toe moves upward but the others do not fan out. This usually is called a *weakly positive Babinski.*

The other reflex, called the *cremasteric reflex,* can be elicited only in men. If you rather firmly stroke the inner side of the thigh, usually from below upward, the testis on that side will move upward.

A final test of complex function is one of *balance.* To carry it out, you have the patient stand with feet together and you stand close enough to grab and steady him. He should be steady with no swaying. You then ask him to close his eyes. A normal person may sway very slightly and visibly right himself promptly. An abnormal test, the *positive Romberg sign,* is one in which the patient with eyes closed begins to fall or sways widely.

EXERCISES

1 Examine the motor, sensory, and complex functions of one or more normal subjects. Pay particular attention to the arm-straightening maneuver for judging muscle tone, the amount of finger and toe movement to reveal position, and the sensitivity to vibration. If time permits, do a general survey of touch and pain sensation. Notice especially how some parts of the body are more sensitive than others. See how effective the subject is in rapid alternating movements, finger-to-nose, and heel-to-knee tests. Practice eliciting the reflexes until this becomes easy to do, and note especially the normal plantar reflex response.
2 If a patient with spastic and flaccid paralysis and another with Parkinson's disease are available, do the neurological examination of the extremities.
3 If possible, watch a demonstration of the signs in a patient with incoordination.

See also Sections 8-1, 8-2, and 9-8.

Chapter 6

Presentation of Clinical Information

6-1 SPECIAL WRITTEN AND VERBAL PRESENTATIONS

The presentations—both written and verbal—discussed in Chapter 3 are in the form used for medical and surgical patients. They can serve for pediatric, obstetrical, or psychiatric patients as well, but each specialty has developed a slightly different order of presentation. Each emphasizes the information of special interest to that branch of medicine.

Pediatric Examinations The pediatrician wants to know immediately, especially for young children, about any trouble that the mother had while she was pregnant with the patient. He also wants to know of any difficulties during and just after the child's birth, how he has been growing, and how he has progressed mentally. He gets useful information from the history of any other pregnancies and deliveries of the mother and of any difficulties experienced by brothers and sisters. The mother's—and father's—intelligence, information, education, and attitude toward the patient may be very important.

The *length* of infants and the *height* of children, as well as their weight, tell a great deal. The temperature may have more significance than it does in an adult. This information starts the report of the physical examination. Very often the circumference of the head and of the chest is included.

Here is a record written in the classical form:

Nov. 11, 1977   GREEN, William ("Spunky") No. 687539
2 yr old Negro boy. Source: Mother—reliable, intelligent, high school graduate, housewife, obvious good relations with child.
No prior contacts here.
PREGNANCY & BIRTH: Normal pregnancy except for nausea in 1st trimester. Duration—"about $8^{1}/_{2}$ mo." Labor—4 hr, no complication. Pt. "just fine" at & after birth.
GROWTH & DEVEL.: Weighed 6 lb at birth, about 24 lb at 1 yr. Breast fed. No feeding problems. Developed normally. Walked at 13 mo. Always very active. Has had 2 "colds" lasting 3–4 d, otherwise well.
SIBLINGS: Sister $4^{1}/_{2}$ yr old. Normal pregnancy & delivery. Normal infancy. Only few acute illnesses. Mother now 2 mo pregnant.
CC: "Fever, 103°; crying"—2 hr.
PI: Spunky was well until 2 d ago when he developed a "cold" with running nose and cough. He did not seem very ill until about 3 hr ago when he became irritable and would not nap. He began crying hard 2 hr ago and his mother found his rectal temperature was 103°. He will not say what is wrong and answers "no" to everything.
PH: Gen'l health excellent.
    CHD: No measles, chicken pox, whooping cough, German measles.
    INJURIES & OPERATIONS: Circumcision at age 3 d. No complications.
    IMMUNIZATIONS: Diphth., tetanus, pertussis, polio, measles—3–9 mo. German measles, 1 yr.
    Medications: None.
    Prev. adm.: None.
FH: F—34, Living & well.
    M—30, Living & well.
    1 sis.—age $4^{1}/_{2}$, living & well.
    Pt.'s grandfather has gout. Great grandparents all living. No known familial dis.
R of S:
    HEAD: Neg. No convulsions.
    EYES: Neg.
    EARS: Neg.
X   NOSE: See PI. Nosebleed after falling on face—6 mo ago.
X   MOUTH: Had thrush as newborn. Responded to treatment in 3–4 d.
    LUNGS: Neg.
    HEART: Neg.

X   DIGESTIVE TRACT: Vomited once or twice, not recently. No diarrhea, constip., or blood.
URINARY: Neg.
GENITAL: Neg.
X   SKIN: Diaper rash repeatedly during 1st yr.
BONES & JOINTS: Neg.
NERVOUS SYSTEM: Neg.
BLOOD: Neg.
ENDOCRINE: Neg.
SH: Born Aug. 2, 1975, Streamview Hosp. Family lives in 6-room apartment. Adequate, comfortable. No financial problems. Now eats all solids, prefers meat to vegetables. 1 pint milk, fruit juice daily, regular vitamins. Usual day—awake at 6–6:30, breakfast 7:30, lunch 12–12:30, nap 1 to 3–3:30, dinner at 6:30, bed 7:30–8. Sleeps soundly.
PE: T 104.2 rectal P 112 R 20 (crying) W 30 lb. H 35 in. Head circum.—50 cm. Chest circum.—50 cm. BP (not taken).
X   Well-nourished & -developed black boy who cries hard and looks acutely ill. Clean, uncooperative.
SKIN: Sweating, hot. Otherwise neg.
X   HEAD & NECK: Skull & scalp norm. Ears: startles on clapping. No discharge. Rt. eardrum infected, dull, pink, bulging. Left normal. Eyes: follows even slight motion. Pupils equal, round, react to light. Movements normal. Conjunctivae injected, crying. Fundiscopic: not done. Nose: bilat. obstruction. Purulent discharge. Mucous membrane red. MOUTH: 18 teeth. Normal tongue, gums, and mucous membranes. Tonsils red but not large. Pharynx fiery red, pus from above.
X   NECK: Soft, tender, movable lymph nodes at angle of jaw and down cervical chain. Neck moves freely.
CHEST & LUNGS: (Pt. crying) Normal fremitus and resonance. No rales or rhonchi.
HEART: PMI in left 5th ICS inside MCL. Heart sounds loud. P2>A2. No murmurs. (poor exam.).
ABDOMEN: No tenderness, organs, or masses felt.
GENITALS: Normal, immature, circumcised male. Both testes in scrotum.
RECTAL: Not done.
BACK: Normal contour.
EXTREMITIES: Symmetrical, good strength. Normal femoral pulses. Knee jerks symmetrical +++.

Summary

2-yr-old boy with normal delivery, infancy, and development. He was well until he developed a "cold" 2 d ago. About 3 hr ago he became irritable and restless; 2 hr ago began crying and had 103° rectally. PE revealed rectal temp. of 104.2 and acutely ill but well-developed and -nourished child, crying hard and perspiring. The rt. eardrum is infected, dull pink, and bulging; left is normal. There is bilateral nasal obstruction with purulent discharge. The tonsils are red but not enlarged, the pharynx is fiery red, and pus is coming from above. There are soft, tender, movable lymph nodes in the superior and anterior cervical groups.

Obstetrical Examination Obstetrical records frequently begin with a tabular summary of the patient's obstetrical history. This includes the *number* of *pregnancies,* counting, of course, the present one, the *number* of *deliveries, children,* and of *abortions,* spontaneous and induced. Usually these are shown as:

"Gravida, 5; Para, 2; Children, 2; Abort. spont. 1, induced 1"

where *gravida* or *G* is the number of pregnancies, *Para* or *P* the number of deliveries, *Abort.* the number of *abortions* divided into *spont.* or *spontaneous* and *induced.* This is often followed by "LMP 3/15/75" or *last menstrual period* with the day the flow began. Sometimes there is an entry of "EDC" or *expected date* of *confinement.* This latter is the date, calculated from all the available data, on which the patient will probably deliver her baby. Even when it appears at the start of the history, it is a professional opinion rather than a symptom or sign.

Psychiatric Examination Psychiatric records include the results of a mental as well as of a physical examination. Various forms of recording are used, but you can use a record of the *mental status.* This can be written in the order given in Section 5-7. It is well to report in this fashion whenever you do a mental status as part of your examination.

The following is the mental status record as part of a general examination:

Mental Status

Mrs. Brown is a tremulous, elderly woman who sits quietly looking at the floor. She does not speak spontaneously, but responds readily. Her facial expression is usually placid but she cries when mentioning her dead dau. (Death occurred 20 yr ago.) She uses no gestures, sitting with her hands in her lap. Her clothing and person are dirty but not foul.

Orientation: Poor recognition of place—"This is a big institution, some sort of store, I guess. It could be a hospital." Of time—"The sun is shining so it's some day. I can't remember which. I haven't looked at my calendar so I don't know the month or year." Of person—"Of course I'm Mrs. Brown. You're a kind of butcher. You've got a white coat. Yes, of course I know you. I remember you from a long time ago." (Never saw pt. before.)

Memory: Immed. recall—very poor, 4-digit span. No recall of name "James Smith" after 30–60 sec. Recent memory—very poor. Cannot say how she got here or that police brought her. Remote memory—fair to good.

Remembers husb.'s full name and that of his father. Recalls end of World War II and son's return home.

Information (college graduate): Recalls earliest 2 of 5 recent Presidents but names all 5 largest U.S. cities. Names 5 European countries & their capitals easily.

Calculations: Subtracts one serial 7, then "I used to be able to do things like that." Cannot add 2 dimes and 1 nickel or two 10's and one 5.

Judgment: Becomes completely confused. "Blue, green, and cat" are "all alike." "Steak, potatoes, and automobiles" are "What you eat, I guess."

Affect: Appropriate but generally seems depressed. Depression excessive (see above) at times. "I get discouraged", but denies suicidal thoughts.

Disordered Thoughts: None elicited. No hallucinations, illusions, or delusions.

Insight: Considerable. "I have inordinate difficulty in thinking things out. My memory has become very bad." "I should eat regularly but I can't remember when it's time to."

Summary

Quiet, passive, depressed elderly woman who is disoriented with very poor recall and recent memory but fair to good remote memory. She has considerable information and good vocabulary but cannot calculate and judgment is severely impaired. Although depressed, she is not suicidal and has no disordered thoughts. She has considerable insight.

EXERCISES

1 Examine, write up, and verbally report on a child under age 4. (Patient need not be ill but parent should be available.)
2 If feasible, determine the mental status of a person with some mental disturbance. Report it verbally and in writing to a physician who has also evaluated the patient.

6-2 OTHER COMPONENTS OF MEDICAL RECORDS

The complete medical record is a summary of what is known, thought, and done about a patient. You have been concerned with only two classes of information entered- in the record—the subjective history and the objective examination to determine his physical and mental status.

The record also contains eventually the results of *chemical* and *microscopic tests* of body fluids—blood, urine, cerebrospinal fluid, bile, and others. It includes *special examinations* such as electrocardiograms, tests of respiratory function, and electroencephalograms as well as x-ray examinations, cultures for bacteria and fungi, and measurements of hearing, sight, pelvic size, and muscle functions. There are the results of *cytological examination* of the body cells and of *biopsies*—examination of tissue removed at operation or by needle. All these findings are considered objective data in the problem-oriented record and they are often recorded under "0" in progress and revisit notes. In either record form they may appear grouped on special sheets.

From the subjective and objective information, including history, physical examination, and the findings of the tests, the *diagnosis* and opinions about the patient are reached. His situation is appraised in this fashion in order to decide what should be done for him. Whether called *impressions, diagnosis,* or *assessment,* this records a step in the decision-making process.

The diagnosis is obviously a critical step, even if it is tentative, because it determines the action to be taken or avoided. This action can be advice, medication, physical therapy, irradiation of various sorts, or an operation. It may include further testing to make a final decision or to check the patient's progress. It may be decided to do nothing because nothing is needed or because no known treatment will help the patient. This does not mean abandoning the patient. Reassurance and support—the nurse's "TLC"—may be all the help needed or available.

The complete medical record contains a report of any treatment given or prescribed, including operations. Records frequently contain notes giving the results of consultations by specialists. If the patient dies and an autopsy is done, it also is reported as the final item in the record.

Most long records have summaries written at intervals during the patient's care and at the end of each period of hospitalization. These summaries are much like those at the end of the initial examination but emphasize the patient's course.

You may already be able to diagnose some simple conditions such as the common cold, menstrual cramps, later stages of pregnancy, or sunburn. Other diseases are much more difficult to recognize and some may mimic simple conditions. Some institutions, therefore, discourage anyone but a physician or dentist from writing an impression, diagnosis, or assessment of that sort in a patient's record. Other institutions will allow or even encourage you to write such opinions as long as you identify yourself and your position on the staff.

Much the same restrictions hold for treatment or relatively hazardous tests. Thus you may find that sections labeled *disposition, treatment, orders* or *recommendations,* or *plan* have certain requirements.

These restrictions on the recording of diagnoses and treatment are not arbitrary or made to protect special rights and privileges. Medical records are potentially legal documents and as such appear in courts. Any irregularities can have important consequences legally as well as medically, and medical institutions have a public obligation to assure their completeness and accuracy. The record must also truly reflect who made decisions as well as what was done.

You must therefore clearly understand what you are authorized to write, as you must understand what you are authorized to do. Beyond this you must recognize your own limitations and, in the last analysis, rely on your own judgment and restrictions of what you are qualified to do and write in the patients best interests.

EXERCISES

1 Review the entire hospital chart of a complicated case. Identify the various kinds of information it contains, how they are recorded, and where. Examine the opinions and diagnoses entered in the record. What actions were taken as a result of these?
2 Look up—with your instructor's help—the earliest symptons and signs of the common cold, measles, and meningococcic meningitis. Also compare the symptoms and signs of severe sunburn and of the cutaneous form of porphyria. What are the symptoms and signs of menstrual cramps and of threatened abortion in early pregnancy?

Chapter 7

Patient Examination in Emergencies

Examination of a patient who needs emergency care is very different from the other examinations. You must keep procedures as brief as you can and still get the essential information. More·important, examination is combined with treatment—the most urgent examination followed by prompt treatment of the immediate threat, then further examination followed by treatment of the next most serious threat, and so on until the emergency is under control. Time is saved by simultaneously questioning and examining, and postponing the usual history and systematic physical examination until later.

Consider a patient spurting blood from a lacerated forearm, with a broken leg and a swollen, abraded cheek. One glance will detect the hemorrhage. It is life-threatening and you treat it without delay. One or two questions or the odd angle of the leg will focus your attention on the fracture. You examine and treat it. Only then do you turn your attention to the cheek; if it is trivial, you question and examine the patient for other injuries before taking care of the face.

This does not finish the job. Later, a more extended history is taken and the physical examination is completed. There may be a complicating disease that will delay recovery.

This all involves decisions on priorities—what to examine and treat first—a process called *triage* (pronounced tree-ahzh), and it establishes the priority for *immediate care.* A condition that is not immediately threatening is postponed for *delayed care.*

Each emergency differs from the one before, and the procedure must fit the situation. This does not mean that you work haphazardly. Each part of your examination is planned and systematic, but the order of the parts changes.

The order is dictated by "first things first." Detect and treat first what most immediately threatens the patient's life. Detect and treat next what threatens his life less immediately. Detect and treat after that what threatens his "limbs." And "threat to limbs" here means anything that will alter or impair his functional ability or appearance. Finally, detect and treat whatever may threaten his recovery.

Two natural questions will get you much of the urgently needed history in any emergency: (1) What happened? and (2) How did it happen? Listen carefully to the replies if they are brief and informative. Learn what you can quickly even if you must seem rude to a long-winded informant. Remember that a seriously ill or injured patient can die while you listen.

Do not let any person who may be a source of information leave without being thoroughly questioned, and be sure that you have names, addresses, and telephone numbers before the informants go. Another trained examiner, if one is available, can question relatives, ambulance attendants, or anyone who accompanies the patient. If you are working alone, these people will simply have to wait until you get the immediate emergency under control.

Never assume that your information is totally accurate or complete. People generally are poor observers in emergencies and even the patient may not know the full story. You may actually learn more from the physical surroundings if you are at the scene of the emergency.

Complete each part of the physical examination promptly. Use the equipment you have at hand and do not delay while you hunt for some instrument. As you become more skilled and efficient, you will be able to accomplish a great deal in a short time without hurrying or being slipshod. You should work thoroughly and carefully, however, even if it takes a little longer before you become efficient.

Reexamine the patient even when things seem to be going well. Some of the most serious conditions are tucked away inside the skull, chest, or abdomen and produce symptoms and signs only after an hour or more.

Do what you know how to do, but get expert help as quickly as you can when things seem beyond your skills. Until someone else takes over, however, you remain with the patient and in charge.

Above all, stay calm. Think what you are doing and plan your next step. This is easier than you may think. Real responsibility steadies most people.

Acute Injury   Injury kills more Americans between the ages of 1 and 36 than any other cause. Many of these lives can be saved if those who first see the injured take prompt and effective action.

Trauma can kill in many ways even when the patient lives long enough for treatment to begin. The first move when faced with an injured patient is to make a survey—a very quick but careful and orderly triage—to guide you in establishing an "order of priority"—deciding what will be done first, second, and so on. The order is determined by what kills most quickly and therefore what bodily functions you need to protect most urgently. The list is especially important in multiple injuries, but you should consider it in any serious situation. The "order of priority" in trauma is as follows:

Immediate Threats to Life

Respiratory difficulties, especially obstructions and apnea
Cardiac arrest
Severe external hemorrhage
Shock
Head and facial injuries

Generally Not Immediate Threats to Life

Neck and back injuries
Abdominal injuries
Injuries to the extremities
Injuries to skin
Other injuries

Respiratory Difficulties   Serious breathing problems must be detected and treated before any further examination is done. You can quickly determine whether the patient has stopped breathing. If you cannot see respiratory movements, listen at the nose and mouth with your face close enough to feel air moving when the patient exhales. Obviously you must provide prompt treatment if respiration has stopped.

You must examine in more detail if the patient is having difficulty breathing. Check to be sure that clothing or jewelry is not strangling the patient. Then start at the mouth by looking and feeling to determine whether the tongue has "fallen back" into the pharynx or whether some object is obstructing the pharynx. If there is, correct the situation and move to the neck. Here you look for bruising or healed scars and gently palpate the larynx, feeling for any crushing. Again, this may have to be treated.

The chest may have to be exposed by cutting away clothing. It can quickly be examined for visible wounds, but you must remember that stab and gunshot wounds may be small and inconspicuous. It is important, also, to note whether one side of the chest moves more than the other, and whether any part of the chest wall moves in while the rest moves out (or the reverse). Rapid palpation of the ribs and sternum for tender points, displacement, or a "gritty" sensation on movement will locate fractures. Quickly percussing the uppermost part of each side will detect the hyperresonance or tympany of pneumothorax. Flatness in the lowermost part may indicate hemothorax.

While palpating the neck and chest, you may feel or even hear a crackling from just under the skin. This is *subcutaneous emphysema*, air which has escaped from the lung and pleural cavity through a wound.

If the patient is coughing up blood, you must try to determine whether it is coming from the chest or from higher up in the nose, pharynx, or mouth. Some patients may be cyanotic even when they are too weak to show much respiratory distress. The blueness may indicate damage to the respiratory tract but may be circulatory, as in shock, or due to changes in the blood itself. If the breathing is reasonably normal, defer any detailed examination of the lungs until you have checked the circulation.

When cyanosis is accompanied by a swollen tongue and protruding, bloodshot eyes, the cause is respiratory. This is *traumatic asphyxia* and requires immediate treatment.

Cardiac Arrest Even cardiac arrest—complete stopping of the heart's contraction—does not necessarily mean death today. It must, however, be diagnosed and treated within 4 min. And treatment must be continuous, so that any further diagnostic procedures can begin only when someone else has taken over the treatment.

You should suspect cardiac arrest and immediately examine any patient who has become unconscious and stopped breathing. Usually unconsciousness occurs first, and the patient takes one or two breaths before stopping. You can feel for the pulse with one hand and open one or both eyelids with the other, if necessary. You will find no pulse and the pupils will be dilating or already fully dilated. You can notice cyanosis, which is usually present in the lips, as you bend down to listen for the heart with your unaided ear. If the heart sounds are inaudible, the patient has cardiac arrest and you begin treatment.

Trauma of the heart itself is suggested by penetrating wounds anywhere in the lower chest and LUQ. Crushing injuries of the precordium are rarely responsible. The pulse is slow, the blood pressure low, and the heart sounds faint or absent. Percussion and auscultation may disclose pericardial effusion. The veins of the head, neck, and arms may be distended. These are important signs; if you suspect but are not certain of them, you should reexamine the patient after a few minutes to determine whether they have become more obvious. If so, prompt treatment is essential.

Severe Hemorrhage   Blood loss kills rapidly if it is brisk, and a good-sized artery spurts blood with each heartbeat. Even a good-sized vein causes considerable blood loss in a short time with its steady flow. Ordinarily, a brief glance will show a bleeder if overlying clothing is cut away or if you cautiously remove a first-aid bandage. The significant bleeder requires first attention.

Check particularly the areas where large blood vessels are near the skin. These are easy to remember because they are where you feel the pulse most easily.

A word of caution about hemorrhage. A little blood goes a long way when smeared over skin and clothing. An abrasion or other injury oozing blood may be messy without being dangerous. You must therefore find the source of bleeding and decide whether it is life-threatening.

Internal bleeding can accumulate blood in the thorax, abdomen, skull, or tissues. Hemothorax is often accompanied by coughing of blood if the lung is injured. Otherwise it will produce only dullness or flatness in the lowermost part of the chest. There is similar flatness in the dependent part of the abdominal cavity when blood accumulates there.

Bleeding inside the skull produces unconsciousness, although many other things do so as well. Intracranial hemorrhage rarely causes shock, so that you should look further if the patient is unconscious and the blood pressure is low. Large accumulations of blood in soft tissue cause large, firm hematomas with or without surface ecchymosis.

Shock   The dangerous drop in blood pressure that occurs in shock can have medical as well as traumatic causes. It is a collapse of the circulation and deprives the entire body of oxygen and other essential materials. You can waste badly needed time in discovering the precise but hidden cause of shock, and a markedly reduced blood pressure calls for prompt treatment.

Shock occurs in many injuries: hemorrhage, severe burns, thoracic damage, crushing injuries, spinal cord trauma—especially in the cervical region, and head injuries where it appears late. Even severe pain can cause shock. Regardless of the cause, however, certain signs appear.

You should suspect shock immediately if the patient seems dreamy, drowsy, "dopey," or unconscious, but he may be restless and anxious. His face is usually pale—"ashy" if he is a black—and often cyanotic. He looks drawn and his breathing is shallow. His skin is cold and clammy with perspiration. He may complain of thirst or of nausea and he may vomit. His pulse is weak—small, soft, and rapid. If injuries prevent your palpating the radial arteries, you can use the carotid or femoral pulses or that at the temple just above the outer corner of each eye.

The blood pressure will confirm the presence of shock with readings below 90/60 and as low as 10/0. But do not waste time hunting for a sphygmomanometer. You should begin treatment immediately.

Head and Facial Injuries   Facial injuries are an immediate threat to life only when they obstruct the nose, mouth, or pharynx so that they interfere with breathing. A fractured mandible can displace the tongue backward or cause it to swell enough to block the pharynx. You can detect the break by palpating along the mandible inside the mouth as well as outside along the jawline and by looking for teeth out of line. This can be coupled with a quick search for broken teeth, dentures, or other debris that may be sucked into the air passages unless removed.

Injuries to the cranium and upper cervical vertebrae are important primarily because they can damage the brain or upper spinal cord. The brain is in less danger if the patient remains conscious or has been unconscious only briefly. Brain damage can, however, appear only later, so you must check the state of consciousness repeatedly over several hours after a skull injury.

In the immediate examination, it takes only a few moments to feel the skull, beginning at the back of the head. Palpate for depressed fractures in which a part of the skull is pushed inward. A fracture along the side of the skull is particularly dangerous, although all are serious. You may feel the sharp edges of the break beneath the scalp, but you should not do more than detect the fracture.

Any hematoma or "goose egg" on the scalp and any laceration should also be noted. The scalp bleeds briskly even though the skull is undamaged, so that the seriousness of the injury cannot be judged by the amount of blood.

The ears and nose can quickly be checked for a watery discharge. This usually indicates a fracture at the base of the skull.

The patient's eyes should be checked to determine whether they deviate or whether they remain aligned with one another. Check the pupils to determine whether they are the same size, whether they are dilated or constricted, and whether they react to light. You can check the light reflex by covering the eyes for a few moments. And remember, the patient may have a glass eye.

Ask the patient to wiggle his fingers, toes, or feet and watch for any movement—it need not be vigorous. You can also ask whether his arms or legs feel odd, numb, or tingling. If he has an obviously painful injury to an arm or leg but feels no pain, there may be central nervous system damage.

If he is unconscious, you can test the reflexes in unbroken arms and legs. Do not waste time hunting for a reflex hammer—use the side of your hand for the legs and the ends of your stiffly bent fingers for the arm reflexes. You can also look for movements when you jab the foot or the hand with a pin, splinter, or sharp point of a penknife.

You can quickly test for flaccid paralysis. Absent reflexes and flaccidity occur in central nervous system damage but in other states as well.

It is particularly important to reexamine a patient with a head injury and to observe him over several hours. Unconsciousness, convulsions, and even increasing restlessness are alarming. So are late changes in the pupils or deviations of the eyes, paralysis, or sensory changes.

Neck and Back Injuries Trauma to the anterior cervical region is most apt to cause immediate problems with respiration or circulation. Injuries to the posterior cervical area and the back are most dangerous because they threaten the spinal cord.

You can examine this area by gently running your hands down the sides and back of the neck, feeling for a displaced vertebra, any bony prominence, or any unusual angling of the neck. This may indicate a dangerous cervical fracture or "broken neck," movement of which can be disastrous.

If the patient is on his back, you can slip your hand under him and feel down the vertebral column, noting any abnormally prominent or depressed vertebral spine, any that is displaced, or any that is tender on pressure. If he is on his side or lying face down, palpate him as he is. But remember that spasm of the large back muscles can obscure serious spinal injury.

Any suspicion of fractures there should be treated promptly. If you must proceed to examine other injuries, the damaged skull or spine must be protected against motion.

Abdominal Injuries Injury within the abdomen may result either from a penetrating wound or from a crushing blow. Stab, puncture, and gunshot wounds almost always enter the abdominal cavity and you can suspect internal injury. A blunt, nonpenetrating blow can cause more serious damage internally with less evidence on the abdominal wall. In this situation, changing signs on repeated examinations may be your best indication of serious trauma.

You should quickly palpate for rigidity and tenderness. If these remain localized and slight without other serious signs such as shock, the injury may be limited to the abdominal wall.

More serious injuries usually involve bleeding into or from solid organs or perforation of the gut. You can detect free blood or fluid in the abdominal cavity by percussing the flanks for shifting dullness and free gas by finding tympany around the umbilicus or over the liver. Short, gasping, labored breathing suggests blood or intestinal contents high under the diaphragm. Hemorrhage near the posterior abdominal wall is serious but may cause few signs other than pain and, later, ecchymosis in the lumbar area.

Bleeding into the liver or spleen may occur slowly. If you find the liver or spleen palpable and tender, you must examine it again at 5-min intervals. Increasing size or tenderness is apt to mean trauma to the organ.

Trauma within the abdomen often paralyzes the bowel, which becomes distended with gas. You will find tympany and a silent abdomen fairly early in such cases. It is important to remember that this can occur with or without intestinal perforation.

On the other hand, tympany over the lower chest with bowel sounds when the area is auscultated suggests a torn diaphragm and intestine within the chest. A penetrating wound of the chest will obscure this picture, but distinct bowel sounds high in the thorax make it likely that the diaphragm is ruptured.

Fractures of the pelvis are often associated with injury to the organs there and with bleeding into structures around the rectum. You should palpate the pelvic bones, feeling for the edges of a fracture, a grating sensation, and tenderness on palpation. You can grasp the iliac crest on both sides and gently try to move them in opposite directions. They should move as a solid unit. Even slight independent motion indicates a fracture.

Bleeding into the pelvis may cause the femoral pulse to disappear on one or both sides. Sooner or later you should do a rectal examination seeking a palpable, tender, smooth mass of blood outside the rectum.

Abdominal injuries are so often subtle that repeated examinations are necessary. They are also so difficult to localize that x-rays and other tests, including exploratory operation, are commonly the only means of diagnosis.

Injuries to the Extremities   You can usually determine quickly the nature and extent of injury to the hands, feet, arms, and legs if you remove the clothing. You may have to cut it away, since you will usually want to move the part as little as possible before you evaluate the damage.

If there is an open wound or laceration, you will have to estimate its depth and determine whether it is a clean incision or a jagged tear. You must detect any foreign matter in it and decide how much damage has been done to the skin around it.

A part may be obviously distorted by a *fracture,* but this is not always so. You will have to look for the less obvious breaks and remember that one fracture often is accompanied by others. Generally there is no serious fracture in an extremity that the patient moves spontaneously.

A fracture may be *incomplete* (see Figure 7-1)—the bone having cracked without breaking all the way through—especially in children and in thin, flexible bones. On the other hand, one broken end may be jammed rather tightly into the other—an *impacted fracture.* Usually any fracture is less painful during the first few minutes, but pain and swelling around the bone begin rather promptly. You can feel the broken ends and detect their motion much more easily before this swelling occurs.

The muscles on one side of a complete break are stronger than those on the other and angulate or bend the broken bone. Either the injury or the muscular pull may displace the fragments so that they slip past one another—called *overriding*—or separate completely in *displacement.* Displacement may be so extreme that one fractured end is driven through the skin—an *open* or *compound fracture.*

An unsplinted compound fracture can be readily identified by the white bone that is seen in the laceration or by palpation of the end. Complete and some incomplete fractures are evident because of the angulation or displacement. Impacted fractures may show neither, but the broken bone is shorter than the corresponding one in the opposite extremity. Displacement, too, can lead to shortening rather than angulation.

Fractures, of course, are painful and tender. You should palpate them and move the part only when you must. You may have to do so in examining incomplete fractures, especially those of the small bones of the hands, feet, ribs, and clavicle. You can feel the gritting or grating of the fragments as you move the bone with a finger over the fracture site. This may be the only way to come to a quick conclusion in an unconscious patient.

Regardless of the kind of fracture, movement of the bone fragments damages surrounding parts. It is important, therefore, to hold broken limbs immobile even during the later examination. The extremity should be *splinted* as soon as you complete its examination.

Dislocations occur when one bone is displaced from the other at a

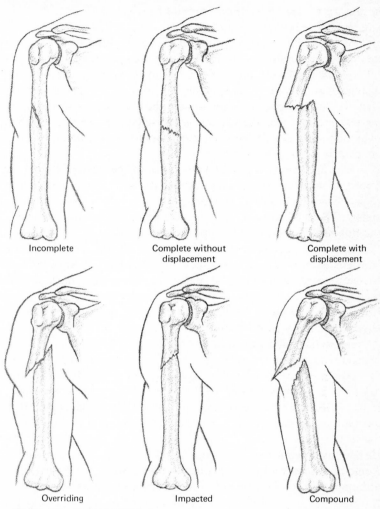

Figure 7-1   Types of fracture.

joint. The resulting distortion can be confused with a fracture near the joint, although you may be able to palpate the smooth, rounded surface of the displaced head of the bone. Swelling about the joint may quickly make this difficult.

You should be able to detect and make a preliminary evaluation of skeletal injuries. Your physical examination will not yield nearly so much information as an x-ray; though you should not attempt to substitute your skill for one, you need the skill nonetheless. When there is no ready access to x-ray facilities, at least first-aid measures will have to be taken without them. Even with facilities available, your initial examination is necessary to decide what part should be x-rayed. In case of doubt about any area, it is best to get a film.

Sprains may cause such doubt. They are tears of the ligaments and tendons which bind joints together and stabilize them. Sprains can be as painful as fractures, and this pain limits motion. They do not cause displacement, however, unless there is also dislocation, fracture, or both. Usually the patient with an uncomplicated sprain will tolerate some passive motion, and there is no gritty sensation. Swelling—which limits palpation—usually develops quite promptly, so that an x-ray is often necessary.

A *strain* is the rupture of a muscle or of the tendon binding it to bone. There is pain, tenderness, and local distortion. Usually the muscle itself feels hard—the typical "charley horse"—and nearby muscles may be in spasm. There is, however, no displacement, gritting, or true tenderness of the bone felt from the side opposite the strain.

Blood vessels can be torn by displaced bony fragments. Fractures can tear even large vessels, especially in the thigh, knee, and shoulder. Vessels may also be injured directly without much damage to the skin. If the vessel is large and the bleeding brisk, a deep bruise or hematoma forms with localized swelling. At times, the pressure of this blood can squeeze nearby vessels closed and block the circulation in an extremity. A hematoma can form rapidly as a somewhat tender lump and blood escape later to appear as a large ecchymosis under the skin.

Nerves can also be damaged without much surface evidence of injury. A conscious patient will tell you that some area below the point of injury feels numb or tingles. You may find painless, flaccid paralysis in the extremity, and you can test the amount of damage by asking the patient to move the part. If he moves his hand or foot, you can test his strength further by having him grip your hand or push against it with his foot. Remember that injury to the muscles may also cause localized weakness, although this is painful unless the nerves are also damaged.

Injuries to the Skin   Injury to the skin is usually obvious if you remove the clothing so that you can see the area. You must be careful not to let superficial wounds distract you from more important, deeper injury.

This is not true of burns if they are extensive or severe. They require prompt treatment. You must, however, quickly determine their extent and severity. If available, you should wear sterile surgical cap, gown, mask, and gloves even for the initial examination.

Burns are described as of three degrees. A *first degree* or *superficial burn* produces only reddening and some thickening of the skin. A *second degree* or *partial-thickness burn* is deeper and usually has a duskier red color. The area will eventually become thickened and blister or, if the vesicles break, will ooze. A *third degree* or *full-thickness burn* extends all the way through the skin and even into the underlying structures. When fresh it may be pale, charred, or have a "cooked" appearance. Later, if untreated, it will slough and scar. Frequently, when fresh, it is surrounded by a bright-red border, and it may be less painful than the more superficial burns.

You must determine the *extent* of first-, second-, and third-degree burns even when one patient has all three. Such estimates are essential in deciding on the treatment to follow. For extensive burns, the percentage of surface burned can be calculated by the "rule of nines." For an adult, each of the following is approximately 9 percent of the total body surface: all of the head and neck, the anterior surface of the thorax, the posterior surface of the thorax, the anterior surface of the abdomen, the posterior surface of the abdomen and the buttocks, the entire right arm, the entire left arm, the anterior surface of the right leg, the anterior surface of the left leg, the posterior surface of the right leg, and the posterior surface of the left leg. The genital area is the remaining 1 percent. For infants and small children, the head and neck is 18 percent of the total area and each leg surface is 7 percent.

Burns caused by *electricity* are usually double—one where the current entered and the other where it left. The entrance burn is usually on a hand; the exit burn is where the body is grounded and so most often on the feet. The surface burn may be small, with the deeper parts severely burned. The current travels along blood vessels and may clot the blood in them. You should check the pulses, therefore, along any affected arm or leg.

Chemical burns from acids or alkalis are common around the face and mouth as well as on the hands. Ultimately you must try to discover what chemical caused the burn, but you should immediately begin treatment by flushing the area with copious amounts of water while you continue your examination.

Burns from *radiation,* such as x-rays, may show changes only late but still be serious. It may be necessary to continue inspection at intervals even for days after the patient was exposed.

Many creatures bite, including man, and some snakes and spiders, of course, inject poison. You should discover, if possible, what animal caused the bite, because the treatment of poisonous bites is directed by that knowledge. Any deep bite from a dog or wild animal should lead you to call the local health authorities to ask about the presence of *rabies* or hydrophobia in the district.

Even insect stings can be fatal to a very sensitive person. They occasionally produce shock that requires immediate treatment.

Other Injuries All injuries to the eyes and eyelids should be considered dangerous. The injured eye should be handled only as much as is absolutely necessary to examine it, since the pain caused by the examination will prompt the patient to squeeze the eye closed, possibly causing further damage.

The cornea can be examined quickly for opacities or foreign objects. In the sclera, look: (1) for a blush of tiny dilated blood vessels immediately around the cornea and (2) for a foreign body, such as a steel sliver, which may penetrate it. Occasionally a blood vessel bursts in the conjunctiva over the sclera and the hemorrhage looks frightening but is not dangerous.

Rather obviously, you should test the vision quickly, even if only by having the patient count fingers. Do not, however, try to clean out the eye in any serious injury to the lids or globe even if your examination is incomplete.

The eardrum can be ruptured by a sharp object in the external canal or by a sudden blow on the ear. Usually the ear bleeds, and this may obscure your view of the eardrum. You may, however, be able to see the hole torn in it.

EXERCISES

List your "order of priority" for examination and indicate each step at which you would treat the patient in the following cases:

1   A 25-year-old man is seen to stumble and fall on his face, striking his forehead. You are called and recognize immediately that he is unconscious and that his right hand is bent abnormally far back at the wrist.
2   A 6-year-old boy is brought in crying and at intervals screaming with pain. His left arm is in a "first aid" sling, tied to a board. The left side of his face is abraded and oozing blood.
3   A 52-year-old woman arrives on an ambulance litter, barely conscious, with a bloody bandage on her right forearm, an emergency splint on her right leg, and obvious bruises and cuts over her right eye.
4   A 16-year-old high school sprinter is carried to you with a swollen, painful right ankle and slightly bloody bandages on his left knee and his hands.
5   A 40-year-old man is brought by ambulance with obvious stab wounds in the left midaxillary line at ICS 5 and in the RUQ of the abdomen. He has labored breathing, is sweating and mumbling.
6   A 65-year-old man arrives assisted by a policeman but walks with ease despite a large "goose egg" on the left side of his head and obvious guarding of his arm.

Nontraumatic Emergencies   The "order of priority" in an emergency not due to trauma is, of course, aimed at preserving life and limb, but it must be a little different from the order when injury has occurred. Hemorrhage, for example, is less common and is internal rather than external. The "order of priority" in nontraumatic emergencies is as follows:

Circulatory problems
Respiratory difficulty
Central nervous system disorders
Abdominal lesions
Metabolic disorders
Other problems

Circulatory Problems   Cardiac arrest presents the same signs in medical as in traumatic emergencies and obviously demands as prompt treatment. It occurs especially in patients with heart disease and can appear even when they seem to be doing well.

Rapidly progressive heart failure is almost as dramatic as cardiac arrest, but you have a little longer to work. The patient usually will be in obvious distress, sitting up or struggling to do so. His respiration will be labored and panting. He usually has a weak cough and his lips may show a bubbly froth. He is cyanotic but his face may be flushed with a cyanotic tinge or ashen, and his eyes may be prominent as he strains to breathe. His hands and feet are usually cold and clammy.

The pulse may be weak—small, soft, and rapid. Such a patient is in shock. On the other hand, the pulse may be bounding—large and hard—with the rate only a little increased. You may find a normal rhythm, a gallop, or total irregularity, but do not take time to study it thoroughly.

You should take a few seconds to auscultate the back of the chest. Start at the top and work rapidly downward. You will hear fine and moderate rales with some rhonchi and often wheezing. This will give some indication of how grave the situation is: the higher the rales on the chest, the more serious is the pulmonary edema and the more urgent is the treatment.

After the emergency has passed, a complete examination of the heart and lungs should be done. The fundi of the eyes, the abdomen, and the venous pressure can be checked when the patient can again lie down comfortably.

Shock occurs in many medical conditions and basically appears as it does in trauma. You should suspect it whenever a patient becomes lethargic or restless, "dopey," drowsy, or unconscious with pallor or "ashy" skin. The most revealing sign is the weak, rapid pulse confirmed by the low blood pressure. You may know that the patient's underlying condition is likely to cause shock. If you do not, you will have to ask quickly about pain and examine the heart, lungs, and abdomen. You should not, however, delay treatment if the blood pressure is falling.

Other circulatory emergencies are urgent but somewhat less so unless they are accompanied by cardiac arrest, acute pulmonary edema, or shock. The patient will appear in less danger of dying immediately and you will suspect circulatory trouble because of chest or precordial pain, increasing breathlessness, arrhythmia, or edema that is rapidly increasing.

You can take a somewhat more thorough history of the episode and what led up to it. Your examination should center on careful evaluation of the pulse, measurement of the blood pressure, thorough examination of the thorax—lungs and heart—upper abdomen, and deep veins of the calf.

Respiratory Difficulties Complete respiratory arrest, like cardiac arrest, allows only about 4 min in which to diagnose and treat. Examination is limited, therefore, to determining that there is no obstruction in the pharynx and no constriction about the neck. Quick percussion of the uppermost part of the chest for bilateral pneumothorax and of the lowermost part for fluid in the pleural cavity is all that should be done before treatment is begun.

Much more often, the patient will be in acute respiratory distress. You have time for few questions but you should watch and listen to the patient breathe. Note the rate and depth of respiration, whether maximal difficulty is in expiration or inspiration, whether there are grunts, wheezes, or whistles with each breath. Also, if the patient is coughing, determine whether the cough is weak and light or hard and deep. You should examine the sputum if any is produced, noting its color, its character, and any evidence of blood. A glance will tell you whether the patient is cyanotic.

Your examination must include the pharynx, especially in infants and children, although you may want to examine it last. Otherwise the child will begin to cry. You also need—for adults as well as children—a rectal temperature, pulse rate, and blood pressure.

Your principal effort should be spent on examining the thorax—heart as well as lungs. This examination should be as thorough as you can make it, but it is also well to get x-ray films of the chest if you can.

In older patients or those with chest pain, it is also wise to examine the deep calf veins for clots. If your examination to this point has revealed no abnormalities, especially in an unconscious or nearly unconscious patient, you will have to embark on as thorough a history and physical examination as possible.

Central Nervous System Disorders and Coma The examination of any patient must include an evaluation of the level of consciousness. Normal responses become evident as you ask the patient questions, even when he is unable to speak, because he will be attentive and react somehow to your questions. A deaf person shows his alertness by reacting to the sight of you or to your touch.

A patient in deep coma is almost equally easy to recognize. He cannot be roused or even made to stir by pain when you squeeze the Achilles tendon. A further test is to tickle inside the nostril with a wisp of cotton or a feather. Normally the patient draws back his head and his nostrils flare. In coma he does not react, but do not waste time hunting for cotton or feathers.

There is a gradual range of consciousness from full alertness to coma, and the patient may wander in either direction along it. You must therefore test him repeatedly until you are certain that his state is not changing.

If the patient is unconscious or nearly so, you must make some quick observations. These include the rate, depth and character of respiration. The rate and characteristics of the pulse together with the blood pressure are important. You should note the color of the skin and mucous membranes of the mouth and eyelids as well as the sclera, looking for pallor, bright "cherry red" discoloration, cyanosis, and jaundice. You should quickly check the chest, face, and arms for any eruption or petechiae. By feeling the chest with the back of the hand, you can detect any significant fever.

It is very important to smell the patient's breath. You can recognize the odor of alcohol, but do not immediately assume that he is simply drunk. Try to identify any fruity odor, a "mousy" one, or a smell somewhat like urine.

You should determine whether the eyes are rolling, deviated to one side, or whether one moves more than the other. Note the pupils' size, any inequality in size, and the response to light. Unless the cause of the unconsciousness is already apparent, the fundi should be examined with an ophthalmoscope. This can be difficult and time-consuming, especially if the eyes are moving. You should not waste time but only try to see the optic discs. You are looking mainly to see whether they are elevated with fuzzy margins.

You can quickly test all the extremities for flaccidity or spasticity, noting any spontaneous movements. Among the tests, try to bend the head forward so that the chin touches or nearly touches the chest. Note that you must be certain that there has been no trauma to the neck before you attempt this. You are looking for rigid neck muscles, not trying to test the joints.

You can then test the reflexes in each extremity, looking for overall responsiveness and for unilateral disturbances. In some instances you may have to follow this with a complete physical examination.

Unconscious patients may vomit, whether they are injured or ill. This carries the risk of choking on—aspirating—the vomitus. Try never to leave the head in such a position that vomitus can collect in the pharynx.

Convulsions, with or without coma, are conspicuous except for very localized convulsive twitching of one hand or even a single finger. You should carefully observe any convulsion, especially if you see it from the start. It can begin as generalized contractions all over the body, face, and extremities. Or it can start in a hand, foot, or one side of the face and progress or "march" to involve the extremity and then one whole side of the body or both.

It is very important to get the history of a patient who is unconscious or having convulsions. Patients with some chronic diseases, such as diabetes or epilepsy, wear special identifying jewelry or carry cards giving the diagnosis and other valuable information. You may have to search out a telephone number or the name of a person to contact by checking the patient's handbag or wallet unless the person who accompanies him has such details.

A patient may become partially paralyzed without losing consciousness, or he may have lost consciousness for a longer or shorter period and regained it before you see him. In these instances you will have adequate time to do a neurological examination and to examine the circulatory system.

The patient who is extremely dizzy, with or without vomiting, should be carefully questioned about true vertigo. Your examination should include looking for nystagmus, testing the hearing of each ear, and inspecting the eardrum.

Abdominal Lesions   Patients with acute abdominal complaints usually have pain, nausea, vomiting, diarrhea, or blood in vomitus, stools, or vagina. They may have several or only one of these. You must do everything reasonable to get an accurate history of these symptoms and of what the patient has eaten or taken as medicine during the past day or two.

Pay particular attention to the onset, course, character, and location of the pain. Often the history is more valuable than the physical examination in deciding on the probable trouble and the course of action.

The physical examination should concentrate on the abdomen, of course, particularly on tenderness and muscular resistance. You should percuss and auscultate as well as inspect and palpate. The rectal and vaginal examinations are intrinsic parts of this abdominal examination. In short, you should examine from diaphragm to pelvic floor as thoroughly as you can.

The examination should then extend to include the pulse, temperature, blood pressure, heart, and lungs. If the patient has been bedridden, is postoperative, or has just borne a child, you should examine the legs carefully, especially the arteries and calf veins.

Metabolic Disorders   The principal metabolic diseases that lead to emergency situations are associated with coma, convulsions, or collapse. These generally develop over several minutes or hours. If the patient seeks help during the early stages, he can usually tell you what the primary problem is. If the patient can no longer communicate at the time he arrives, you will have to proceed as you would in the case of convulsion, coma, or shock. Laboratory tests are usually the shortcut to discovering the cause and status of the difficulty. It is for this reason that they are so widely used in characterizing coma and shock.

Other Problems Most other emergencies are handled more nearly like ordinary illnesses, with complete histories and physical examinations. Two situations—drug intoxication and severe mental disturbances—require special consideration.

Drug intoxication following abuse of narcotics, hypnotics, stimulants, or hallucinogens is apt to be complicated if the patient has used two or more drugs within a brief period. You will have to decide quickly the respiratory, circulatory, and mental status of the patient, treating immediately any threat to his life. As soon as possible you should try to get a complete drug history from the patient or his companions, especially to determine what drugs he has taken during the past 12 hr or so. You will probably get the "street name" of the drug, and even this is often inaccurate. If possible, get a sample of any drug he has taken. Remember that you are not a policeman. Convince your informant that what you learn is confidential and that the information will be used only for the patient's own good.

Mental disturbances may appear alone, but they often accompany drug abuse, withdrawal from alcohol or other drugs, and physical illness. They may be complicated by disruptive, abusive, destructive attacks on others—including you—or by suicide attempts. In any event you will have to evaluate the mental status as an emergency procedure.

Your ability to do this quickly will improve with experience, but certain questions will help you verify what you see and what the patient volunteers. If you have any doubt as to the patient's orientation, you should ask him where he is, who he is and who you are, how long he has been where he is, and the date. You can test his recent memory by asking when, where, and what he last ate, his more remote memory by asking about where he grew up and his early schooling. You can get some idea of his current intellectual capacity by getting him to do a simple addition or subtraction, often in calculating the time since a certain date. With skill you can weave these questions naturally into a series of sympathetic inquiries without alarming the patient or arousing his resentment.

From this you can go on to his affect by asking how he feels at the moment, what his mood generally is, whether it has changed recently, and whether he has been feeling that life is generally just not worthwhile. This can lead naturally into asking about despondency and suicidal thoughts.

You can ask about how he is sleeping, whether he dreams, has night-mares, has feelings of unreality, hears or sees things that other people do not, and whether there is any external voice, power, or force commanding him to do certain things.

You will, of course, be noting his reactions as well as his answers to your questions and watching for bizarre or unusual actions and speech patterns. You should be able to describe his mental status fairly accurately, if superficially, after 10 or 15 min with him. Most importantly, you should be able to judge whether he is apt to be disruptive or suicidal during the next few hours.

EXERCISES

List the "order of priority" for your examination and indicate each step at which you would treat the patient in the following cases:

1   You are called at 2 A.M. to the bedside of a 63-year-old woman who woke up breathless, and you find her sitting upright and fighting to get her breath.
2   A 12-year-old boy arrives with a "stomachache" of increasing severity that began 3 hr ago.
3   As you pass the bed of a 50-year-old man admitted the day before with a heart attack, you see his hand go limp so that he drops a magazine he was holding, and his head drops back against the pillow.
4   A 70-year-old man is brought by ambulance accompanied by his daughter, who says she found that she could not rouse him when she tried to wake him from a nap; he still has neither wakened or moved except to breathe.
5   A young man and woman help a 20-year-old man into the room, announce that "he has had an overdose," and turn immediately to leave. The patient seems barely conscious and is breathing only about five or six times a minute.
6   A fat, 43-year-old woman comes in with abdominal pain and vomiting of 2-hr duration.
7   A 26-year-old woman is brought by her husband because she has been crying most of the past 2 weeks, has not slept more than 2 or 3 hr a night, and has just torn up most of her dresses.
8   A healthy-looking 47-year-old man complains of pain on the right side of the small of his back. The pain comes in waves so strong that he doubles over and cries out. It began 1 hr ago.

Signs of Death   Not all parts of the body lose the signs of life at the same time. Despite this fact, there is a point in time beyond which nothing can revive the patient. This is the time of death in a medical and social sense.

The usual signs of death are loss of motion and consciousness so that nothing arouses the patient, absence of respiration, absence of signs of cardiac action, and fixed, usually dilated pupils that are unreactive to light. All these occur in cardiac arrest, and yet the patient can be revived if effective resuscitation is begun within about 4 min. It is equally certain that persistence of the signs for 10 to 20 min means that the patient is dead.

You may have to determine quickly whether a person is dead. This frequently occurs during triage when there are several victims in the same disaster and the living need attention. The examination is essentially that of looking, listening, and feeling for signs of respiration, of feeling and listening for pulse and heartbeat, and of inspecting the pupils especially for response to light. You can add an attempt at arousal by squeezing the Achilles tendon.

Some time after death, the blood settles to the lowest part of the body, so that the area usually becomes a mottled, dull reddish-purple. The blood drains from the uppermost parts, leaving them pale. If the eyes are open even slightly, the cornea dries and becomes cloudy. The presence and rate of appearance of these signs depend upon several circumstances, but if they are present, they confirm your opinion that the person is dead.

Later still, the muscles stiffen for a period in rigor mortis and then relax. The body cools to room temperature after death. Again, the rate of such changes varies with circumstances, but their presence makes your evaluation simple.

The muscles of the extremities, trunk, or face may twitch slightly or shiver soon after death. Occasionally the abdomen may rumble for a brief period or on shifting the body. When the body is moved, air may be forced from the lungs, even producing a rasping or grunting sound. These are sometimes considered signs of life by the uninformed, but a skilled observer will recognize them as insignificant.

Part Three

Basis for Findings in Health and Disease

Anatomy, physiology, and pathology provide background information necessary to understand the symptoms and signs discovered during a medical examination. Each is a broad subject offering several approaches that depend upon how you intend to use it. You will use each to improve your ability to examine patients rather than to learn in detail how each organ is constructed, how it functions, and how it goes wrong.

In *anatomy,* you need to know how to locate various parts from outside the body. This is *surface* or *projection* anatomy and takes up the body region by region rather than system by system. It is applied gross anatomy.

The physiology you need is often called *organ* or *system* physiology. It deals with the functions of organs such as the stomach or systems such as the urinary tract and can guide your review of systems.

Pathology describes abnormal structure and function. The science includes innumerable details of all the known diseases, but you can appreciate much of what you find by knowing in general how disease and injury change the body.

Chapter 8

The Anatomical Basis

Anatomical descriptions are more understandable if you use specific terms that locate the body's parts. "Top" and "bottom" mean little when a man may be standing, lying down, or even standing on his head. It is customary, therefore, to use all terms as though the person were standing on both feet, his head in a normal face-front position, and his arms hanging at his sides, palms facing inward (see Figure 8-1).

A line drawn down the center of the body—in front through the nose and the umbilicus and in back along the spinous processes—is the *midline*. A plane passing through this midline is called the *median plane*. Obviously it separates the right from the left side of the body. Any other plane dividing the body in the same front-to-back direction is a *sagittal plane*.

A plane drawn at right angles to the sagittal plane so that it separates the front half from the back half is the *midfrontal plane*. It passes roughly through the external auditory canal and runs downward through the tip of the shoulder and hip joints. It thus separates the front (*anterior* or *ventral*) from the back (*posterior* or *dorsal*) parts.

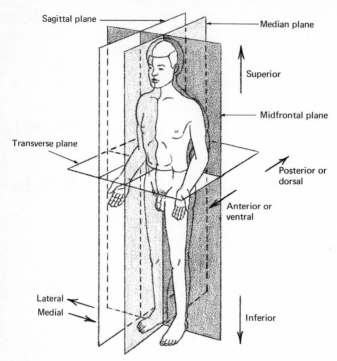

Figure 8-1 Anatomic position with planes and directions.

A plane at right angles to both of these and therefore across the body is a *horizontal* or *transverse plane.* Although there is no recognized midplane, any part above a certain transverse plane is *superior* to it, any part below is *inferior.*

Within the head, neck, trunk, and extremities, a thing which lies near the middlemost part is *central,* anything toward the surface is *peripheral.* *Superficial* is almost the same as "peripheral," and *deep* is roughly equivalent to "central."

In the extremities, a structure can be central, as is the thighbone, or peripheral, as are the muscles around it (see Figure 8-2). A part along the limb that lies closer to the body is *proximal,* one farther from it is *distal.* Thus the wrist is distal to the elbow and the ankle is proximal to the toes.

Since "to flex" means to bend and "to extend" means to straighten, extremities have *flexor* and *extensor* sides. The inside of the elbow is properly the flexor surface and the knuckles are on the extensor surface of the fingers.

Another pair of terms you may already know. *Medial* means near the median section and *lateral* means away from it.

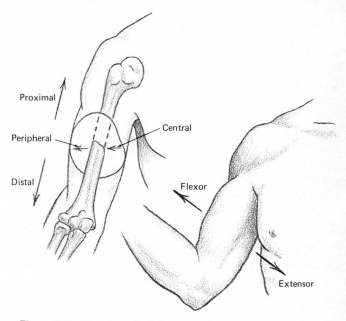

Figure 8-2 Directions in limbs.

EXERCISES

1   What bone lies in the midline of the anterior chest? What transverse structure separates chest from abdomen? What kind of plane passes through the midclavicular line (MCL)? Through the left ear canal and the right shoulder?
2   Describe the location of the palm of the hand in reference to the back of the wrist. Describe the location of the umbilicus. Describe the anatomical location of the eyelids when the eye is open with reference to the cornea and of the inner corner of the eye with reference to the nasal septum.
3   What is the anatomical location of the skin? Of the bones with reference to it? Of the hair? Give the anatomical location of a stab wound that was delivered straight from the side into the midaxillary line, entering the chest on the level of the nipples.

8-1 HEAD AND NECK

Head   The head consists essentially of two parts: the *cranium* or skull, with its contents and coverings, and the face. The two parts obviously merge with one another and with the superior structures of the neck.

Skull   The cranium lies superior and posterior to the face. The base as seen from the side begins at the eyebrows and extends posteriorly and inferiorly to include the *mastoid process* behind the ear (see Figure 8-3). From there the base continues posteriorly and superiorly to the back of the skull as you palpate it. The anterior, superior, posterior, and lateral surfaces are largely palpable except where they are hidden behind the facial bones. Except in the facial area and at its base, the cranium is covered by the skin of the forehead and scalp. Laterally, it provides the broad attachment for the *temporal muscle,* which you can feel by clenching your jaws. There are smaller, more superficial muscles above the eyebrows and about the ears. These structures are supplied by several arteries, the largest being the *temporal arteries,* which run upward anterior to each ear. You can feel one branch of the temporal artery superior and just posterior to the lateral end of the eyebrow. Several large veins drain blood from the scalp, the largest *temporal vein* running with the artery of that name.

Cranial Contents   The cranium is lined internally with a tough sheet of tissue, the *dura mater,* except where openings allow the spinal cord, nerves, and blood vessels to enter. Running within the dura are large veins which drain the surface of the brain and some of the arteries which supply blood to it.

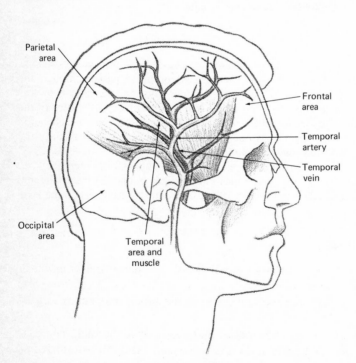

Figure 8-3   Cranial areas with temporal structures.

Central to the dura mater are two thin, connected membranes—the *meninges*—covering the brain. Between these two and outside them is *cerebrospinal fluid,* or *CSF,* forming a watery cushion over the surface of the brain.

Brain For practical purposes you can consider the brain as having four principal parts: paired *cerebral hemispheres,* a *cerebellum,* and a *brainstem.* All these interconnect with one another, and the brainstem continues inferiorly into the spinal cord (see Figure 8-4).

The right and left cerebral hemispheres make up approximately 85 percent of the brain. They occupy the superior, anterior part of the cranium, resting on its base anteriorly and joined in the central portion to one another and to the superior part of the brainstem. The surface of each hemisphere is thrown into folds, the deepest of which divide it into four regions or lobes.

Each *frontal lobe* lies behind the forehead—the frontal area—back almost to the midfrontal plane through the ear. Each *parietal lobe* lies posterior to the frontal lobe, extending to about the area of the smaller fontanel in a baby or the slight irregularity which remains there in the adult. Its posterior boundary extends from that point downward toward the mastoid bone behind the ear.

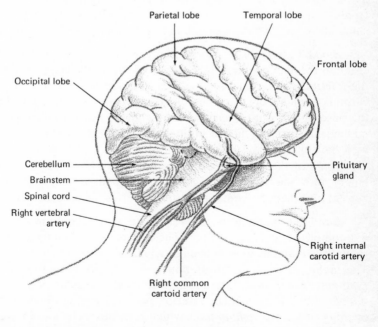

Figure 8-4 Brain and principal arteries from below and from right.

The *occipital lobe* lies posterior to this boundary. The *temporal* lobe is on the lateral surface of the brain. It lies more or less horizontally beneath the posterior part of the frontal and the anterior portion of the parietal lobe. The lower edge of the temporal and occipital lobes forms a horizontal plane that passes just above the auditory canal from about the joint of the lower jaw to the *occiput* or most posterior point of the skull. The base of the frontal lobes is also almost horizontal but is about on the level of the eyebrows.

Brainstem   The brainstem lies centrally between and beneath the cerebral hemispheres. It is an irregularly shaped mass, larger above and tapering to the smaller spinal cord. The cord continues downward through the large opening or *foramen magnum* at the base of the skull and into the *cervical vertebral column.* The brainstem contains the vital centers for control of respiration, circulation, and other autonomic functions. The cranial nerves also have their central endings in it.

Cerebellum   The cerebellum lies posterior to the brainstem beneath the occipital lobes, from which it is separated by a shelf of dura. Its tightly folded surface is roughly egg-shaped and it lies across the width of the occiput just posterior to the foramen magnum.

The cerebellum connects to the brainstem, and so does the *pituitary gland,* which lies in the median plane at the base of the cranium about in a frontal plane through the joints of the jaw. The gland occupies its own small bony cup or *sella* beneath the brainstem.

Blood Vessels   The arteries and veins of the brain enter or leave the cranium through openings in the base of the skull. The chief arteries are the *internal carotid* on either side and the *vertebral arteries.* The internal carotids branch from the *common carotid arteries* in the neck. They enter the base of the skull after a winding course which brings them near the midline and anterior to the pituitary gland. The vertebral arteries enter with the spinal cord.

Some of the veins leave the cranium with the spinal cord, but most empty into the *internal jugular veins* which accompany the internal carotid and then the common carotid arteries deep in the neck.

Ear   The cranium in its inferior, lateral portion contains the small but complex cavities of the ear. These begin superficially as the *external auditory canal,* the outer portion of which is formed of cartilage or gristle. The inner part is bounded by bone and ends in the fibrous eardrum or *tympanic membrane.* Interior to this is an irregular bony cavity, the *middle ear.* At its medial, inferior portion, this narrows to form the opening of the *eustachian tube,* which provides a channel for air to enter the middle ear from high in the pharynx (see Figure 8-5).

The bone around the middle ear, especially below and behind it, is

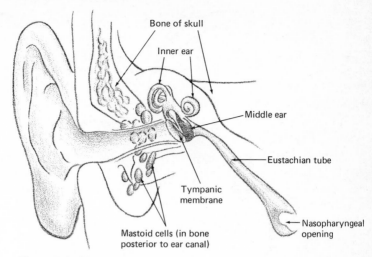

Figure 8-5 Right ear.

honeycombed with small, interconnecting, air-filled cavities. These are the *mastoid cells,* all of which communicate with the middle ear.

The middle ear contains a chain of three tiny bones, the outermost of which attaches to the tympanic membrane and the innermost of which connects to the *inner ear.* This inner ear lies in an interconnecting series of small cavities. One, coiled like a snail shell, is called the *cochlea* because of that. Three others are *semicircular canals.* The cochlear cavity contains the organ of hearing; the semicircular canals, together with a tiny cavity where they join, contain the organs of balance.

The middle and inner ear chambers are located largely superior and posterior to the tympanic membrane. Because of this, there is only a thin layer of bone between some of the cavities of the middle ear and the dura covering the brain.

Facial Skeleton   The skeleton of the face consists of many fused bones, including those of the anterior part of the base of the cranium. There is only one jointed, movable bone—the lower jaw or *mandible.* Several of the fused bones serve as landmarks, since they can be readily felt.

The rim of the eye socket or *orbit* forms a solid ring of bone (see Figure 8-6). Superiorly, the edge is the anterior inferior edge of the frontal part of the cranium. Above the orbit, this bone contains within its thickness the irregular and variable *frontal sinuses,* which open by a narrow *duct* or tube into the nasal cavity on either side (see Figure 5-5). These sinuses usually do not form until about age 9.

Laterally, the frontal parts of the cranium join the cheekbone, or *zygoma,* which forms most of the lateral and inferior rim of the orbit. The

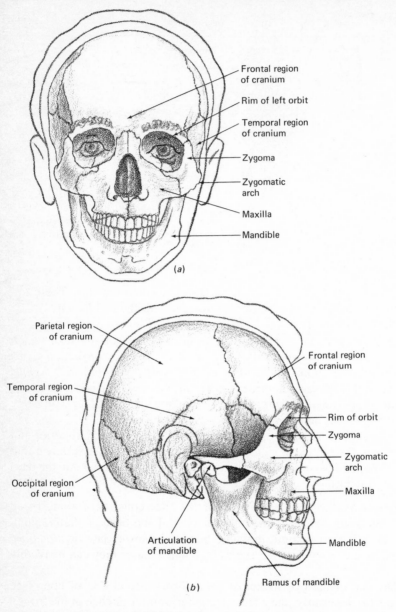

Frontal region
of cranium

Rim of left orbit

Temporal region
of cranium

Zygoma

Zygomatic
arch

Maxilla

Mandible

(a)

Parietal region
of cranium

Frontal region
of cranium

Temporal region
of cranium

Rim of orbit

Zygoma

Zygomatic
arch

Occipital region
of cranium

Maxilla

Articulation
of mandible

Mandible

(b)

Ramus of mandible

Figure 8-6 *(a)* Frontal and *(b)* lateral view of skull.

maxilla or upper jawbone completes the rim, meeting the frontal parts on either side of the nasal bridge.

The zygoma and part of the maxilla swing laterally, and the zygoma then angles posteriorly to join a process from the *temporal* part of the cranium. This forms an arch in front of the mandibular joint—the *zygomatic arch*—which stands out away from the more central facial bone.

The maxillary bones of the two sides fuse along the midline under the nose and along the *hard palate*. They form most of the bony rim of the nasal opening, the lateral walls and floor of the nasal cavity, and the front part of the bones below the eyes. Within each maxilla is the large *maxillary sinus,* which opens through the lateral wall of the nasal cavity (see Figure 5-5). This sinus is tiny at birth and grows as the face becomes larger, until it occupies much of the maxilla in the adult. The upper teeth grow from the horseshoe-shaped lowermost part of the maxilla.

The lower teeth grow from corresponding sockets in the mandible. The body of this bone is shaped like a deep horseshoe lying horizontally. At each posterior end the mandible bends sharply upward to form an almost upright *ramus.* The bend is the *angle of the jaw,* and the upper end of the broad ramus has an *anterior* and *posterior process.* The posterior process bears the knoblike head which fits into a socketlike cup on the base of the skull just anterior to the external auditory opening. This is the *hinge joint* of the jaw. The anterior process fits inside the zygomatic arch and provides a leverlike attachment for the temporal muscle, one of those that close the jaw.

The roof of the nasal cavity is formed by one of the bones—the *ethmoid*—which is part of the base of the cranium in the midline. The irregular ethmoid forms the bony part of the upper and middle nasal turbinates. It also contains air-filled *ethmoid sinuses* and is perforated from the cranial cavity to the nasal cavity by small holes. Through these the olfactory nerves (cranial nerve I) pass to carry the impulses of the sense of smell from the nasal mucous membrane to the brain.

The ethmoid is relatively weak; if it breaks, CSF can escape into the nose. A break can occur from a crushing blow to the nose, since the anterior-superior part of the nasal septum is a sheet of bone extending downward from the ethmoid. This plate can be pushed upward by the blow and so crack the ethmoid part of the cranium.

Facial Muscles, Blood Vessels, Nerves The bones of the face provide attachments for numerous muscles which move the skin in changing expressions, open the eyelids, move the eyes, and provide motions to the jaws, tongue, soft palate, fauces, and pharynx. Running among these muscles and through openings in the bones are the blood vessels and nerves of the face. Most of the arteries arise from the *external carotid artery,* and the veins empty into both *external* and *internal jugular veins.* The nerves of the face are the cranial nerves, especially I through

X, except that the auditory nerve (VIII) really stays within the cranium to reach the inner ear.

Eye The eye includes the deep bony *orbit* or socket, the *globe* or eyeball, the muscles which move the globe, the eyelids which cover it, and the *lacrimal* or tear *glands* which wash and lubricate it.

The *ocular globe* is a nearly perfect sphere of tough white *sclera* with a circular opening in front. This opening is covered by the bulging, transparent *cornea*. A smaller round opening behind admits the optic nerve (cranial nerve II), with a small artery and veins running in its center (see Figure 8-7). The sclera is lined by a thin black, pigmented layer, the *choroid coat,* which forms a thicker ring around the inside of the corneal opening. Part of this ring continues on into the corneal region as the *iris.* The more posterior part of the ring, hidden from outside view by the iris, is the muscular *ciliary body.*

Short, transparent fibers run from the inner edge of this ciliary body to the circumference of the *crystalline lens.* The diameter of this lens is a little smaller than that of the cornea but larger than that of the pupil at its widest. When the muscles in the ciliary body relax, pressure within the eyeball tenses the fibers to the lens. This—despite its name—is elastic and then flattens in the center, making it a weaker lens. When the ciliary muscles contract, they counteract the pressure within the eyeball by

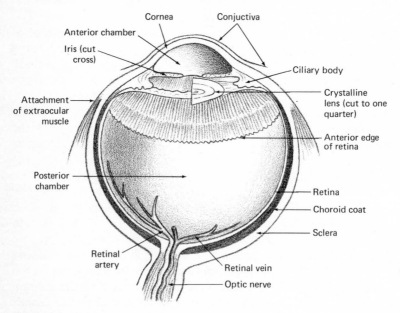

Figure 8-7 Ocular globe cut through optic disc.

pulling the choroid toward the lens, relaxing the fibers, and allowing the lens to bulge in the middle. Thus it becomes a more powerful magnifying lens.

The *retina,* a yellowish, thin membrane, lines the choroid from the optic nerve's ending—the optic disc—nearly to the ciliary body. The retina contains not only the tiny cells that sense light but also nerve cells and their fibers running into the optic nerve. Exactly opposite the pupil lies a small *macula,* with a shallow central pit which has a high concentration of visual cells.

The interior of the globe posterior to the lens and its circle of fibers is filled with a transparent, jellylike mass, the *vitreous humor.* The *anterior chamber* communicates freely with the larger *posterior chamber* through the fibers surrounding the lens.

Orbit   The globe rests in the orbit, surrounded by loose cushions of fat except in front. Six small muscles attach to the sclera and run from it to the walls of the orbit. These *extraocular muscles* move the globe within the orbit and are controlled by the oculomotor, trochlear, and abducent nerves (cranial nerves III, IV, and VI). The entire anterior surface of the globe is covered by a thin membrane, the *conjunctiva.* This is thrown into loose folds at the edge of the visible part of the globe so that it can move freely in any direction. Beyond the folds the conjunctiva continues as the lining of the eyelids.

The lacrimal gland lies within the orbit and above the conjunctiva at the superior, lateral part of the orbital rim (see Figure 8-8). Its short ducts, however, penetrate the conjunctiva there, so that the tears enter the conjunctival "sac"—which really is saclike only when the eyelids are

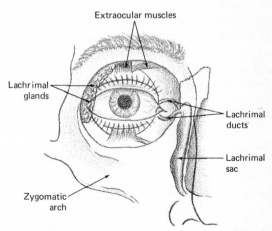

Figure 8-8   Right orbit and contents.

closed. The tears are moved, chiefly by blinking, into the inner corner of the eye, lubricating and washing the eye on the way. On the inner edge of both upper and lower lids near the nasal angle of the eye is a tiny but visible opening. These two openings are the start of ducts which drain the tears into a somewhat larger *tear sac* within the maxillary bone. The bottom end of this sac opens into the nasal cavity under the anterior end of the inferior turbinate.

Each eyelid contains a tough, flexible, flattened, but curved plate which stiffens it. Small muscles move these plates together or apart to close and open the eyes. The plates slip into the orbit when the eyes are wide open, the loosely fitted conjunctiva and skin folding back out of the way. The free edge of each lid is blunt with eyelashes along its outer part and small glands streaking away from its inner edge. These are visible as yellowish streaks against the red conjunctival background, especially on the inside of the upper lid.

Nose   The external nose is shaped in part by two small, thin, fused *nasal bones* jutting out like a small steep roof from the frontal part of the cranium (see Figure 8-6). They are rather short, and most of the nose is supported by a firm but flexible set of *cartilage* plates. The most anterior part of the nasal septum is also shaped by a cartilage plate which joins the bony septum posteriorly. Thick skin covers the outside of the nose, and its interior is part of the *nasal cavity.*

This cavity extends on each side from the nostril posteriorly to the *nasopharynx.* The posterior boundary of the cavity is a bony ridge which swings upward on either side at about the posterior edge of the hard palate. The nasal septum also ends at this depth.

The roof of the nasal cavity is about on a level with the nasal *bridge,* the indentation between the eyes that marks the superior limit of the external nose. The floor of the nose is about on a level with the posterior rim of the nares. At its widest point, near the floor, each nasal cavity extends laterally to about the full width of the hard palate. The cavity narrows considerably from below upward so that, seen from the front, the two sides and the floor almost form a triangle. The width of the cavity is further narrowed by two or three shelflike *turbinates* running along each side. The free edge of each turbinate curls more or less downward and laterally. Air makes its way along the floor below the lower turbinate, between the septum and the turbinates, or between the turbinates as they lie one above the other.

The mucous membrane lining the nasal cavity and covering all its walls contains many small blood vessels which can fill with blood to increase the membrane's thickness. Water easily leaves these vessels to form edema and further thicken the membranes. There are plentiful small glands throughout the membrane which can produce watery or mucous secretions in abundance. Because the air passages are narrow, swelling of the membranes or an excess of secretion can stop completely the flow of air through the nose.

Nasal Sinuses   Swollen nasal mucous membranes can also block some or all of the openings to the three sets of *paranasal sinuses:* the frontal, maxillary, and ethmoid sinuses. Another sinus, the *sphenoid,* is often grouped with the latter. It lies in the midline, above the naso-pharynx, but it opens into the posterior part of the nasal cavity.

Mouth   The mucous membrane of the mouth swells less obviously than that of the nose and, when the mandible is dropped open, the oral cavity greatly exceeds the size of the nasal cavity. The mouth is lubricated principally by saliva secreted from three pairs of *salivary glands.*

Salivary Glands   Each *parotid gland* lies external to the mandibular ramus and so is anterior to the external ear, extending from just below the level of the zygomatic arch to the angle of the jaw. Stensen's duct empties it into the oral cavity.

Each *submaxillary* gland is smaller and lies farther forward inside the lower edge of the mandible. It can be located by palpating for the pulse at the mandibular edge. The gland lies just anterior to the artery but medial to the bone. Its duct runs forward and medially to open beside the *frenulum* of the tongue.

The *sublingual glands* lie even more medially. Their anterior ends can be seen beneath the mucous membrane of the floor of the mouth. When the tip of the tongue is raised, the gland is visible as a pink ridge running on each side, converging toward the frenulum and the opening of the *submaxillary duct.* Usually the *sublingual duct* empties into the submaxil-lary duct near this opening (see Figure 2-3).

Tongue   The tongue itself is composed of complex bundles of muscles, some attaching to the mandible, some to other bones of the skull, and some to the small *hyoid bone* in the neck. The mucous membrane on the superior surface or *dorsum* continues posteriorly and inferiorly to form part of the anterior wall of the pharynx. Fine and broader papillae make a velvety surface over the body of the tongue, and a row of several much broader papillae appears far back on the surface. These papillae form a V-shaped row, the apex of the V being posterior. From there downward, the tongue is in the pharynx, and most of its surface is cobbled with the *lingual tonsil.*

On either side of the tongue the *fauces* or pillars and the lower edge of the *soft palate* with the *uvula* mark the posterior opening of the oral cavity into the pharynx. Contraction of muscles within the fauces and elevation of the posterior end of the tongue close off this opening (see Figure 2-4).

Pharynx   The pharynx really begins superior to the part seen through the oral cavity and ends below the visible level. The superior part is behind the nasal cavity, the inferior part ends in the esophagus at the level of the larynx.

The pharynx is a tube whose *posterior wall* is nearly vertical when the head is upright. This wall follows closely the anterior surface of the cervical vertebrae. The mucous membrane is separated from the spine only by a rather thin layer of muscle and the coverings of the vertebrae. The side walls are muscular and are closer together below than above, so that the pharynx looks somewhat funnel-shaped when seen from behind.

The *anterior pharyngeal wall* is much more varied and provides the landmarks that divide the pharynx into three segments, one above the other (see Figure 8-9). The *nasopharynx* begins at the base of the skull as a direct continuation of the nasal cavities. Below, it opens into the *oropharynx,* whose upper limit is marked by the elevated soft palate.

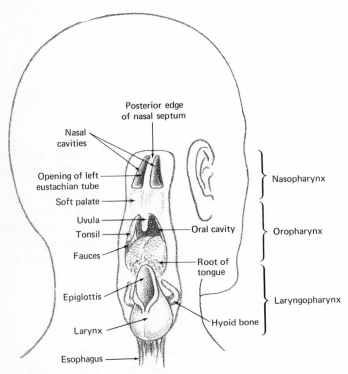

Figure 8-9   Pharynx from behind and from right posterior.

During swallowing, the soft palate swings up and backward and completely closes off the nasopharynx. The lowermost part, the *laryngopharynx,* begins at a level a little above that of the angle of the mandible and extends downward until it opens into the *larynx* anteriorly and continues as the *esophagus* posteriorly.

The anterior area of the nasopharynx is almost completely taken up by the nasal opening. The posterior wall is largely covered by the *adenoids* or *pharyngeal tonsils,* and the lower ends of the eustachian tubes from the middle ear open into the side walls. These openings lie about on a level with the lowest end of the cartilage in the external ear.

The anterior wall of the oropharynx is the posterior surface of the soft palate above and the lingual tonsil on the back of the tongue below. The opening of the oral cavity, with the fauces on either side, lies between the two.

The anterior wall of the laryngopharynx is more complicated. Much of it consists of the opening of the larynx. This opening slopes downward at an angle, so that its anterior edge lies above its sharp posterior lip. Rising above the anterior edge is a cartilage-stiffened lid—the *epiglottis*—which closes the open top of the larynx during swallowing. It sticks upright against the lingual tonsil during breathing. During swallowing, the tip swings downward and posteriorly to form a smooth slope over which food and water can slide into the esophagus. Below the laryngeal opening, the posterior surface of the larynx forms the anterior wall of the lowermost part of the laryngopharynx. The side walls of the pharynx stand away from the side walls of the larynx, so that there is a blind pouch on either side. The blind ends of the pouches mark the lower limits of the pharynx.

The *tonsillar tissue*—the tonsils of the fauces, the lingual tonsil, and the adenoids—forms an irregular ring around the pharynx. This tissue is related to that of lymph nodes, and similar tissue occurs in many small nodules over the posterior and lateral walls of the pharynx.

EXERCISES

1 Examine a skull and identify the cranium. Identify the frontal, parietal, temporal, and occipital regions, the ethmoid bone and the cuplike fossa for the pituitary gland (if the skull is opened), as well as the foramen magnum at the base. As you recognize them, palpate as much as possible of these bones on your own head or that of your partner (you cannot feel the ethmoid bone, of course). Identify the external auditory canal and the cup-shaped joint socket immediately anterior to it. While clenching and relaxing your jaw, feel the large temporal muscle on the side of the cranium. Can you identify where this attaches on the bones of the skull?

2 On the skull, identify first the region of the face and then find the zygomatic

bone and arch, the maxillary and nasal bones, and the mandible. Palpate these on yourself or your partner while orienting yourself on the skull. What bones form the rim of the orbit? Which edge forms the bony nasal orifice? Identify the nasal septum and bony turbinates as seen from in front and behind. If the skull is divided in the midline, identify the ethmoid bone and the sphenoid sinus below the pituitary fossa. Name the parts of the mandible and determine how it is joined to the cranium. How far back does the hard or bony palate extend? Can you visualize where the nasopharynx and oropharynx are with respect to the bones?

3   Examine x-rays of the skull—beginning with a lateral view and then a posteroanterior view. Identify the regions of the cranium and the facial bones you have studied. Note especially the sinuses. In the lateral film, can you recognize the pharynx? Try to identify its three regions.

Keep several things in mind when you examine x-ray films. They are negatives, so that the most dense structures appear lightest. You are looking *through* everything, including bone, so you see one thing superimposed upon another. The densest (and thus brightest) substance is bone, the next is flesh (muscles, glands, brain, and liquids), next is fat, and gas is the least dense (and darkest) of all.

4   If models or specimens are available, examine the nasal cavity and pharynx. Identify the structures you know and visualize their relations to what you can see with a nasal speculum and using a tongue blade. Could you reach the epiglottis with your finger? Could you reach a foreign body anywhere in the pharynx?

Neck   The neck begins above the base of the cranium posteriorly and on a horizontal plane with the angle of the jaw anteriorly. The lower boundary is the sternal notch and the superior edge of the clavicles anteriorly and the level of the lowest cervical vertebra posteriorly. This posterior point is marked by the prominent spinous process of the seventh cervical vertebra, which is higher than the sternal notch.

Cervical Skeleton   The column of seven *cervical vertebrae,* deep in the neck and reaching from the base of the skull to the first thoracic vertebra, are the only bones in the neck with one exception. The small, delicate *hyoid bone* is at the top of the neck anteriorly. It is shaped like a horseshoe opening posteriorly and is near the anterior surface of the neck almost within the rim of the mandible.

The first and second cervical vertebrae are not typical, but the lower ones are. Such a typical vertebra consists of an anterior cylindrical *body* which bears the weight of the parts above it (see Figure 8-10). Posteriorly, the *neural arch* of more slender bone attaches to it. This arch, with the posterior surface of the body, forms a ring. Stacked one atop the other, these rings provide the skeleton for the *vertebral canal,* in which the spinal cord runs vertically. At its most posterior point, the arch extends as the *spinous process,* the tip of which may be palpable beneath the skin.

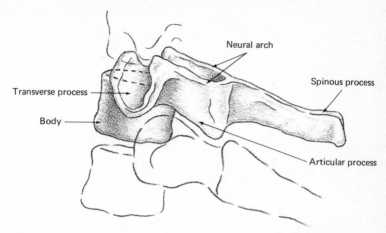

Figure 8-10 Sixth cervical vertebra from left side with articulations of fifth and seventh vertebrae.

This process points downward as well as posteriorly on vertebrae above the eleventh thoracic one. In all, the palpable tip of the spine lies somewhat below the body of its vertebra. From either side of the neural arch, a *transverse process* extends laterally except in the thoracic vertebrae, where they point more posteriorly and form one of the joints with the ribs. Each neural arch also has processes on either side pointing up and down. These *articular processes* meet the corresponding ones from the vertebrae above and below to form joints that enable the spine to bend. This is possible because the bony vertebral bodies are not in contact with the ones above or below. The tough but springy *intervertebral discs* separate them from one another.

The cervical spine is the most flexible part of the entire column and is surrounded, except on its anterior surface, by long and short muscles which move it and the head. Anteriorly, these muscles are more laterally placed and less densely packed (see Figure 8-11). This allows room for the respiratory tract, the esophagus, the thyroid gland, the carotid artery, the internal jugular, and several important cranial nerves.

Airway In the anterior region of the neck, beneath the skin, runs the middle part of the respiratory tract. The top of the *larynx* is inferior to the hyoid bone by a variable distance which depends on the position of the head. Its support is a cylinder of cartilage, four irregular pieces joined by tough membranes. One piece on either side is moved by small muscles; in moving, they relax or tighten the *vocal cords* within the larynx. These "cords" are really thin shelves of tissue protruding from each lateral wall on the interior of the larynx. They are relaxed and the posterior ends are swung apart during breathing. During speaking, these ends are moved

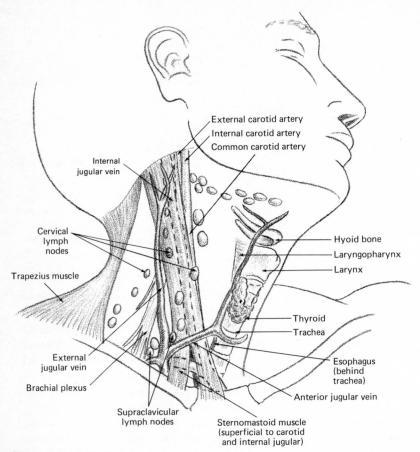

External carotid artery
Internal carotid artery
Common carotid artery

Internal
jugular vein

Cervical
lymph
nodes

Trapezius muscle

Hyoid bone
Laryngopharynx
Larynx

Thyroid
Trachea

External
jugular vein

Brachial plexus

Esophagus
(behind
trachea)

Anterior jugular vein

Supraclavicular
lymph nodes

Sternomastoid muscle
(superficial to carotid
and internal jugular)

Figure 8-11   Lateral and anterior regions of neck.

together, the edges of the shelves are tense, and air sets them vibrating as it comes up through the larynx.

The lower end of the larynx opens into the *trachea,* whose walls are formed of cartilaginous rings, one above the other. These rings may feel complete, but each has a posterior gap, so that the wall there is formed by a tough membrane which also joins the rings with one another. The topmost ring is similarly joined to the inferior edge of the larynx.

The thyroid gland lobes on either side of the inferior part of the larynx and the superior part of the trachea are joined across the trachea anteriorly. Usually this isthmus is only a thin strand of glandular tissue across the upper trachea.

Esophagus   Just posterior to the air-filled trachea and just anterior to the vertebral bodies, the upper part of the esophagus descends. This muscular tube is usually collapsed, flattened from front to back, when it is empty. The trachea and esophagus run downward together in the median plane to enter the superior portion of the thorax.

Blood Vessels The *common carotid artery* runs upward on either side close to the esophagus from thorax to pharynx, where it divides into its internal and external branches. The *internal jugular vein* accompanies the artery, lying lateral to it above and anterior to it below. Accompanying them is the long *vagus nerve* (cranial nerve X).

The muscular lateral region of the neck is roughly triangular, since the *sternomastoid* (also called the sternocleidomastoid) *muscle* forms its anterior boundary. Its posterior boundary is the edge of the large *trapezius muscle.* This edge becomes prominent when the muscle shrugs the shoulders. The large *external jugular vein* just beneath the skin angles backward and downward across the midportion of the sternomastoid. The smaller *anterior jugular vein* courses downward on the anterior surface of the neck and crosses the sternomastoid nearer its inferior attachment.

Lymph Nodes The chains of *cervical lymph nodes* chiefly follow the sternomastoid muscle, most of them lying deep to it but some superficial, especially along its posterior edge. Another important group lies rather deep behind the upper edge of the clavicle, just posterior to the attachment of the sternomastoid there. These lower nodes, like this entire region, are called *supraclavicular.*

Nerves The cervical portion of the spinal cord occupies the verte-bral canal of the cervical spine. Between the skull and the first cervical vertebra and between each vertebral junction below that, the cord gives off the *roots* of a *spinal nerve* on either side. There are thus eight cervical nerves on either side to form a complicated interchange, the *cervical plexus.* From this plexus come the large nerves of the arm. The plexus emerges from deep in the neck, posterior to the lower part of the sternomastoid muscle, and angles laterally and downward deep in the supraclavicular space toward the *axilla* or armpit.

EXERCISES

1   Examine x-rays of the neck in lateral and anteroposterior views. Identify the cervical vertebrae, hyoid bone, larynx, and trachea. If an esophagram is available, determine the position of the esophagus relative to the cervical spine, larynx, and trachea. Remember that the gullet lies flatter against the spine when it is empty.
2   Examine one of the lower cervical vertebrae (or another typical one). Orient it with respect to your own body and then identify the parts. If the adjacent vertebrae are available, determine how they articulate. When you palpate the carotid pulse, you press the artery against a cervical vertebra. Which part of it

are you pressing against? Can you palpate the spinous processes of the cervical vertebrae? If so, which ones?

3 Follow the entire course of the sternomastoid muscle, both anterior and posterior boundaries, on a subject. Is the anterior region of the neck wider superiorly or inferiorly? Follow the entire superior border of the trapezius muscle. Is the lateral region of the neck wider superiorly or inferiorly?

4 Determine the course of the carotid artery and the internal, external, and anterior jugular veins in a subject's neck. The internal jugular is neither visible nor palpable, but you should be able to visualize it. Where does the vagus nerve run in the neck?

8-2 THORAX AND SHOULDER GIRDLE

Skeleton   *Thoracic Boundaries*   The superior border of the *thorax* proper is a bony ring composed of the superior edges of sternum, first rib, and first thoracic vertebra, but of these only the sternum is palpable. The reason is, of course, that the bones and muscles of the shoulder are closely applied to the upper parts of the rib cage, so that the thorax usually is considered to include what lies below a tilted plane passing through the sternal notch and the last cervical spine as well as the lateral ends of the clavicles at the shoulder.

The inferior border of the thorax is the *diaphragm* and therefore movable. It usually lies at about the level of the tenth thoracic vertebra posteriorly and of the lower end of the sternal body anteriorly.

Shoulder Girdle   The bony *shoulder girdle* consists of the two *clavicles* and the two *scapulae* (see Figure 8-12). They join the thoracic skeleton only at the *sternoclavicular joints,* which are palpable just lateral to the sternal notch. The clavicle runs a slightly S-shaped course laterally to join the scapula above and anterior to the shoulder joint. It is palpable for its entire length.

The scapula is more complex and less completely palpable. Its triangular body is almost flat, with its anterior surface applied to the posterior wall of the rib cage over which it moves. About three-quarters of the way up from the lower pole a shelf of bone—the *scapular spine*—projects posteriorly. This spine continues laterally and superiorly free of the scapular body's surface to end in the blunt *acromion*—the tip of the shoulder. The acromion wraps around the lateral end of the clavicle, which forms a joint with its medial surface. Below the level of the acromion, the lateral edge of the scapular body broadens out to form the cuplike *glenoid cavity,* into which fits the head of the *humerus* or armbone. The body also gives rise, at the upper rim of the glenoid cavity, to the *coracoid* process, which arches anterior to the cavity. This process with the acromion and the lateral end of the clavicle then partially surround the shoulder joint.

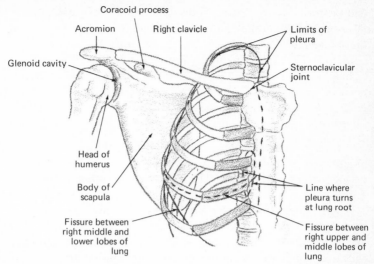

Coracoid process

Acromion   Right clavicle   Limits of pleura

Glenoid cavity   Sternoclavicular joint

Head of humerus

Body of scapula   Line where pleura turns at lung root

Fissure between right middle and lower lobes of lung   Fissure between right upper and middle lobes of lung

Figure 8-12   Right half of shoulder girdle with pleural margins in upper chest.

Most of the scapula lies beneath the heavy muscles of the shoulder girdle, which move it and the arm. The large *trapezius muscle* posteriorly attaches to the scapular spine and acromion as well as to the lateral part of the clavicle. These attachments are palpable, as are the spine and acromion. The tip of the coracoid process can also be felt anteriorly: the median border, lower pole, and lateral border of the scapula can be felt posteriorly.

Thoracic Cage   The ribs, the sternum, and the thoracic vertebrae make up the *thoracic cage.* All provide attachments for muscles which move the shoulder girdle and upper arm. On the anterior chest wall the *pectoralis major* muscle is easily felt as it arises from the inferior margin of the clavicle's medial half, the manubrium and body of the sternum, and part of the rib cage. It runs laterally to attach to the upper part of the humerus (see Figure 8-24).

Internally the thoracic cage with the diaphragm forms an almost conical space, with its base below. This, in turn, is subdivided into four spaces by the *pleura* and the *pericardium.* On either side is a *pleural space* containing a lung, medially the *mediastinum,* and within it the pericardial sac containing the heart.

Contents   *Pleural Spaces*   The pleural spaces extend upward as dome-shaped areas embraced by the first ribs (see Figure 8-12). In the anatomical position, the top reaches above the plane of the clavicles and almost to the level of the seventh vertebral spine. Anteriorly, laterally, and posteriorly, the spaces follow the inner surfaces of the rib cage and inferiorly of the dome-shaped diaphragm. Medially the boundary follows the bodies of the thoracic vertebrae posteriorly and then begins to approach the median plane as the mediastinum narrows anteriorly. The right pleural space continues forward beneath the sternal margin. The pericardium occupying the anterior inferior mediastinum pushes the medial border of the left pleural space outward from about the second intercostal space to the diaphragm.

Lungs   Since the lungs with their bronchi and vessels fill the entire pleural space, their boundaries are the same and their projections match on the surface of the chest. The lungs, however, are divided into lobes and their separations are projected onto the chest walls (see Figure 5-8).

The plane dividing the *left lower lobe* from the *left upper lobe* slopes from high posteriorly downward anteriorly. The line marking the boundary at the chest wall begins medially just below the level of the *second thoracic spine (T 2)* and runs laterally and downward to cross the midaxillary line at the *fourth intercostal space (ICS 4)*. It reaches the diaphragmatic level at ICS 6, well inside the midclavicular line. The left upper lobe then occupies most of the anterior as well as the superior part of the surface; the lower lobe lies under most of the posterior and inferior surface.

The upper boundary of the *right lower lobe* mirrors that on the left. The upper boundary of the *right middle lobe,* however, projects as an almost horizontal line leaving the upper lobe boundary at the midaxillary line. From this point in ICS 4, it more or less follows the anterior course of the right fourth rib to the sternum. It never projects onto the back at all.

Superior Mediastinum   The superior part of the mediastinum begins above as the trachea, esophagus, carotid arteries, and jugular veins passing behind the sternal notch. The trachea courses somewhat posteriorly as it continues downward, so that it lies in the midfrontal plane by the time it reaches the level of the *sternal angle.* Just below the angle, the trachea divides in the *right* and *left bronchi,* which continue laterally and inferiorly to enter each lung at its *hilum.* The level of this division or *bifurcation* is at the fourth thoracic spine posteriorly (see Figure 2-6).

The esophagus enters the mediastinum posterior to the trachea and remains between it and the vertebral bodies until the trachea divides. The large *descending aorta* then displaces the esophagus somewhat to the right and moves to a position between it and the vertebral bodies until they penetrate the diaphragm almost in the median plane.

In infants an organ called the *thymus* lies immediately behind the manubrium (see Figure 8-37). It somewhat resembles a lymph node and gradually shrinks until, in later childhood, it is very small. In adults a lobe of the *thyroid* may extend downward into the superior part of the mediastinum as a *retrosternal thyroid.*

Great Vessels   Much of the superior mediastinum is occupied by the great blood vessels (see Figure 8-13). The *internal jugular veins* run downward and are joined by the large veins from the arms—the *subclavian veins*—behind the medial ends of the clavicles. The subclavian veins have already received the external and anterior jugulars.

The body's *lymphatic system* also ends in the subclavian veins. The *right vein,* just as it joins the internal jugular, receives the thin-walled *lymphatic trunk,* into which have emptied the lymphatic vessels on the right side of the head and neck, the right arm, and some of those from the right side of the chest wall.

The *left* subclavian *vein* at its junction with the internal jugular is joined by the larger but still thin-walled *thoracic duct.* The lymph from the remainder of the body passes through this duct into the vein.

The vein formed by the juncture of each internal jugular and subclavian is the *anonymous vein.* The short right anonymous runs almost straight down, the longer left anonymous vein crosses obliquely downward through the anterior region of the mediastinum behind the manubrium. The two anonymous veins join to form the large *superior vena cava,* which opens into the superior part of the right atrium.

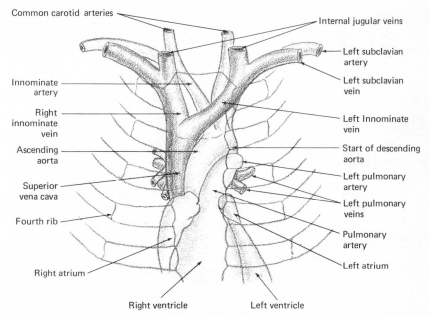

Figure 8-13   Great vessels of upper mediastinum.

The aorta arises from the left ventricle adjacent to the superior vena cava and slightly anterior to it. The *ascending aorta* lies almost exactly in the median plane up to about the level of the second ribs. Here it turns posteriorly and slightly to the left as it forms the *aortic arch.* This arch hooks over the left bronchus in the mediastinum and, turning downward, becomes the *descending thoracic aorta.* As such it continues downward behind the esophagus and just anterior to the vertebral body, penetrates the diaphragm, and enters the abdomen.

As the aorta begins to bend into the arch, it gives off a large branch, the *anonymous artery.* This runs upward and to the right where, behind the medial end of the clavicle, it divides into the *right common carotid,* running up in the neck, and the *right subclavian artery,* which supplies the right arm and shoulder.

Near the top of the aortic arch, the *left common carotid artery* leaves its superior surface, running upward and laterally until it reaches the medial end of the clavicle, where it turns upward. The *left subclavian artery* arises a little farther along the arch and runs upward and laterally to follow the line of the clavicle. All these aortic branches lie posterior to the great veins.

Besides these large vessels, the *thoracic aorta* has smaller branches. Just beyond the aortic valves at its origin, the ascending aorta gives off a *right* and a *left coronary artery* to supply blood to the myocardium (see Figure 8-14). The left coronary promptly divides into a *descending* and a *circumflex branch.* The former runs down the front of the heart in a groove, separating the left from the right ventricle. The right coronary and the circumflex arteries circle the base of the heart externally in the superficial depressions separating the atria from the ventricles.

Blood is drained from the myocardium by veins accompanying the arteries but running around the heart to its inferior surface. Here they form a pouchlike *sinus* lying in a deep superficial groove. This sinus empties into the right atrium.

The descending thoracic aorta supplies small arteries to the chest wall and thoracic organs. One pair of *bronchial arteries* runs into the lungs through the hila. They supply blood only to the bronchi and their branches and not to the alveoli, which receive blood from the pulmonary artery.

The large *pulmonary artery* arises to the left of the aorta, although it comes from the right ventricle. It runs upward and posteriorly to the left of the aorta until it reaches about the level of the tracheal bifurcation. Here, beneath the aortic arch, it branches sharply into the *right* and *left pulmonary arteries,* which accompany the bronchi into the hila of the lungs.

The *pulmonary veins* emerge from the hila, and two or more open directly into the left atrium. In doing so, they remain posterior to the superior vena cava, the aorta, and the pulmonary artery.

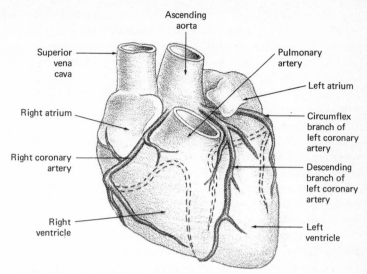

Figure 8-14   Coronary arteries seen from in front and above.

In the inferior posterior part of the mediastinum is the *inferior vena cava.* This large vein, draining blood from the entire lower part of the trunk and the legs, enters the chest through an opening in the right leaf of the diaphragm. This opening is slightly posterior to the midfrontal plane and about in the same sagittal plane as the medial end of the right clavicle. After it passes the diaphragm, the vein curves somewhat anteriorly and medially to enter the right atrium from below (see Figures 8-18 and 8-20).

Lymphatic System   The mediastinum contains, besides the structures mentioned above, numerous *lymph nodes* and *lymphatic vessels* as well as *nerves.* The lymph nodes form an especially prominent group at the hilum of each lung.

In the posterior part of the mediastinum runs the *thoracic duct,* the major lymphatic vessel of the body. It enters the thorax from below, where the aorta penetrates the diaphragm. The duct continues upward along the right side of the descending aorta to the arch. Above, it inclines to the left and accompanies the esophagus into the neck, where it turns farther to the left and slightly downward to join the subclavian vein at its union with the internal jugular.

Along its course it receives the lymphatic vessels of the thorax and, above the clavicles, those from the left side of the head and neck, the left arm, and the left chest wall. Before entering the thorax, it has drained lymph from all of the lower body.

Despite its extensive connections, the thoracic duct is inconspicuous, thin-walled, and takes up little space in the mediastinum. The greatest part is occupied by the heart within the pericardial sac.

Heart   The heart lies upon the diaphragm when a person stands, and much of its anterior surface is in contact with the lower half of the sternal body. More of its anterior surface is thrown into contact with the chest wall as the ventricles' contractions rotate them forward during systole.

When projected onto the anterior chest wall, the lateral wall of the *left ventricle* forms almost the entire left border of the heart (see Figure 5-10). The *aorta* arises behind the sternum at about the level of the third rib. The *right ventricle* extends as a band, broader below, obliquely across the heart. Its right margin approaches the angle of the heart with the diaphragm, but it does not make up any part of the right heart border as seen from the front. Its oblique course upward ends with the origin of the *pulmonary artery* at about the left sternal margin in ICS 2. Just below that point, the right ventricle makes up a fifth to a quarter of the left cardiac border at its superior end.

The left ventricle then lies to the left of and behind the right ventricle. Blood leaves the left ventricle by passing upward and to the right. It leaves the right ventricle by passing upward and to the left.

The *right atrium* makes up the lower part of the right cardiac border. The superior part of the border of dullness above the third rib is formed by the superior vena cava. The right atrium also lies posterior as well as lateral to the right ventricle.

The *left atrium* cannot be seen from in front. It lies superior and largely medial to the right atrium and superior and posterior to the left ventricle, centered behind the origin of the aorta.

Spinal Cord   The *spinal cord* runs, of course, posterior to the vertebral bodies in the vertebral canal (see Figure 8-15). The neural arches forming the skeleton of this canal have notches on their superior and inferior surfaces near the body. When one vertebra rests atop another, the notches match and form a hole through which nerves can enter or leave the canal. As the spine bends or rotates, these holes remain open.

The spinal cord itself is flexible and fairly tough, as are the nerves, so that they bend easily with the bones. The cord is further protected by tough dura mater, finer membranes, and the cerebrospinal fluid surrounding it.

In the adult, the spinal cord is not so long as the vertebral column and its canal. The cord extends through the cervical and thoracic regions but, at the level of the first or second lumbar vertebra, it tapers down to a threadlike *terminal filament* that extends to the coccyx. This filament serves as an anchor and is not nerve tissue at all.

In fetal life, the spinal cord runs the entire length of the vertebral canal, and in infancy it extends down as low as the fourth lumbar vertebra. One result of this relative shortening of the spinal cord is that the nerve roots arising from it have to travel downward to reach the intervertebral levels at which they exit from the spine. The vertebral canal of the lumbar spine is chiefly occupied by such descending roots, in the middle of which runs the terminal filament.

Nerve Roots The spinal cord is said to be *segmental*, built up of similar areas one atop the other. Each segment of the cord gives off two pairs of symmetrical *nerve roots*. On each side is an *anterior* or *ventral root* which contains only *motor nerve fibers* and a *posterior* or *dorsal root* of *sensory fibers*. Each posterior root has a *ganglion*, a collection of nerve cells outside the central nervous system (see Figures 9-8 and 9-9).

Spinal Nerves Peripheral to this sensory ganglion, the anterior and posterior roots unite to form the *spinal nerve,* which thus contains both sensory and motor fibers. Soon after it leaves the vertebral column, each nerve gives off a *posterior branch* going to the back. The *anterior branch,* which is much larger except in the three first cervical nerves, remains independent of the ones above or below in the thoracic nerves. In the cervical, lumbar, and sacral nerves they have numerous cross connections with the nerves above and below. These cross-connected nerves form the *cervical, brachial,* and the *lumbosacral plexuses.*

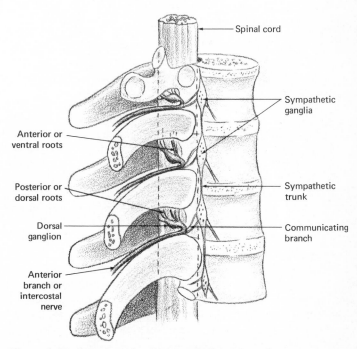

Figure 8-15 Spinal cord and nerves in thoracic region.

Autonomic Nervous System   Whether or not it forms a plexus, each anterior branch gives off one or two *communicating branches* which run anteriorly to a *sympathetic ganglion.* This ganglion is part of the autonomic nervous system and in the thorax lies near the junction of rib and spine on each side but within the rib cage. Each ganglion is connected to the ones above and below by a *sympathetic trunk.* From the ganglia arise nerves going to the blood vessels and organs within the thorax.

The other part of the autonomic system, the *parasympathetic,* arrives in the thorax chiefly through branches of the *vagus nerves.* Some parasympathetic fibers come, however, from the spinal cord, accompanying the sympathetic nerves.

EXERCISES

1   Identify on a skeleton the bones of the shoulder girdle and the parts of the scapula. Pay particular attention to the clavicular joints. Palpate on a subject as much as you can of shoulder girdle, positioning the arm to give you access to as much as possible of the bones.

2   Palpate the limits of the trapezius muscle and of the pectoralis major.

3   Examine the bones of the thoracic cage. Identify each vertebra and rib by number. Note especially the joints of the ribs to the vertebra and their attachments to the sternum. Does the chest cage have the same anteroposterior diameter in each sagittal plane? Where is the AP diameter greatest? Identify the location of the great vessels, the heart, and the lung hilum on the skeleton and then on a subject. Remember that this must be in three dimensions.

4   On a subject, percuss and mark the diaphragmatic levels and the cardiac dullness. Then mark the projected boundaries of the lobes of the lung. What lobe borders the cardiac dullness in each intercostal space on either side?

5   Examine first a PA x-ray film of the chest and then a lateral view. If possible have available a set of contrast angiocardiograms and an esophagram. Identify as many as possible of the structures of shoulder girdle and thorax. Relate these to the structures on the skeleton and in the living subject.

If available, study a model or dissection of the thorax and its contents, relating these to their position in the x-ray and in the living subject.

6   Examine a model or dissection of the thoracic spinal cord, its roots, sensory ganglia, and nerves. If available, study the arrangement of the segmented thoracic sympathetic chains and identify the parts.

8-3 ABDOMEN AND PELVIS

Walls   *Diaphragm*   The *diaphragm,* forming the upper boundary of the abdomen and the floor of the chest, is a broad, kidney-shaped dome dividing the trunk in half (see Figures 8-16 and 8-18). Its central portion is a sheet of tough tendon from which the muscular portion radiates peripherally to its attachments or *origin.* This origin begins anteriorly from the posterior surface of the xiphoid process. On either side it continues around the chest wall, involving in turn ribs seven through twelve. Posteriorly the origin follows the twelfth rib until it reaches the anterior surface of the lumbar vertebral bodies.

This attachment projects on the body surface well below the level of diaphragmatic dullness at full inspiration, especially posteriorly. The reason is that posteriorly and laterally the diaphragm runs sharply upward to form the high domes, and as it descends in full inspiration, it can never pull the dome completely down to the level of the origin. The upper abdominal organs, then, are located within the lower portions of the rib cage.

Abdominal Walls   The forward curve of the five large lumbar vertebral bodies gives the diaphragm its kidney shape and below the diaphragm partially divides the abdominal cavity into right and left halves. The posterior, lateral, and anterior abdominal walls between ribs and pelvis are formed of muscular sheets and thicker straplike muscles

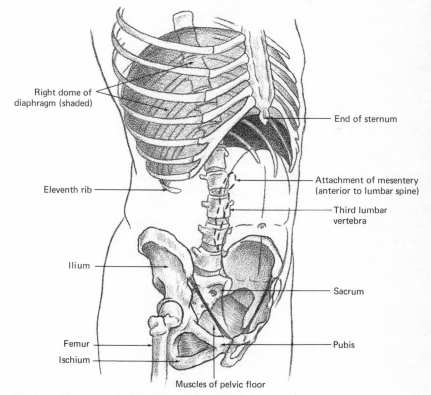

Figure 8-16   Walls of abdomen.

except where the transverse processes of the lumbar spine extend laterally. Internally the posterior wall, divided by the spine, bows posteriorly on each side, forming a depression called the *gutter.*

Large strap muscles run along the spine on either side internally and externally and, with some long muscles running up from the legs internally, give the back a rather thick muscular wall. The broad, medial, straplike *rectus abdominis* muscle thickens the anterior wall where it runs from the xiphoid sternum and lower ribs down to the pelvis. Three much thinner muscular layers form the lateral wall as well as the more lateral parts of the anterior and posterior walls.

Pelvic Skeleton   The pelvis and sacrum contain the lower part of the abdomen. The *sacrum* forms from five or six vertebrae which fuse together into a broad bone on which the fifth lumbar vertebra rests. It curves backward and then forward so that it is concave anteriorly. At its lower end, a chain of four or five small fused vertebrae, called the *coccyx,* continues the forward curve of the sacrum (see Figure 8-16).

On either side the sacrum has an irregular joint surface formed by the fused transverse processes of its two upper vertebrae. These lateral surfaces make an immovable joint with the pelvis.

The pelvis has two symmetrical halves, each half formed from three fused bones—the *ilium, ischium,* and *pubis.* Together with the sacrum, they form a large open-bottomed bowl to the sides of which the *femurs* or thighbones are jointed.

Each joint includes a cuplike structure, the *acetabulum,* on the lateral surface of the pelvis. The three pelvic bones fuse into a single structure at that point.

Above and posterior to the acetabulum, the ilium rises and flares laterally. Posteriorly it joins the sacrum. The superior rim of this ilium, palpable as the "hipbone," is the *iliac crest.* Its anterior end is the blunt *anterior superior iliac spine.*

Below the acetabulum, the ischium turns downward and then forward to meet the pubis. At its posterior inferior extremity, just where it turns forward, the ischium broadens into the *ischial tuberosity.* The tuberosity on either side bears the body's weight when a person sits. It is readily palpable, especially in the sitting position.

Anterior to the acetabulum, the pubis extends anteriorly and medially, then turns downward to fuse with the forward end of the ischium. In effect, the fused pubis and ischium form an irregular ring of bone anterior to and below the acetabulum. The most medial part of the pubis reaches almost to the midline and there forms a firm, immovable, but not fused joint—the *pubic symphysis*—with the pubis of the opposite side. This bone is palpable above the genitalia.

The sacrum and pelvis seen from above and in front form a broad ring of bone. Through this ring the baby is born. The inferior opening and the entire ring are larger in the female pelvis than in the male. Seen from the side, the sacrum and pelvis are somewhat funnel-shaped internally. This funnel is wider and slightly shorter in women than in men (see Figure 8-17).

The sacrum and the pelvis are bound together by tough *ligaments,* and the cordlike *inguinal ligament* runs from the iliac spine to the pubic bone near its medial end. Except for the passages of the urethra, vagina, and rectum, the lower opening of the pelvis is closed by muscular sheets which make up the *pelvic floor.* Large muscles of the back and thigh also attach to the interior of the pelvis chiefly along the sides. The external surfaces also provide attachments for muscles of the legs, back, and buttocks.

Contents   *Stomach*   The greatest part of the abdominal cavity is occupied by organs of the *digestive tract*—the stomach, intestines, liver,

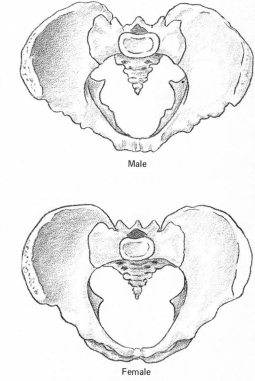

Male

Female

Figure 8-17   Male and female pelvis seen from above.

and pancreas. The esophagus passes the diaphragm almost in the median and midfrontal planes. It bends sharply to the left and almost immediately opens into the stomach at the valvelike *cardia* (see Figure 8-18).

The stomach is a pliable sac with muscular walls and so assumes different positions and shapes depending upon its contents and the body posture. Generally speaking, it is somewhat J-shaped but larger at the superior end or *fundus*. This end bulges above the cardia and occupies most of the left dome of the diaphragm, lying to the left of the cardia.

From its fundus the stomach curves downward, somewhat anteriorly and to the right, where it turns upward to end at the *pyloric valve.* This valve, a thick circular ring, marks the start of the small intestine, the segment called the *duodenum.* The stomach narrows as it approaches the pylorus, and the part immediately before the valve is called the *pyloric region.*

Duodenum   The *duodenum* turns posteriorly and somewhat to the right as it leaves the pylorus. It sweeps downward, then to the left and up, forming a loop and ending in the *jejunal segment* of the small intestine. Most of this loop is firmly fixed to the posterior abdominal wall, the start of the descending limb of the loop lying to the right of the first lumbar vertebral body. The downward sweep carries it to the level of the third lumbar vertebral body which it crosses, and then it ascends to end to the left of the second lumbar vertebral body. At its most inferior point, where

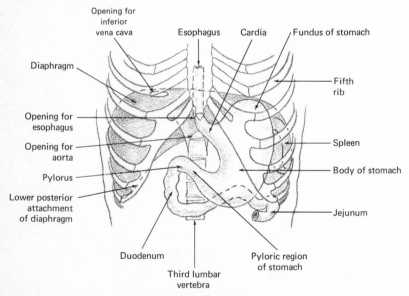

Figure 8-18   Upper abdominal organs and diaphragm.

it crosses the vertebra, it is about in the transverse plane through the lowest part of the tenth rib. The duodenum is the only part of the small intestine fixed in one position; all other parts can move about to a considerable degree.

Liver and Gallbladder This immobility may be related to the entrance of ducts from the two largest digestive glands about halfway down the descending duodenal segment. The *liver,* by far the largest gland in the body, is connected to the intestine directly only by its *bile duct* (see Figure 8-19).

The liver occupies the entire dome of the right half of the diaphragm and extends across the upper abdomen beneath the heart anteriorly. Its anterior inferior edge slopes from the left downward to about the level of the eighth rib laterally on the right. The superior surface curves upward as it follows the diaphragm. The inferior surface also curves upward.

On this inferior surface, just to the medial side of the midclavicular line, the *gallbladder* lies in a groove. It extends from just beyond the anterior edge of the liver back about halfway below the lower surface. It is a thin-walled blind sac whose only opening is near its posterior end, where the *cystic duct* enters. This cystic duct runs from the gallbladder toward the left to form one member of a three-way junction. Running anteriorly from this junction is the *hepatic duct,* which breaks up and enters the substance of the liver. The posterior member of the junction is the *common bile duct.* It bends downward behind the highest part of the duodenum and continues down the posterior surface to its opening into the intestine.

The liver forms green bile, which it empties into tiny branches of the hepatic duct. These branches unite until they leave the liver. At the junction with the other two ducts, the bile may continue down the common duct and enter the intestine. There is, however, a muscular valve around the lower end of the common duct. This is contracted and closed most of the time, and the bile can leave the junction only by way of the cystic duct. From the cystic duct it enters the gallbladder, where it is stored. During active digestion, the common duct's valve opens and the muscular wall of the gallbladder contracts, forcing its contents back out through the cystic duct to flow down the common duct.

Hepatic Blood Vessels Blood enters the liver through its inferior surface near the junction of the ducts. Some blood arrives through the *hepatic artery,* but most reaches the liver through the *hepatic portal vein.* This vein is unusual since the blood in it does not go directly to the right atrium. The hepatic portal vein arises in the capillaries of the intestines, spleen, and pancreas. Blood there is collected in larger and larger veins

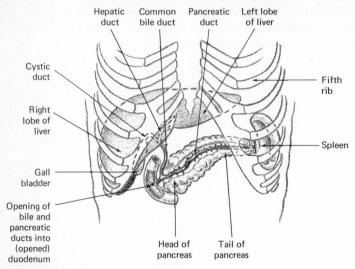

Hepatic   Common   Pancreatic   Left lobe
duct   bile duct duct   of liver

Cystic
duct
                                                  Fifth
                                                  rib

Right
lobe of
liver
                                                  Spleen

Gall
bladder

Opening of
bile and
pancreatic
ducts into   Head of   Tail of
(opened)   pancreas   pancreas
duodenum

Figure 8-19   Upper abdominal organs.

until it enters the liver. Here the hepatic portal vein again divides repeatedly until it forms a second set of capillaries.

Blood in the liver, whether from the hepatic artery or the hepatic portal vein, is collected by the *hepatic veins.* These empty into the *inferior vena cava* just below the diaphragm, often within the substance of the liver. This is possible because the inferior vena cava coming from the lower abdomen passes the posterior edge of the liver in a groove or is completely surrounded by liver just below the diaphragm.

Pancreas and Spleen   The *pancreas,* the second largest digestive gland, is more closely associated with the duodenum (see Figure 8-19). The gland lies transversely across the posterior wall of the abdomen about on a level with the first lumbar vertebral body. Its broader part, called the *head,* nestles within the duodenal loop. From this head, the narrower *tail* of the pancreas stretches out to the left about as far as the midclavicular plane.

The *pancreatic ducts* run within the gland from the tip of the tail through the head. They empty into the duodenum either through a single opening very close to that of the common bile duct or through the same opening as the bile duct.

The *spleen* is not a digestive organ but is closely associated anatomically with the pancreas and stomach. Rather bean-shaped, the spleen has a rounded superior and lateral surface which fits up under the diaphragm in the left superior, posterior corner of the abdominal cavity. The indented right surface accommodates the left kidney medially and the stomach more anteriorly. The tip of the pancreatic tail touches the spleen, and the splenic vein runs toward the right along the superior edge of the gland, receiving smaller veins from it. This splenic vein forms part of the hepatic portal system.

Jejunum, Ileum, Mesentery, and Peritoneum The *jejunum* begins at the duodenum's end and continues into the *ileum*. These two parts of the small intestine coil irregularly in the abdominal cavity, the jejunum tending to be in the left upper quadrant and the ileum terminating in the right lower quadrant. With the duodenum, they form a hollow muscular tube some 22 ft long. Unlike the fixed duodenum, the jejunum and ileum are anchored only by a wide, thin double membrane—the *mesentery*—attached along one edge of the tube. This membrane ends posteriorly along the anterior surface of the vertebral bodies, which are much shorter than the intestine (see Figure 8-16). The mesentery is, therefore, fan-shaped.

The mesentery is formed by the *peritoneum* lining the abdominal cavity when it turns inward from right to left as the double membrane. The peritoneum then continues around the intestine to cover its surface. Through the mesentery run the large branches of the aorta on their way to the intestine and the branches of the hepatic portal vein coming from it. Nerves to and from the intestine as well as lymphatic vessels also course through it (see Figure 10-3).

The duodenum, lying against the posterior abdominal wall, is covered by peritoneum with no mesentery. The reflections of the peritoneum over the freely movable stomach are more complex, and from the organ's lateral and inferior surfaces hangs an apron of double membrane—the *omentum*. This contains more or less fat and is the most anterior structure within the abdominal cavity, lying against the anterior wall.

Large Intestine The ileum ends in a valve which opens into the *colon* or large intestine (see Figure 8-20). The first part of the colon lies against the right lateral and posterior abdominal wall. It extends downward as a short, wide, blind pouch—the *cecum*—below the entrance of the ileum. At its blind end is a second, much smaller blind tube, the *appendix*. Above the valve, the intestine climbs as the *ascending colon* into the right upper quadrant. There, deep behind the liver, it bends rather sharply forward, to the left and somewhat downward. This bend is the *hepatic flexure.*

Past the hepatic flexure the *transverse colon* runs across the abdomen to the left. It has a membranous *mesocolon* and so is movable. It lies anteriorly for most of its length, with only the omentum between it and the abdominal wall. Often it swings downward well below the umbilicus before rising and turning posteriorly to the region of the spleen, which it touches. Here, at the *splenic flexure,* it turns sharply downward.

The *descending colon* follows the left lateral and posterior wall

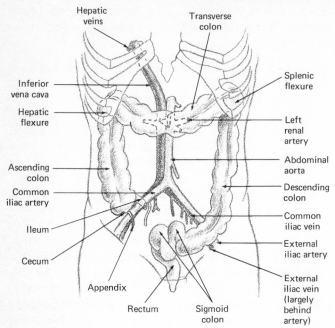

Figure 8-20 Large intestine and great vessels of abdomen. Hepatic portal vein not shown.

downward below the iliac crest, where it turns medially and becomes the *sigmoid colon.* The sigmoid has a mesocolon, and so its position varies. Usually it is somewhat S-shaped as it curves to the median plane just anterior to the sacrum. There, it turns sharply downward to become the *rectum.*

The entire colon has a much greater diameter than the small intestine. Its muscular wall is not much thicker, however, and forms a series of rounded outpocketings that make it look rather coarsely puckered.

Abdominal Blood Vessels   The *descending aorta* comes through the diaphragm just in front of the vertebral bodies and remains there as the *abdominal aorta* until it reaches the lower margin of the fourth lumbar vertebra (see Figures 8-20 and 8-21). Just after it enters the abdomen, it gives off the first of three large arteries that go to the organs of the digestive system. The lower two of these arteries run anteriorly in the mesentery to the small intestine. On either side, at the level of the first lumbar vertebral body, the short *renal arteries* go straight laterally to the kidneys. Other smaller arteries leave the aorta going to the abdominal wall and to the other organs.

The aorta divides like an inverted Y to form two *common iliac arteries* at the level of the fourth vertebral body. This is about at the level of the iliac crests. A little below this point, each common iliac gives off a large posterior branch, the *internal iliac artery,* which supplies most of the posterior muscles of the pelvic region and the pelvic viscera. It then continues downward, laterally, and forward to become the *external iliac artery.* As this passes the inguinal ligament to enter the leg, it becomes the *femoral artery.*

The *femoral vein* lying medial to the artery becomes the *internal iliac vein* and accompanies the artery of the same name. It receives branches from the pelvic region and becomes the *common iliac vein* until it unites with the corresponding vein of the opposite side. This occurs just below and to the right of the aorta's division. The *inferior vena cava* so formed courses upward to the right of the aorta, receiving *renal veins* on the way. Although it drains the pelvic organs and the abdominal wall, it does not receive any large branches from the digestive organs until the *hepatic veins* enter just below the diaphragm.

Lymphatic Systems The abdomen contains many lymph nodes associated with almost every organ. The lymphatic vessels from these nodes and those from the legs reach the large blood vessels and follow them to and up the aorta. Numerous lymph nodes lie along these chains, close to the aorta and posterior vena cava.

About the level of the kidneys, lymphatic vessels converge to form the single *thoracic duct.* This duct then accompanies the aorta upward through the diaphragm.

Autonomic Nervous System The autonomic nervous system in the abdomen is more complicated than in the thorax. The segmented sympathetic ganglia connected by the sympathetic trunk continue down to the coccyx, lying on the lateral surfaces of the lumbar spinal and sacral bodies. As in the thorax, they receive communicating branches from the spinal nerves and send branches to the viscera. The parasympathetic supply reaches the upper organs by way of the vagus nerves, which accompany the esophagus through the diaphragm. The pelvic organs receive their parasympathetic fibers through the sacral spinal nerves and their communicating branches.

What makes the autonomic system more complicated is the presence of autonomic plexuses and ganglia closely associated with the organs, in the mesentery, and about the great vessels. Associated with these plexuses are numerous ganglia of the parasympathetic system, the whole supplying autonomic nerves to control visceral function and to transmit visceral sensations.

Spinal Nerves The *lumbosacral plexus* is formed by the anterior branches of the spinal nerves from the twelfth thoracic through the third sacral. It is part of the peripheral rather than the autonomic nervous system and supplies nerves to the pelvic region and the legs. Above, it lies among the internal muscles of the back, and lower down, it is interior to the muscles lining the pelvis where it joins the sacrum. Nerves from the plexus leave the interior of the pelvis by several paths. The largest, the *sciatic nerve,* leaves posterior to the acetabulum. Here it enters the posterior part of the thigh (see Figure 8-32).

Kidneys   The *kidneys* lie in the gutters on either side of the vertebral bodies (see Figure 8-21). They, like the great vessels and lymph nodes, are behind the peritoneum or are *retroperitoneal.* The higher left kidney has its upper *pole* about on the level of the eleventh thoracic spinous process and its lower pole about the level of the third lumbar process. The right kidney's upper and lower poles are about one spinous process lower. Both extend below the costal margin. On the superior, medial part of each kidney's upper pole is the small, roughly triangular *adrenal gland.* It is not connected with the kidney and, being an *endocrine* gland, has no duct.

On the medial surface of each smooth, bean-shaped kidney there is a puckered indentation, the *hilus.* Through this the renal artery enters and the renal vein leaves. The duct which carries urine from the kidney also emerges at the hilus. It is a downward-directed, thin-walled funnel which narrows to form the *ureter.*

Ureters   The urinary bladder, with its thick muscular wall, lies collapsed behind the pubic bone when empty. When full, its dome rises

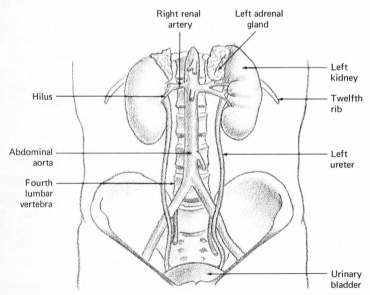

Figure 8-21   Urinary organs.

above that level and its wall extends farther laterally and posteriorly. The *ureters* enter through its posterior wall well above the lowest point and on either side of the median plane (see Figure 8-23).

At its lowest point the bladder narrows to form the upper end of the *urethra*. A ringlike muscular valve or *sphincter* contracts around the urethral neck to keep it closed except during urination, when the sphincter relaxes and the bladder wall contracts.

Urethra In the woman, the short urethra passes behind the pubis downward and forward to open through the meatus in the vulva (see Figure 2-18). Just inside the meatus, several small urethral glands open onto the posterior walls.

In the man, the urethra is much longer, passing downward, then forward and downward again, in an S-shaped curve (see Figure 2-15). It traverses the penis in its ventral part to reach the meatus in the glans. The initial descending portion of the male urethra is surrounded by the *prostate gland* (see Figures 2-18 and 8-23).

Scrotal Contents Each *testis* in the *scrotum* has a tough capsule which is penetrated by several small tubules or ducts near its upper pole. These short tubules collect sperm formed in the testis and unite to form the *epididymis,* a larger coiled duct. The epididymis runs laterally and posteriorly over the surface of the testis from its upper to its lower pole. There, it turns abruptly upward as the *vas deferens,* the smooth tube carrying the sperm to the prostate (see Figure 8-22).

Vas Deferens To reach the abdomen the vas travels in the *spermatic cord,* which also contains the artery and the tortuous veins of the testis. A sheath surrounds these structures in the scrotum and in turn is surrounded by a loose network of muscle which can retract the testis upward.

The spermatic cord enters the medial end of the *inguinal canal* above the inguinal ligament, and its contents traverse this canal laterally, upward and inward to the pelvic cavity. Here the vas turns downward, backward, and toward the median plane (see Figure 8-23). It crosses the iliac vessels and the ureter as it follows the lateral and posterior walls of the bladder. On the posterior wall, it turns sharply downward as it approaches the median plane, so that it almost touches the vas from the opposite side as they enter the superior part of the prostate.

Seminal Vesicles and Prostate A coiled blind sac, the seminal vesicle, lies lateral to each vas on the posterior wall of the bladder. This vesicle empties into the vas as it enters the prostate. Each vas continues through the prostate to enter the urethra on its posterior wall. The prostate completely surrounds the first, descending portion of the urethra,

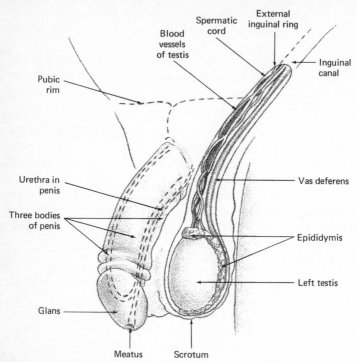

Figure 8-22 Male external genitals with left scrotal contents.

and its many small ducts empty into that tube. Both seminal vesicles and prostate are glands whose secretion, together with *sperm* arriving from the vas deferens, form the *ejaculate* during the male orgasm.

Female Pelvic Organs In the woman, the internal sex organs lie posterior and superior to the urethra and bladder (see Figure 2-18). The ureter as it descends passes beneath the ovary and lateral to the uterus on its way to the bladder.

The roomier lower female pelvis allows an extension of the peritoneal cavity to continue downward posterior to the uterus. This may contain a few loops of small bowel, or the uterine fundus may bend backward into it rather than forward over the bladder. Such a *retroflexed uterus* is a normal variation.

Rectum The most posterior pelvic organ in both men and women is the *rectum.* From its upper junction with the sigmoid colon, it runs downward in the midline—following the curvature of the sacrum and coccyx—until it turns posteriorly just above the anus. Its anterior wall in the man is in contact with the urinary bladder, the vasa deferentia, the seminal vesicles, and the prostate. In the woman, the anterior wall is

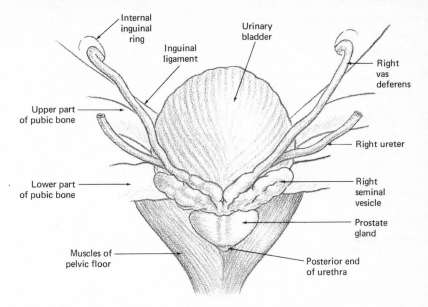

Figure 8-23   Urinary bladder and male internal sexual organs, seen from behind.

adjacent to the peritoneal pouch and its contents above, with the uterus and vagina below.

EXERCISES

1   On a model or dissection, examine the diaphragm, noting its shape, composition, and the positions of the three openings. Name the passengers through each opening. Note also its attachments and relation to the abdominal viscera. Which viscera would you expect to descend when the diaphragm contracts? Locate the diaphragmatic attachments on your partner or subject.

2   Examine the lumbar spine on a skeleton, noting the relative transverse plane of each vertebral body and its spinous process. Note also the curve followed by the anterior surfaces of the vertebral bodies and the angle at which the lowest vertebra joins the sacrum.

3   Examine the sacrum, pelvis, and coccyx of a skeleton. Is it male or female? How do the sexes differ in pelvic structure? Palpate on your partner the lumbar spine, sacrum, coccyx, iliac crest and anterior spine, and the ischial tuberosities and pubic bone. Can you detect the pubic symphysis?

4   Identify in AP and lateral x-rays the various bones of the lumbar and pelvic regions. What occupies the acetabulum?

5   In a model or dissection, study the arrangement of the muscles of the abdominal wall, the back, and the pelvis, including the pelvic floor and inguinal canal. Identify and describe the rectus abdominis. In late pregnancy, the enlarged uterus separates the two halves of the rectus in the median line. Would this tear the muscle itself?

6 In a model or dissection, examine each of the abdominal viscera. Note shape, color, blood supply, and the position of each. Which are hollow and contain some air or gas? Which contain fluid? Note carefully the position of each organ in relation to the anatomical landmarks on the body's surface.

7 If available, examine x-ray films of the stomach and small intestine, the rectum and colon, the gallbladder, the kidneys and ureters. Locate these dye-filled organs with respect to the skeleton.

8 Using a ballpoint pen or wax pencil, mark the location on your partner of the liver, gallbladder, stomach, spleen, pancreas, duodenum, colon, and kidneys. Use palpation and percussion to check your findings.

9 On a model or dissection, identify and note the position of the abdominal blood vessels. If possible, examine angiograms of the aorta. Locate these vessels on your partner.

10 Examine the male and female pelvic organs on a model or dissection. If available, examine an excretory cystogram and contrast x-rays of the uterus and fallopian tubes. Note especially the anatomical relations of the organs to the skeleton and to one another.

8-4 EXTREMITIES

Although the arm and leg of the human seem very different, their structure is basically the same. Each joins the trunk at a highly movable ball-and-socket joint. Each has a single bone in its proximal part, and this bone ends in a hinge joint allowing movement in only one direction. Each has a double-boned segment below this hinge, terminating distally in a flexible region of several small bones. Beyond this, the extremity consists of five more or less parallel bones, from the distal ends of which arise jointed *digits.*

The resemblance between arms and legs goes beyond this. Each receives most of its blood through a single artery from the aorta, and this artery divides into two large branches below the hinge joint of the elbow or knee. These two arteries form arching connections proximal to the digits of each extremity. The veins of each extremity, however, form a double system which unites to form a single vein before the limb's junction with the trunk.

The movement allowed by a joint dictates the arrangement of muscles in and about the extremity. Since muscles can pull by *contracting* but never push by pressing, each joint has one or more sets of *opposing* muscles. Thus one or several muscles will *flex* a joint and are called *flexors;* other muscles in the group will *extend* or straighten it and are called *extensors.* Thus also *abductor* muscles will move an extremity away from the median line, and opposing *adductors* will move it toward or across the median line. Every set of *rotator* muscles has an opposing set to rotate or turn the extremity in the opposite direction on its long axis.

Upper Extremities *Humerus* The skeleton includes the *humerus* of the upper arm, with a spherical joint surface at its proximal head. This *articular surface* is directed medially, somewhat upward and more posteriorly than anteriorly (see Figures 8-12 and 8-24). The bone's distal end is widened laterally and narrowed anteroposteriorly, with a *spindle-shaped* joint surface jutting below it. A deep indentation on both the front and back of the bone, just above this spindle, increases the forward and backward range of motion at the joint. The flared distal ends of the humerus on either side are readily palpable, and the medial one has the name *epitrochlea*. The lateral flare has a smooth *spherical* articular surface directed forward and somewhat downward.

The surface of the humerus has spiral ridges along its shaft and two knobs or *tubercles* at its proximal end, near the articular surface. These provide attachments for the muscles of the shoulder girdle and upper arm.

Proximally the humerus articulates with the *glenoid cavity* of the shoulder girdle. Distally it joins the two bones of the lower arm at the elbow. The medial of these, the *ulna*, articulates with the spindle-shaped surface, and the lateral, the *radius*, with the spherical knob.

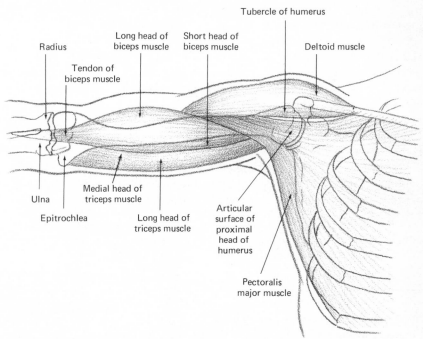

Figure 8-24 Skeleton and some muscles of upper arm, seen from in front.

Muscles of the Upper Arm   The humerus, almost surrounded by muscles, is located centrally in the upper arm. One of these crosses the top of the shoulder, surrounding the lateral, anterior, and posterior boundaries of the glenoid cavity and the humeral head. This *deltoid muscle* has its broad *origin* from the shoulder girdle and narrows to *insert* about halfway down the lateral aspect of the humerus. When it contracts, it *abducts* or lifts the upper arm, although it can rotate it forward or backward as well, since its anterior and posterior parts oppose each other in this rotation.

The two-headed *biceps muscle* is large and superficial on the anterior surface of the arm. Its *shorter* head arises from the coracoid process of the scapula. Its *longer,* more lateral head arises in a long, cablelike tendon which runs from the superior lip of the glenoid cavity across the head of the humerus and downward in the groove between the two tubercles of that bone. This tendon is surrounded by a thin, fluid-filled sac or *bursa,* as are similar mobile tendons crossing bone. Below the bursa the tendon joins the belly of the long head, and in the lower part of the upper arm, the two heads fuse. Just above the elbow, the belly of the muscle narrows to form a thick tendon that is easily palpable where it crosses the elbow to insert at the upper end of the radius. The muscle thus can lift or abduct the arm and flex the elbow.

The opposing muscle, the three-headed *triceps,* occupies the superficial part of the posterior surface. The *long* head, the most median, arises on the lower lip of the glenoid cavity, another head on the lower posterior surface of the humerus, and the *lateral* head from higher on the posterior surface. The three heads fuse into a broad flat tendon which inserts primarily on the most proximal part of the ulna, the *olecranon process.* The long head adducts the arm and draws it backward, while all the heads extend the forearm.

Other muscles are in the upper arm or attach to the humerus; but the deltoid, biceps, and triceps provide readily recognizable landmarks. They are important in tracing the vessels and nerves.

Blood Vessels of the Upper Arm   The *axilla* or armpit provides a common path for these structures. As the subclavian artery passes between the lateral head of the clavicle and the underlying ribs, it assumes the name of *axillary artery* (see Figure 8-25). It continues distally high in the axilla, passing in front of and just below the joint and humeral head. After it passes beneath the insertion of the pectoralis major on the humerus, it changes its name again to the *brachial artery.* The level of this change can be found by tracing the distal end of the pectoralis major where it crosses the biceps and ducks beneath the deltoid muscle. At about this point the pulsation of the axillary artery can be detected by

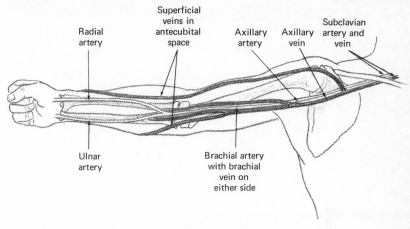

Figure 8-25   Large blood vessels of arm and axilla.

deep palpation from in front, beneath the inferior border of the pectoralis major.

The brachial artery can be palpated more superficially as it passes down the medial surface of the arm in the groove which separates the short head and belly of the biceps from the long head of the triceps. As it approaches the elbow, it swings anteriorly and can be felt along the medial side of the biceps tendon in the *antecubital space,* which is the anterior or flexor surface of the elbow. Here it turns deeper into the muscles of the forearm and is lost to palpation.

In their course the axillary and brachial arteries give off branches to the muscles and other structures around them. This blood is, of course, returned by the veins of the arm. These veins are variable and have frequent interconnections.

A large *superficial* and palpable *vein* in the antecubital space lateral to the biceps tendon can be followed upward and laterally for some distance on the biceps. An even more superficial vein medial to the tendon runs upward and medially. There are usually two *brachial veins* deep in the arm, following more or less parallel paths. These brachial veins unite at the level of the pectoralis major and form the *axillary vein,* which accompanies the artery until it becomes the subclavian vein beneath the clavicle.

Nerves of the Upper Arm   The nerves of the arm cross the axilla like a net around the axillary artery, since the *brachial plexus* extends down to the level of the pectoralis major insertion. At that level three main nerves are distinct, one having already separated somewhat more proximally (see Figure 8-26). This one, the *radial nerve,* loops deep from the medial to the

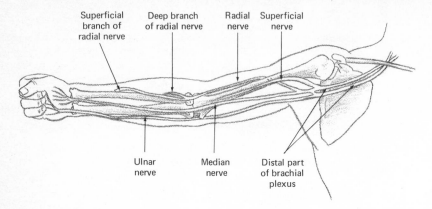

Superficial branch of radial nerve	Deep branch of radial nerve	Radial nerve	Superficial nerve

Ulnar nerve	Median nerve	Distal part of brachial plexus

Figure 8-26   Major nerves of arm and axilla.

lateral side of the humerus, passing posteriorly beneath the triceps muscle. It then passes the elbow on its lateral or radial side anterior to the head of the radius.

The other two main nerves, the *ulnar* and the *median,* accompany the brachial artery until about two-thirds of the way to the elbow. Here the median nerve swings around the lateral surface of the arm and crosses the antecubital space beside the artery. The ulnar nerve, however, swings medially and crosses the elbow just inside the epitrochlea. It can be palpated there and is the source of the pain and tingling when you hit your "funny bone."

The brachial plexus as well as the three large nerves give off numerous branches to the muscle and skin. The first are chiefly motor branches, the latter sensory.

Lymphatics of the Upper Arm   Lymphatic vessels from the hand and forearm cross the elbow to continue up the arm. There is a collection of lymph nodes, the *epitrochlear group,* just above the epitrochlea on the medial side. An even more important group of *axillary nodes* lies high in the axilla and drains most of the arm as well as the upper chest wall.

Skeleton of the Forearm   The two bones of the forearm are so arranged that the distal end of one—the *radius*—can swing across the other—the *ulna.* This structure allows the hand to rotate palm up or palm down (see Figure 8-27 and 8-28).

The *ulna* is a long, thin bone that looks like a wrench. The proximal end—the wrench's head—has a deep notch on its anterior surface with curved "jaws" above and below it. The notch is the surface which hinges around the spindle on the end of the humerus. Lateral to the lower lip of the groove is a second, more cuplike *articular surface* to receive the head of the radius. The most proximal part of the ulna is a process—the *olecranon*—which forms the upper part of the "jaws." The olecranon juts out on the posterior or extensor surface when the elbow is bent. When the elbow is extended, it fits up into the posterior indentation on the humerus. When the elbow is flexed, the lower lip of the "jaws" fits into the anterior indentation.

The shaft of the ulna is smaller than the proximal end and terminates distally in a *double articular surface*. One surface is at the extreme end and looks toward the wrist. The other almost completely surrounds the first as a wide rim which articulates with the radius alongside it.

The *radius* has a similar double surface at its small proximal end. At its extreme end it has a concave surface which fits the small articular knob on the lateral side of the humeral head. The broad, smooth, lateral surface circling the end rotates in the cuplike surface on the lateral side of the proximal ulnar head (see Figure 8-24).

The distal head of the radius is broader than its shaft. Its extremity has two concave articular surfaces in the direction of the wrist and another looking sideways on its medial or ulnar surface. When the two bones of the forearm are fitted side by side, the two proximal joint surfaces provide a wide, stable hinge articulation with the humerus. The elbow joint can only swing open and closed. The two bones provide a wide distal surface in which the wrist bones can rock side to side as well as bend backward and forward in extension and flexion.

While maintaining these joint surfaces, the broad distal head of the humerus can roll back and forth over the surface of the distal ulnar head. At the same time the proximal head of the radius turns in place as its surface moves in the lateral articular surface of the ulna.

The heads of the two bones and much of their shafts are palpable. Their relative motion during rotation is easy to appreciate by feeling up and down the forearm during this motion.

Muscles of the Forearm   The forearm contains numerous muscles, most of them spindle-shaped, with long tendons running across the wrist to the hand and digits. Some have their origin on the humerus, others on the radius or ulna. One muscle on the flexor surface of the forearm, the *long palmar muscle,* has a long, prominent tendon running just lateral to the long axis of the lower forearm and into the palm. It crosses the wrist slightly toward the radial side, where it serves as a landmark.

Blood Vessels and Lymphatics of the Forearm   The *brachial artery,* as it swings deep behind the biceps tendon's insertion, divides into two. The *radial artery* curves laterally and then runs anterior to the radius straight to the wrist; the *ulnar artery* swings medially and runs to the wrist along the ulna (see Figure 8-25). Both arteries give off numerous branches and remain deep among the muscles and tendons until they near the wrist. Their pulsations can be palpated, however, along the lower part of the

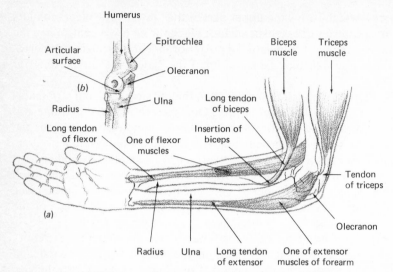

Figure 8-27 (a) Skeleton and some muscles of forearm, seen from ulnar side with elbow flexed. (b) Elbow extended, same view, in insert.

course. Usually the radial artery is larger and more easily felt, but the ulnar may be as large or larger.

Paired *radial veins* accompany the radial artery and a pair of *ulnar veins* accompany the ulnar artery. Both empty into the *brachial veins* below the elbow. These deep veins are comparatively small because much of the blood from the forearm and hand is returned through the network of *superficial veins* just below the skin.

Lymphatics accompany the blood vessels up the forearm. There are, however, no significant groups of lymph nodes distal to the elbow.

Nerves of Forearm and Hand   The *radial nerve* divides at the elbow into a deep branch which spirals around to the dorsal side to reach the extensor muscles of the forearm and a superficial branch which runs down the lateral surface of the forearm (see Figure 8-26). Near the wrist it and its branches swing around to the back of the hand, ultimately reaching the tips of the thumb and first two fingers dorsally and laterally.

The *ulnar nerve* runs down the medial side of the forearm, crossing the wrist anteriorly to supply the *palmar surface* of the last three fingers. A branch spirals around the ulnar side of the wrist to supply the same three fingers dorsally and laterally.

The *median nerve* runs deep down the middle of the anterior aspect of the forearm and crosses the wrist near the long palmar tendon. Its branches then run distally to the thumb and first three fingers.

Radial, ulnar, and median nerves give off branches to the muscles and skin along their courses. They also interconnect with one another.

Wrist The wrist consists of two rows of four *carpal bones* each. These fit snugly together to form a plate of bones, narrower at the proximal end. At this end, three of the bones make a rounded surface that articulates with the radius and ulna (see Figure 8-28).

At the broader distal side of the plate, the carpals have articular

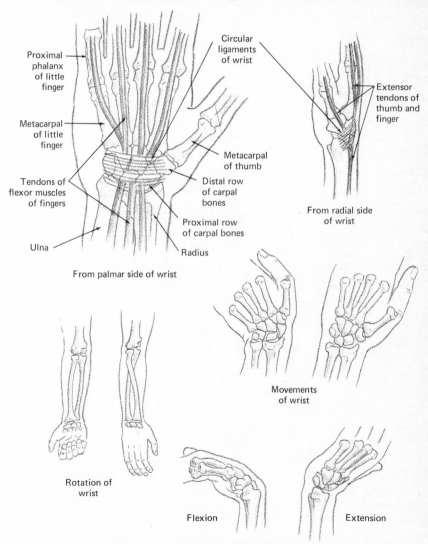

Figure 8-28 Structure and movements of wrist.

surfaces for the five bones of the hand. The resulting joints except for the thumb allow much less movement than do the carpal joints with the radius and ulna.

Like all joints, the wrist bones are bound together by tough ligaments. These may be bands, broad sheets, or cords and allow any movement of which the joint is normally capable. The wrist is further covered by a broad, circular band of ligament just under the skin. It encircles, like a wristband, the heads of the radius and ulna as well as the proximal row of carpal bones. Beneath it pass the tendons, arteries, deep veins, and nerves.

Skeleton of the Hand   The palm contains five slender *metacarpal* bones whose dorsal surfaces can be felt running from the wrist to the digits (see Figure 8-29). Each has an articular head at either end of the shaft, and the rounded distal head is the prominent knuckle of each digit.

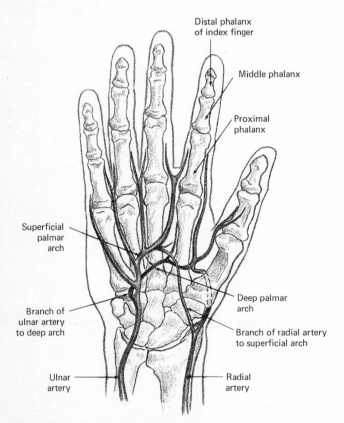

Figure 8-29   Skeleton and chief arteries of hand, seen from palmar surface.

Each finger contains three shorter *phalanges*—called the *proximal, middle,* and *distal phalanges*—each shorter than the more proximal one. The first two have articular surfaces at either end; the distal phalanx ends in a bony tuft.

The thumb is different, with a highly mobile *carpometacarpal joint* and only two phalanges. The base of the thumb contains a muscle on its palmar surface, and this forms the *thenar eminence* on the palm.

Muscles and Blood Vessels of the Hand The hand contains other small muscles between and on the sides of the metacarpals. Most of the force of the hand's and fingers' movements comes, however, from the forearm muscles, whose long tendons insert on the metacarpals and phalanges.

The *radial artery,* as it leaves the wrist, loops around the thumb's metacarpal and swings into the deep layers of the palm. Here it forms an *arch,* joining a deep branch of the *ulnar artery.* The ulnar artery continues into the palm, forms a more superficial arch, and joins a superficial branch of the radial. These cross connections allow blood to pass freely into the radial artery when the ulnar is blocked, and vice versa. The loops give off branches into the fingers and thumb, so that their blood supply is assured by the connections.

Most of the blood is returned from the fingers and hand by the network of veins on the dorsal surface. These are readily visible. The deep veins and those on the palmar surfaces are equally netlike but carry less blood.

EXERCISES

1 Examine the humerus, radius, and ulna. Identify their parts and their articulations with one another and with the glenoid cavity. Determine especially the motions allowed at each joint by the skeletal form.
2 If available, examine the bones and joints of the arm in x-rays, identifying the various parts. Note especially the articulations at the shoulder, elbow, and wrist. It is better to have views of the joints in several positions.
3 On your partner, identify the humerus and its parts. It is easiest to begin with the shaft, feeling the medial side of the relaxed arm. Similarly palpate and identify the accessible parts of the radius and ulna. Palpate the joints in several positions, relating what you feel to what you see in the skeleton and x-rays.
4 Identify the deltoid, biceps, triceps, and pectoralis major muscles on your partner. Find the insertion tendon of the biceps in the antecubital space and palpate more proximally where the muscle divides into two heads. Try to identify the origins and insertions of the biceps and triceps on a skeleton.
5 Palpate the axillary and brachial arteries on your partner. Palpate as much as you can of the course of the brachial artery, paying particular attention to its relation to the humerus and the elbow joint.

6   If a dissection or model is available, trace the course of the radial, ulnar, and
    median nerves from the axilla to the hand. Note the relation of the nerves to
    landmarks and plot the course on your partner's arm. In the dissection or
    model, follow the radial and ulnar arteries in the forearm and hand.
7   Palpate as much of the course of the radial and ulnar arteries as you can,
    beginning at the wrist and feeling upward. Then examine the superficial veins
    on all aspects of the hands and arms of one or more subjects. You can
    exaggerate their size by constricting the upper arm.
8   Examine the bones of the wrist and hand, identify each one and determine how
    they articulate with one another. If available, examine and identify the wrist
    and hand bones in an x-ray. Then palpate as many as you can and for as much
    of their surface as you can on your partner.

Lower Extremities   *Femur and Patella*   The *femur* or thighbone is
massive, with a heavy shaft and prominent heads. The complex proximal
end has a *spherical articular surface* joined to the shaft by a narrower
neck. This neck angles upward, medially and slightly posteriorly from the
shaft (see Figures 8-16 and 8-30). Where the neck joins the shaft, it is
almost surrounded by blunt processes. The shaft broadens below and
terminates in three articular surfaces. Two lie side by side, are largely
posterior, extend onto the dorsal surface, and are separated by a deep
groove. The third forms a shallow concave surface where the groove
extends onto the anterior surface. The paired surfaces articulate with the
lower leg bones, the third with the *patella* or kneecap.

The patella is a separate bone with a rounded anterior surface and
two concave articular surfaces posteriorly. These surfaces are in contact
with the round surfaces on the distal end of the femur when the knee is
flexed.

The largest process on the femoral shaft can be felt on the side of the
hip. The femoral head fits into the acetabulum somewhat above this level.
The lateral surface of the shaft can be felt rather indistinctly for a
distance below this level if the leg muscles are relaxed.

The flared lower end of the femur can be felt on either side just above
the knee and, when the knee is flexed, the outer parts of the articular
surfaces are palpable on either side of the patella. The anterior surface
and lateral edges of the patella are easily felt when the leg is extended and
relaxed.

Muscles of the Thigh   The thigh muscles are large and numerous,
many attaching to the femur, the bones of the lower leg, and the inner and
outer surfaces of the pelvis, sacrum, and coccyx. The large posterior,
superior muscles, together with the fat overlying them, form the *buttocks*.

One thigh muscle formed by the union of four heads, the *quadriceps
femoris muscle,* makes up the anterior mass on the lower part of the thigh

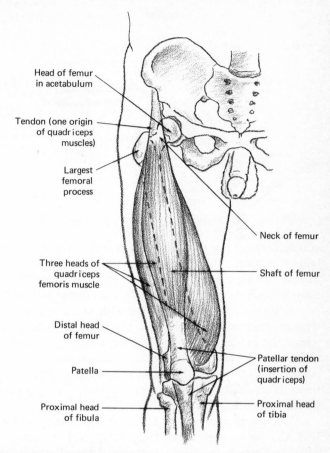

Head of femur
in acetabulum

Tendon (one origin
of quadriceps
muscles)

Largest
femoral
process

Neck of femur

Three heads of
quadriceps
femoris muscle

Shaft of femur

Distal head
of femur

Patella

Patellar tendon
(insertion of
quadriceps)

Proximal head
of fibula

Proximal head
of tibia

Figure 8-30 Skeleton and one muscle of hip, thigh and knee. Fourth head of quadriceps muscle lies deep to other three.

and continues up its lateral aspect. The major *insertion* of this muscle is the *patellar tendon*. This tendon, an important landmark, runs from above to insert along the upper and lateral surfaces of the patella but passes in part anterior and lateral to it. These direct fibers, with others from the lower patellar edges, continue downward to insert on the anterior surface of the upper part of the *tibia,* the larger bone of the lower leg. The patella, then, is a bone within a tendon.

Blood Vessels and Lymphatics of the Thigh The *femoral artery* is palpable in the *femoral triangle* as it emerges from beneath the inguinal ligament (see Figure 5-14). It can then be felt a short way down the thigh as it swings medially. It continues deep in the muscles, spiraling to the posterior surface of the femur above the knee (see Figure 8-31). During its

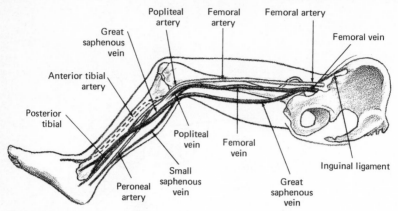

Figure 8-31 Large blood vessels of leg, seen from median side.

course through the thigh, it gives off branches chiefly to the muscles, the largest arising not far below the triangle. As the femoral passes deep behind the knee joint, it assumes the name of *popliteal artery,* since the distinct pocket on the flexor surface of the knee is the *popliteal space.*

A single *popliteal vein,* lying with the artery, comes from the lower leg and continues upward as the *femoral vein* to become the external iliac within the pelvis. As in the arm, the *superficial veins* are important. The largest is the *great saphenous vein,* which extends from the ankle on the medial surface past the knee and upward on the medial surface of the thigh. It gradually becomes more anterior, to empty into the femoral vein at the triangle.

The lymphatic vessels from the lower leg and foot course upward with the veins, and those from the posterior parts enter the popliteal space, where there is a deep group of lymph nodes. Lymphatic vessels from the remainder of the leg and foot follow the veins to the femoral triangle, where the other group of lymph nodes is located.

Nerves of the Thigh   The *sciatic nerve* supplies most of the innervation of the muscles and skin of the leg. It arises from the lumbosacral plexus and leaves the pelvis through the large notch on the dorsolateral aspect of the pelvis, about on the level of the acetabulum. It rather promptly turns downward to run deep in the buttock and back of the thigh. It passes about midway between the ischial tuberosity and the palpable process at the upper end of the femur (see Figure 8-32). At the *gluteal fold,* the deep crease that marks the lower edge of the buttock, it is almost centered on the posterior aspect of the thigh, and it maintains this position as it continues downward.

The sciatic nerve divides in the middle or lower third of the thigh into the *tibial nerve,* which continues downward on the centered course, and

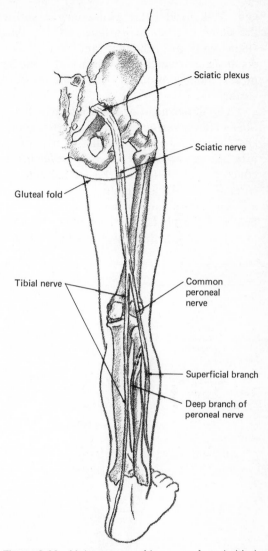

Figure 8-32   Major nerves of leg, seen from behind.

the *common peroneal nerve,* which runs laterally to cross the popliteal space just inside the tendons which make up its lateral wall.

Skeleton of the Lower Leg   The lower leg contains two bones which form essentially immovable joints with one another. The larger bone, the *tibia* or shinbone, lies medial and anterior to the smaller *fibula* (see Figure 8-33).

The *tibia* forms all of the knee articulation at its wide, flattened upper end. This head bears two concave surfaces side by side to receive the convex articular surfaces of the distal femoral head. Its heavy shaft—with a prominent anterior ridge—widens again to form the distal head, which also bears a concave articular surface. On its medial side, a process—the *medial malleolus*—extends below the joint surface.

The upper head of the *fibula* articulates with that of the tibia on the tibia's lateral surface, below the articular surface of the knee. Its thinner shaft runs downward parallel to that of the tibia and ends in a wider process, the *lateral* or *external malleolus,* which extends below a small concave articulation on the medial side. Together, the tibia and fibula form an archlike articulation at the ankle.

The entire anterior-medial surface of the tibia is palpable, as are the heads of the fibula. The fibular shaft, however, is buried in the lateral muscles of the calf until it reaches the narrowed part of the lower leg.

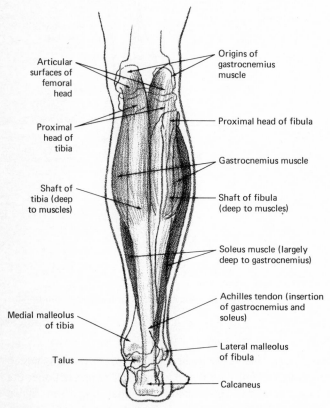

Figure 8-33 Skeleton and large muscles of lower leg, seen from behind.

Here it can be traced to the lateral malleolus. The medial malleolus on the tibia is equally palpable.

Articulations The knee joint, like other movable joints, has articular surfaces covered with tough, smooth cartilage or gristle. The joint proper is surrounded by a membrane, the *synovial membrane,* which attaches to the bones beyond the articular surfaces. The membrane secretes a *synovial fluid* which lubricates the joint surfaces.

The bones are attached to one another by tough *ligaments* so arranged as to stabilize the joint but to allow its motion. In the knee—a hinge joint—the arrangement of these ligaments is complex.

The *tendons* crossing the joint further stabilize it and, as the muscles contract during motion, can allow movement in a selective fashion. The tendons would encounter friction, however, if they were not cushioned by fluid-filled *bursae* and *tendon sheaths.* The *patellar bursa* under that bone and its tendon is large and extends on either side of and well proximal to the patella.

Muscles of the Lower Leg The muscles of the leg are roughly divided into a dorsal group, the *calf,* and an anterolateral group. The dorsal group consists principally of the more superficial *gastrocnemius* and the deeper *soleus muscles.* The former arises from the distal end of the femur, the latter from the proximal ends of the fibula and tibia. They insert below, through the large prominent *Achilles tendon* at the back of the ankle. This tendon runs down to insert on the heel or *calcaneus* bone.

Blood Vessels of the Lower Leg The *popliteal artery* extends just below the knee joint, where it divides into the *posterior* and *anterior tibial arteries.* The *posterior tibial* runs under the gastrocnemius muscle, angling somewhat medially until it lies deep to the medial edge of the Achilles tendon behind the medial malleolus. Below this point, it turns forward into the sole of the foot (see Figure 8-31).

The *anterior tibial artery* swings anteriorly between the upper part of the shafts of the tibia and fibula. It then runs downward, still deep in the muscles, on the lateral side of the tibia. As it descends, it angles medially and crosses the ankle to the dorsum of the foot, just about midway between the two malleoli but still deep among the tendons.

A pair of *deep veins,* the *anterior tibials* and the *posterior tibials,* accompanies each of the two arteries at the ankle. These four veins run with the arteries until they unite to form the popliteal vein.

The *superficial veins* of the lower leg form a complex network. Those on the anterior and lateral surfaces empty into the *great saphenous vein,* which crosses the ankle just anterior to the medial malleolus. It then runs up along the "bare" face of the tibia, swings further laterally in the upper part of the lower leg, and crosses the knee to continue on the thigh.

The *small saphenous vein* drains the calf region. It usually forms just below the belly of the gastrocnemius muscle and continues up the midline of the calf, crosses the popliteal space, and swings deep to join the popliteal or femoral vein. It generally is visible or palpable over much of its course.

Nerves of the Lower Leg and Foot   The *tibial nerve,* after crossing the popliteal space, continues downward deep in the calf almost in the midline. It gradually slopes toward the medial side and lies deep to the medial edge of the Achilles tendon at the ankle. It then passes medial to the calcaneus, dividing as it goes to supply the *plantar* or sole surface of the foot and toes (see Figure 8-32).

The *common peroneal nerve,* after crossing obliquely in the popliteal space, passes just under the tibial head and lateral to the fibular head. Here it divides into *deep* and *superficial branches* which run almost parallel courses downward among the muscles and tendons of the anterior muscle group. The more lateral *superficial peroneal nerve* goes to the great toe and the two adjacent toes on the dorsal surfaces. Both peroneal branches and the tibial nerve send branches to the muscles and skin along their courses.

Ankle   The ankle contains two large *tarsal bones,* the *talus* and the *calcaneus.* The remaining five tarsal bones functionally form part of the foot. The *talus* is a rather block-shaped bone whose superior surface bears a saddle-shaped articular surface. This forms the hinge joint with the lower leg bones. On either side of this large surface are concave areas which articulate with the inner surfaces of the malleoli. In the joint, the talus fits up into the archlike space formed by the tibia and fibula. It can rock back and forth in extension and flexion of the ankle, but it cannot shift sideways (see Figure 8-34).

The inferior surface of the talus has a concave articular area posteriorly and a smaller flat one anterior to it. These make the joint with the *calcaneus.* The anterior surface of the talus has a knob for articulation with another tarsal bone.

The calcaneus forms the heel by means of a rough posterior knob. Above this knob and well anterior to it, the superior surface has a convex surface and a flatter one, both for articulation with the talus. More anteriorly, it has a concave surface where another tarsal bone joins it. In place, it supports the talus above it and—as it juts out behind and below—provides the bony support of the heel.

The ankle joint is stabilized by numerous ligaments and further strengthened by the numerous tendons which cross or end there. As at the wrist, these are encircled by a broad ligament running around the ankle.

The posterior tibial artery can usually be felt as a pulse at the ankle, where it passes in the hollow just behind the medial malleolus. The anterior tibial lies too deep to be felt in this region. A considerable extent of the posterior part of the calcaneus can be palpated and the insertion of the Achilles tendon felt on its superior surface.

Skeleton of the Foot The five tarsal bones other than the talus and calcaneus fall into two groups. One bone of a group of four articulates with the anterior face of the talus, where the broad proximal tarsal forms a movable joint. Its distal face articulates with three tarsals arranged side by side, and each of these forms a joint with one of the medial three *metatarsals.* The largest of the tarsal and metatarsal bones go to the *proximal phalanx* of the great toe. This medial group of tarsals and metatarsals together with the phalanges of the first three digits bears most of the weight placed on the anterior part of the foot (see Figure 8-34).

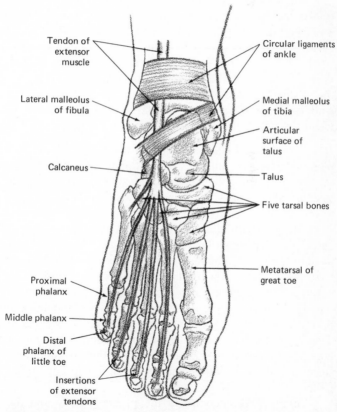

Figure 8-34 Skeleton of foot and ankle with ankle straightened as far as possible. Circular ligaments and tendon of one extensor muscle shown.

The lateral group of bones consists of a large, broad tarsal which articulates with the anterior face of the calcaneus and with the proximal heads of the two lateral metatarsals. These, with the phalanges of the last two digits, supplement the weight bearing of the heel, and the proximal head of the fifth metatarsal is enlarged on its lateral and plantar surface.

As in the wrist, the tarsal bones form a compact group. The metatarsals all lie parallel with one another but not in a plane. Rather, they form an arc, the medial one being higher than the lateral one, where they articulate with the tarsal bones.

The *phalanges* of the toes also parallel one another. Like the thumb, the great toe has only two phalanges; the other toes have three. The phalanges are distinctly palpable, the dorsal surfaces of the five metatarsals less so. The lateral prominence on the proximal head of the fifth metatarsal can be felt on the outer side of the foot.

The ligaments of the tarsal and other joints of the foot are strong and reinforced by the tendons from the muscles in the lower leg. Together with the bony structure, they form arches in two directions. The *plantar surface* and—less distinctly—the *dorsum* of the foot arch from front to back. They also arch from the lateral to the higher medial side. Together, these arches form the instep, so that weight is borne on the heel, across the distal heads of the metatarsals, and along the lateral surface. In walking or running, the medial three digits momentarily bear the body's weight, most of it on the great toe.

Muscles and Blood Vessels of the Foot   There are muscles on both plantar and dorsal surfaces of the tarsal and metatarsal bones, principally on the dorsum. Other smaller muscles lie between and lateral to the metatarsals. Most of the power of the foot is delivered, however, by the lower leg muscles through their long tendons.

The *posterior tibial artery* enters the sole on the medial side of the calcaneus. It swings laterally as the *lateral plantar artery* until it passes inside the proximal head of the fifth metatarsal. A little distal to this point it forms an arch, the other end of which includes a branch from the anterior tibial. The arch, in turn, gives off branches to the toes.

The *anterior tibial artery* continues from the ankle along the dorsum of the foot, among the tendons, as the *dorsalis pedis* artery. Usually it runs just lateral to the first metatarsal bone and to the prominent tendon going to the great toe. At the level of the proximal metatarsal heads, it forms an arch, the other end of which is another branch of the dorsalis pedis.

Small veins accompany the plantar artery and the dorsalis pedis. Each pair bears the name of the artery it accompanies. There is as well a network of *superficial veins* easily seen on the dorsum. These can be traced upward to the great saphenous vein. A similar net is visible only in the instep but occurs elsewhere in the sole as well. Most of these veins drain upward to the dorsum, but some go posteriorly to join the small saphenous vein.

EXERCISES

1 Examine the femur, tibia, and fibula, identifying their parts. Note how the femur articulates with the pelvis and how the bones, including the patella, join at the knee. What motions do the bones allow at hip and knee? What prevents this full range in the living person?

2 If available, examine x-rays of the thigh and leg. Identify each bone and its parts, noting especially the articulations.

3 On your partner, identify the palpable superior process of the femur and trace the shaft as far down as you are able. To do this, the leg must be completely relaxed. Resume the palpation just above the knee. Feel the patella with the knee fully extended to relax the tendon. Then palpate the knee, especially the femur, with passive flexion. Palpate the tibia for its entire length, the two heads of the fibula, and as much of its shaft as you can at the lower end.

4 Identify the quadriceps and gastrocnemius muscles on your partner. Palpate the tendon of insertion for each, identifying the bones passed by and fastened to these tendons. What active movements of the leg or foot tenses these tendons?

5 Palpate the femoral triangle and the artery there. How far can you trace the pulsations? Palpate the popliteal artery, the posterior tibial at the ankle, and the dorsalis pedis. How far can you trace each of these vessels? Identify and trace the great and small saphenous veins.

6 If a model or dissection is available, trace the course of the arteries, deep veins, and nerves of the leg. Name the various vessels and nerves and note their relation to the landmarks.

7 Examine the bones of the ankle and foot, identifying each bone and its parts and noting how they articulate. If available, examine x-rays of the ankle and foot, identifying the parts and their joints. Palpate and identify as much of these bones as you can on your partner. How much active and passive motion is allowed in each part?

8-5 NORMAL VARIATIONS IN ANATOMY

Just as the face differs from person to person, so the internal anatomy varies among normal individuals. Some differences—size, sex, body type—are obvious; others are subtle.

Many normal variations have medical significance; women and men get different diseases of the sex organs. Some abnormal conditions are exaggerations of normal variations, as extreme obesity is an exaggeration of normal plumpness.

You can consider normal variations as falling into several categories, realizing that each person is in several categories at the same time. Age, sex, race, environmental factors, congenital or inborn differences whether hereditary or not, and miscellaneous conditions all produce individual differences. Even a change of posture shifts some anatomical relationships.

Changes with Age   As life is change, so the same individual changes greatly as he grows and ages. Passing from babyhood to adulthood involves much more than simply increasing in size.

A person alters anatomically by a continuous series of small changes, but it is convenient to name certain periods in the life-span. The *newborn* or *neonatal period* extends from birth to the age of about 2 weeks. *Infancy* covers the time to the age of 1 year, when the baby is weaned and walking. *Early childhood* spans the period from age 1 to 5 or 6, when the baby teeth begin to be lost. *Late childhood* extends from that age to puberty. In girls, puberty usually begins between the ages of 11 and 14 and between 12 and 15 in boys. *Adolescence* extends from puberty to about age 17 for girls and 19 for boys. *Young adulthood* spans the period from that age to about 23 for women and 25 for men. *Mature adulthood* continues to the menopause in women, usually between ages 40 and 50, and to a less sharp point some 5 years later in men. *Middle age* lasts until the mid-sixties, to be followed by *old age.*

Changes are rapid in the neonatal period and infancy, somewhat slower in childhood. They become rapid again in adolescence and thereafter are gradual.

Head and Neck   The newborn has a relatively enormous cranium and brain which grow rapidly until they reach almost adult size when he is 6 years old. In contrast, his face is small and broad, tucked under his large cranium. His maxilla and mandible are narrow and shallow; the orbits are relatively tiny. His nose is broad and his chin recedes. His cheeks are plump because he has a *buccal fat pad* among the muscles on either side. His lips show a distinct line where the mucous membrane ends and the thin red skin of the lips begins. This mucous membrane bordering the mouth opening is roughened by tiny projections which help him retain the nipple when he nurses.

His tongue is short and blunt at the tip, so that he has no pointed end and cannot lick his lips. Indeed, the tongue is used to create a vacuum during sucking, and the buccal pads prevent his cheeks from being drawn in as he does so.

His palate is arched high and, with the squat maxillary bones, reduces the volume of his nasal cavity. Added to this is his small nasopharynx, so that nasal obstructions occur easily.

At birth the external auditory canal is short and straight. The outer opening is small, but the canal widens to a large chamber that ends in a tympanic membrane of adult size. The middle ear is relatively large, but it and the eustachian tube contain a semisolid substance rather than air.

The neck looks short and almost absent, but in fact the cervical vertebrae are relatively the largest of the whole spinal column. The pharynx, however, is short from top to bottom and narrow from front to back. The epiglottis is relatively large and broad; the larynx is small.

During infancy and early childhood, the face develops gradually (see Figure 8-35). The mandible deepens, teeth erupt, and the facial bones

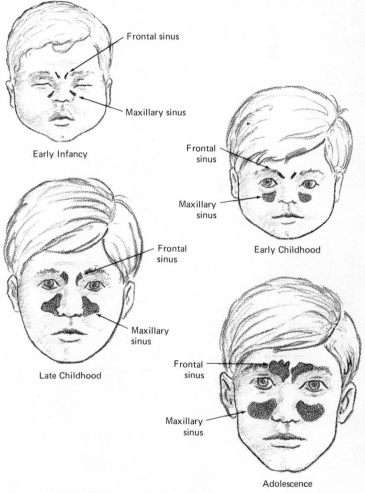

Figure 8-35 Development of nasal sinuses.

increase in size. Maxillary sinuses grow into the maxillary bones but remain small, and the buccal fat pads persist. The face continues to look broad, but the chin becomes more prominent.

The palatal arch begins to flatten and the pharynx to increase in size. This is partially offset by the growth of tonsillar tissue, especially the adenoidal mass, which reduces the depth of the nasopharynx (see Figure 8-36).

The tip of the tongue develops more than its body, so that it becomes more mobile and able to manipulate food. The laryngopharynx remains relatively shallow but gradually lengthens until the organs of the neck

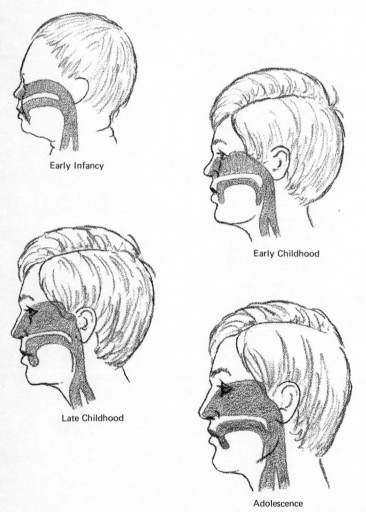

Early Infancy

Early Childhood

Late Childhood

Adolescence

Figure 8-36 Changes in nose, mouth and pharynx during growth.

reach their adult levels. The middle ear becomes air-filled and the auditory canal begins to deepen.

These changes continue into childhood as the neck becomes more distinct and the ramus of the mandible assumes the angle that it lacked earlier. The maxilla grows as its sinuses enlarge, lengthening the face. The apparent narrowing is heightened as the fat pads gradually disappear. Growth of the larynx more or less parallels that of the body, but the epiglottis assumes its adult narrow and peaked form.

During adolescence, the facial bones and the sinuses assume their adult proportions and the external ear canal its final depth and shape. The external nose increases in size but becomes relatively narrower. In boys the larynx becomes larger and the beard appears. The skin and hair become coarser and more oily in both sexes but especially in the boy.

The head and neck change relatively little from the later part of adolescence throughout young and mature adulthood. In middle age the normal skin furrows deepen into wrinkles and the face again begins to shorten from above downward. This is due in part to wearing away of the teeth.

In old age the face shortens farther as the chin decreases in height, especially if some teeth are lost, and the angle of the ramus decreases. The oiliness and coarseness of the skin and hair become less and the hair becomes thinner in both sexes. The skin not only loses fat but its tougher fibrous layers thin, so that it develops fine wrinkles. As the cheeks and chin become less prominent, the nose becomes more so, and loss of fat in the orbit may make the eyes recede behind thinned lids. The upper lids tend to droop and the lower lids to sag. The iris color may fade and the pupils become smaller. The external ears seem larger and more prominent because the fat, and to some extent the muscles, of the face and neck diminish.

The larynx drops lower in the neck. Its cartilages become less elastic and develop thin plaques of bone. The intervertebral discs narrow, particularly on their posterior areas, so that the cervical spine bows forward and becomes shorter.

Trunk Everything about the trunk of the newborn is displaced toward his head. The shoulders are high, the relatively small chest and its organs are above the adult level, and the tiny pelvis will not accommodate the organs that later occupy it.

The thoracic cage is almost round in the transverse plane and the first rib is truly horizontal, the remaining ribs almost so. The newborn's diaphragm is so high that the central part reaches to the level of the seventh or eighth thoracic vertebrae. The heart is relatively larger than in later life and the right ventricle almost equals the left in size (see Figure 8-37).

Not only the heart is large but the *thymus,* in the superior anterior mediastinum, is almost as large. There is little room for the lungs, and the trachea, only 1 $^1/_2$ in long, is less than 1/4 in in diameter. The horizontal ribs do little to assist respiration, and the newborn depends on his diaphragm during inspiration.

The newborn's liver is relatively twice as large as the adult's and takes up nearly half the abdominal cavity. It extends below the umbilicus and well over into the LUQ, where it touches the spleen. The adrenal glands are very large as well.

The newborn's bladder is long and spindle-shaped. It and the tiny uterus and ovaries in the female are above the pelvic brim and lie within the abdomen. The pelvic brim is horizontal, reflecting the straight but very flexible spine.

During infancy there is only a gradual change in these characteristics, but as the child begins to walk the spine assumes the lumbar lordotic curve and the normal kyphotic curve in the thorax. The pelvis begins to tip forward and the buttock muscles develop. The child's lumbar spine remains relatively short, the pelvis is small, the liver large, and the baby fat still remains. The result is the protuberant abdomen or "potbelly" that is normal during early childhood.

At the same time, the rib cage has begun to descend anteriorly and the heart continues to grow. In fact, the left ventricle has outgrown the right to about adult proportions by the age of 6 months. Despite the large heart and thymus, the lungs have become relatively larger. The trachea, however, remains narrow, less than 1/2 in wide at age 2, so that it is easily obstructed.

In late childhood, slow, steady growth of the thorax widens the chest, the pelvis widens and tips farther forward, and the lumbosacral spine becomes relatively longer. All these changes allow the viscera to assume their adult positions. The shoulder girdle also drops, and baby fat is lost. The trunk, therefore, more closely resembles that of an adult.

A year or two before puberty, the growth spurt starts and the girl's pelvis noticeably broadens. Her breasts begin to become prominent chiefly as fat is laid down. The boy, however, usually becomes leaner. Internally, the girl's ovaries and uterus increase in size. This uterine growth is chiefly in the fundus, which has been only about half as large as the cervix. At puberty it becomes about twice the size of the cervical portion, and *menarche* occurs as the girl begins to menstruate.

The boy's penis, testes, and scrotum enlarge rather rapidly. His prostate and seminal vesicles grow even more dramatically. In both sexes pubic and axillary hair appear.

At the same time the thymus, which has gradually increased in absolute but not in relative size, begins to regress. Lymphatic tissue and tonsils also begin to be less prominent.

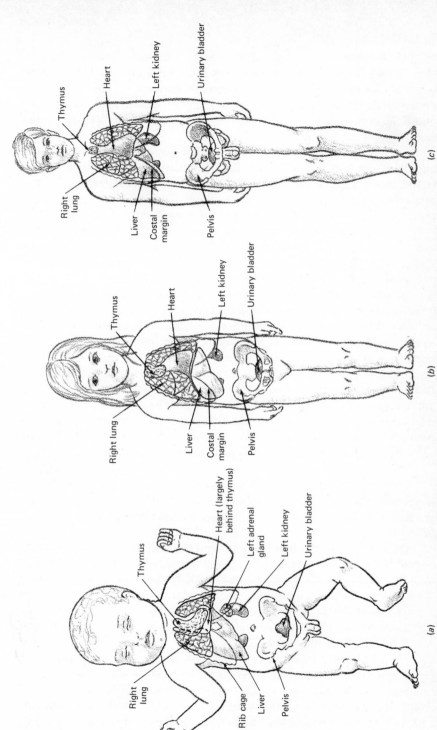

Figure 8-37 Changes in viscera with growth. Early infancy (left), early childhood (middle), and late childhood (right).

Adolescence lasts longer than puberty. During it there is growth of the internal organs as height increases. The girl's breasts develop more glandular tissue. The boy replaces the baby hair on his trunk with darker, coarse body hair, first above the pubic area and then often over the chest and lumbar area. In girls such changes, if they occur, involve only a few hairs around the nipple.

During adulthood the normal trunk changes little, and even in middle age the alterations are relatively slight. An increasing amount of calcium is laid down in the rib cartilage and the bones of the trunk become heavier and coarser. The vertebrae begin to show *"lipping;"* new bone is laid down around the anterior upper and lower margins of the body.

The greatest change occurs in women at the menopause, which ushers in middle age. At this time the ovaries and uterus regress in size as menses cease. The breasts lose glandular tissue but not necessarily fat and so retain their adult configuration in large part.

In old age the spinal column usually decreases in height as the intervertebral discs lose substance. This loss is most marked on the anterior side of the disc in the thoracic region, accentuating the normal kyphosis. It is less evident in the lumbar region, where the posterior side thins slightly, accentuating the normal lordotic curve.

The internal organs show comparatively little gross change. The heart muscle becomes browner, the liver and pancreas decrease in size, and the prostate may either shrink or enlarge. The intestinal and stomach walls thin somewhat, but most of the changes reported in the aged are probably the result of disease. The arterial walls do thicken and develop calcium deposits, but this may occur in younger people as well.

Extremities   At birth the arms and the legs are of equal length and the feet of the newborn are held soles together. The muscles of the arms are better developed and have a more complete nerve supply than those of the legs.

During infancy the legs lengthen and the feet turn outward or *evert*, so that the soles are more nearly flat on the ground when the child begins to walk. In general, the ligaments and tendons about the joints are rather slack and the infant is naturally "double jointed."

The bones of the extremities continue to lengthen and thicken during childhood, those of the legs particularly. Long bones lengthen by growth at a cartilage plate—the *epiphysis*—where the head at either end joins the shaft. The bones thicken as new bone is formed just under the outer covering of the shaft and head. At birth, the heads of many bones are all cartilage, and the time each ossifies or becomes bony differs from bone to bone. The ossification of the heads and the state of the epiphyses of various bones determines the skeletal age of the child (see Figure 8-38).

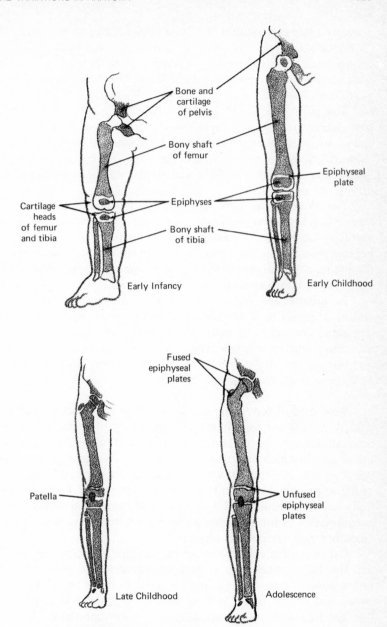

Figure 8-38 Development of skeleton of leg.

In early childhood, the talus not only enlarges but changes position and shape. These changes bring it into line under the tibia and fibula to form an ankle joint of the adult type. At the same time the acetabulum deepens while the femoral head and neck change to make the adult type of hip joint, capable of bearing the body's increasing weight. These changes, with the continuing development of buttock and leg muscles, limit somewhat the motions of the joints but make possible the upright posture of man.

The periods of rapid growth before and after puberty are marked, particularly in the boy, by a relative lengthening of the leg bones. By the end of adolescence many epiphyses have stopped growing and *ossified* or "closed." Some, however, do not close until the end of young adulthood, specifically those of the tibia and fibula, so that some growth occurs during this period.

The skeleton remains relatively stable during adulthood, although there is a gradual and continuous decrease in the thickness of the articular cartilages covering the joint surfaces. This is particularly true in weight-bearing joints, where the bone next the cartilage becomes dense and that around its edges grows outward to form lipping. These normal changes do not seem to interfere with the joints' function.

In middle age these joint changes are more evident, and they continue in old age. In advanced years some joints have detectably decreased motion. The ligaments become less elastic and usually the muscles gradually weaken. The bones also lose calcium, become lighter and thinner, and have less "give." Loss of bone strength and increased brittleness make fractures more likely.

Sex and Race   The sexual differences in normal anatomy are usually considered as primary and secondary. The primary sexual characteristics are those of the internal and external genitals. The secondary are all others which distinguish the typical normal man and woman. These are generally evident and well known: the greater height and longer legs of the adult male, his larger larynx with deeper voice, his beard and coarse body hair; the breasts and wider pelvis of the normal woman, the greater accumulation of fat about her buttocks and thighs, her finer head hair and smoother skin are equally obvious.

Other anatomical differences may escape casual notice. The cranium and the facial bones of a woman are smaller than those of a man. His bones generally are heavier and his muscles more bulky. He has less fat over most of his body, making him more angular in appearance. The internal organs of women are usually smaller than those of men, but the woman's thyroid gland is larger than a man's and her stomach and adrenals are the same size as his.

Even the tendency of men to get bald in the area above the forehead and on the crown is a secondary sexual characteristic. Pubic and axillary hair, however, are not different in the two sexes.

Women have a wider "carrying angle" at the elbow. This is the lateral deviation of the forearm when the arm hangs loosely at the side, palm forward.

Racial differences also tend to be superficial and obvious: the color of skin, hair, and eyes; facial characteristics of eyes, nose, and lips; differences in height (which are partly nutritional); and differences in hair texture. More subtle variations occur in head shape, with Orientals and central Europeans tending to have rounder, broader heads. The short stature of Orientals is largely due to relatively shorter legs; the tall Africans and Scandinavians have relatively longer legs. Scant facial hair in men of Oriental, American Indian, and some African groups, as well as differences in the amount of male body hair, is also racially determined.

Aside from differences in the size of internal organs that parallel those of the body size, there are few racial distinctions in internal anatomy. The differences seen are generally due to disease or environmental effects.

Environmental Factors Size, within the normal range, results from both heredity and nutrition, especially the diet before adulthood. An undernourished or improperly nourished child may grow into a small but normal adult. The amount of body fat depends upon many factors, but food intake is the principal one.

The environment apart from diet also alters normal anatomy. Foot shape is changed by certain types of shoes. The right arm and shoulder are usually larger and more heavily muscled in right-handed people. The difference is usually less marked in left-handed people who must live in a right-handed world.

Specific occupations are reflected in anatomical changes. There are typical calluses on the hands of carpenters, guitar players, and fishermen. Those who habitually go barefoot have thickened soles. Glassblowers and horn players have muscular cheeks. The facial and hand skin of outdoor workers and larger areas of skin of devoted sunbathers often show premature changes of aging.

Congenital Differences Apart from familial and racial characteristics, people show individual anatomical variations. If these are extensive or critical enough to interfere with health or happiness, they are considered abnormal and called *congenital defects, malformations,* or *congenital diseases.* If the variation is of little or no consequence, it is an *anomaly,* which is not considered abnormal. The difference is one of degree and the line often is a fine one.

Blood vessels are very variable. The radial artery is usually larger than the ulnar, but an individual may have so small a radial that no pulse is palpable while the large ulnar artery is readily felt. In this anomaly the arterial arches in the hand distribute the blood and no ill consequence results. Similar anomalies are even more common in the posterior tibial and dorsalis pedis arteries.

A major artery or vein may follow an anomalous course. Veins are especially variable and, while occasionally troublesome to someone drawing blood, the anomalies do not handicap the person.

Bony anomalies are less common, but extra ribs can occur on the seventh cervical or first lumbar vertebrae, and the fifth lumbar vertebra may fuse with the sacrum. Sixth fingers and similar *supernumerary* toes, with or without an extra metacarpal or metatarsal, are usually removed for cosmetic reasons but are really anomalies.

A person may live a long, healthy life with an extra pulmonary lobe or with his appendix in an anomalous position, tucked up behind the cecum. He may have a single kidney fused across the midline at what would be the lower poles, or he can have two ureters coming from a single kidney. One kidney may have two rather than one renal artery.

A much more extreme anomaly may not interfere with his life or be noticed until he has a physical examination or routine x-ray. This major anomaly is called *situs inversus,* and in it the organs are reversed, so that the heart and aorta are on the right. The "left ventricle" is really to the right and all valvular areas of auscultation are in mirror-image positions. The situs inversus may or may not involve the abdomen. If it does, the liver is in the LUQ and the appendix in the LLQ. The stomach and spleen are in the RUQ and the sigmoid colon in the RLQ.

It is fair to say that the internal anatomy varies as much as the external appearance within the normal range.

Chapter 9

The Functional Basis

The medical history deals largely with the patient's bodily functions, the everyday evidence of physiology. The examiner guides the patient into reporting that evidence so that abnormalities can be detected. You will find this easier if you use your own knowledge of the body's functions, backed up by some less obvious details.

The review of systems provides a framework for an organization of functions. You can then use any or all of this organization in framing questions about the present illness and other parts of the background history.

9-1 HEAD, BRAIN, AND SENSE ORGANS

The central nervous system with the sensory organs, peripheral nervous system, and autonomic nervous system makes up one of the two chief control mechanisms of the body. The other is the endocrine system, whose effects generally come on slowly and last for a long period. The nervous system, in contrast, quickly detects and promptly responds to changes.

Central Nervous System   The brain itself neither feels nor moves. It is, however, truly the center of the nervous system, into which flows the information and from which emanate the responses of all parts of the body. Its functions are so complex that its many parts reflect an intricate organization.

In one sense the brain is arranged into separate centers to deal with information coming to it over the cranial nerves, the spinal cord, and even the bloodstream. It has other centers which send out impulses and chemicals prompting the various bodily parts to action. Still other centers are intermediate between these two—interpreting the incoming information, determining the action to follow, modifying that reaction by orders to other parts of the body, coordinating the resulting action, and storing memories of the event.

Functional Levels   Rather obviously, the highest parts of the brain involved with conscious thought cannot participate in all the responses. The brain, therefore, is organized into various levels of function.

The lowest levels on the *sensory* side receive the incoming *nervous impulses* or messages from the sense organs of the head and body, arrange these for interpretation, and pass along the modified impulses. The lowest levels on the *motor* side relay the impulses from sensory centers or from higher levels to appropriate *effectors*, the muscles and glands. At least one set of lower centers can convert blood-borne hormones into sensory impulses and another can make hormones to act on effector glands. These centers provide a link between the central nervous and the endocrine systems.

Somewhat higher levels are able to interpret more or less *automatically* incoming sensory impulses and send out responsive motor impulses over autonomic and peripheral nerves. These levels regulate such automatic functions as respiration and circulation.

One level, on receiving both sensory impulses and motor impulses from higher centers, *coordinates* the motor response. To do this, it initiates impulses to opposing muscles and more distant ones, thus assuring smooth reactions with a stable supporting base. This coordination is the basis of grace and balance in movement.

Another level interprets *emotional* reactions and orders responses to them. While modified by impulses from higher levels, these centers of emotional reaction are not dependent on them.

The levels so far described all have centers in the spinal cord and brainstem. The cerebellum contributes centers for muscular coordination.

None is involved in conscious perception, interpretation, memory, thought, or voluntary action.

The complex higher functions are performed by the cerebral hemispheres. In their outer layer or *cortex* are more or less distinct areas which contain the centers for these higher functions.

Central Nervous System Defects   Injury to or disease of the brainstem, then, can interfere with essential bodily functions; in fact, destruction of some small areas controlling vital functions can be immediately fatal. Injury or disease has a less devastating effect if it involves a small area of the cerebral cortex. A person with extensive damage to the cortex can be kept alive for months or years even though comatose.

Although the brain itself is insensitive, head injuries are painful and headaches may arise from inside the cranium. This is because the blood vessels and the membranes or meninges covering the brain have sensory nerve endings. Most headaches, however, are caused by abnormal though transient changes in the blood vessels of the skull outside the cranial cavity or by alterations in the muscles of the neck and jaw, in the eyes, or in the sinuses.

Sense Organs   *Refractive Errors of the Eye*   The eye receives light through the curved cornea and lens. If properly shaped, these parts focus the light sharply on the retina, particularly on the macular area. An improperly shaped cornea or an eyeball that is too long or too short can make a sharp focus impossible. A spectacle or contact lens can correct such defects. The ciliary body adjusts the shape of the eye's own lens to focus on near and far objects. Impulses from the brain, initiated automatically or consciously, bring about this focusing.

The lens of the aging eye becomes less elastic and variable and the muscles of the ciliary body probably also weaken. The result is a loss of ability to focus on near objects, which most people experience during their forties. This loss of near focus is corrected by lenses, usually bifocals. These difficulties that are correctable by lenses are called *refractive errors* or defects, because *refraction* or bending of light is responsible for all focusing.

Defects in the Media   The cornea with its conjunctiva, the aqueous humor, the lens, and the vitreous humor all transmit light to the retina. Normally they are almost perfectly clear and transparent. The *media* can be made opaque by injury or disease to produce *media defects*. The conjunctiva is extremely sensitive, so that most defects there are accompanied by pain. The cornea itself, however, may become cloudy with no symptom except foggy vision. The aqueous humor and vitreous humor become cloudy when some substance like pus or blood gets into them.

This can be painless but often accompanies a painful condition. The lens is the most frequent location of a media defect called a *cataract*. The lens is insensitive, so the cataract is not painful.

Glaucoma   The aqueous humor is secreted into the eye constantly by the ciliary body. It passes through the pupil from the posterior into the anterior chamber and its only exit from the eye is by way of a tiny circular canal system running just where the cornea joins the sclera and iris. Since the eye is a closed globe, anything which blocks removal by way of the canal raises the pressure within the eyeball. This is *glaucoma*. If it rises suddenly, increased pressure causes pain; but there is no pain if the rise is gradual. The high pressure may also injure the cornea, causing it to fog slightly, so that the patient sees colored halos around bright lights. When the pupil enlarges, the iris bunches in the area of the canal and rapidly increases any blockage there. A patient with slight glaucoma then experiences acute pain when he goes into dim light.

Retinal Lesions   The retina, which converts light waves into nerve impulses, is a complex organ, actually an outlying center of the brain. Like the brain, it cannot repair or regenerate itself, so that any destruction causes a permanent defect. Since different parts of the retina receive light from specific parts of the view seen by the eye, it is possible to map the location of a partial retinal injury by determining localized areas of blindness. Each eye has one normal *blind spot* corresponding to the optic disc or nerve head. This area, made up of optic nerve fibers and central blood vessels, interrupts the retina. When glaucoma stretches the retina by expanding the eyeball, this normal blind spot enlarges and the optic disc can be seen to cup posteriorly.

The Ear   The ear converts sound waves into nerve impulses and simultaneously senses the position or motion of the head. It is a double sense organ: the *auditory* part is concerned with hearing, the *vestibular* with balance.

Sound waves in the air pass through the external auditory canal to set the tympanic membrane in motion. This, in turn, vibrates the small chain of three bones in the middle ear, and the other end of the chain moves a small membranous window to the inner ear. Anything that interferes with the passage of sound waves and vibrations up to this point causes partial or complete deafness of the *conductive type*. Some causes of conductive deafness, especially with an acute onset, are painful. Others are not.

Each eustachian tube normally opens during the pharyngeal movements of swallowing. This briefly connects the air in the nasopharynx with that in the middle ear, so that the pressure is the same on both sides of the tympanic membrane. If the pressure of the surrounding air suddenly increases or decreases, that in the middle ear will not change as quickly, so that the tympanic membrane bulges painfully outward or inward and transmits sound waves poorly. Similarly, fluid under pressure in the middle ear can cause pain and conductive deafness.

The true auditory organ lies bathed in fluid within the spiral cochlear part of the inner ear. Vibration of that fluid by the bony chain at the window sets a specific part of the sense organ in motion, and this part initiates a nerve impulse. The impulse then passes over the auditory nerve to the brainstem. Any defect of the auditory organ, the nerve, or its connections within the brain causes *sensorineural deafness*. Usually such defects are present from birth or develop slowly and painlessly.

The vestibule which houses the sensory organs of balance lies close to and connects with the cochlea. The vestibular apparatus itself consists of two fluid-filled parts, the *semicircular canals*—which convert head motion in any direction into nerve impulses—and a system of tiny chambers. Sense organs in these chambers initiate nerve impulses which reflect the head's position at rest. The nerve impulses from the vestibule pass over a separate part of the auditory nerve to the brain.

Disturbances of the vestibular apparatus cause true vertigo. This is often so severe that the patient cannot stand and frequently vomits. Since the vestibule and cochlea are connected, there is usually some disturbance of hearing at least during the episodes of vertigo. The disturbance may be a sensation of sound (*tinnitus*), partial deafness, or both.

Olfactory Organ   The sense of smell is located in the olfactory organ, a patch of specialized mucous membrane located on the ethmoid bone at the most superior part of the nasal cavity. After the sensory cells have converted the airborne chemicals' reaction into nerve impulses, these pass through the olfactory nerves to the brain. Any obstruction of the nasal cavity, defect of the olfactory organ, or injury to the ethmoid bone through which the nerves pass can impair the sense of smell.

Taste Organs   The true organs of taste are located chiefly on the dorsum of the tongue and detect only chemicals dissolved in water. They respond by creating nerve impulses to only four categories of substances—sour (or acid), salt, sweet, and bitter. All other "flavors" are detected by their odor, which can reach the olfactory organ by passing through the oro- and nasopharynx. The nerve impulses of true taste reach the brainstem through the facial nerve from the anterior two-thirds and through the glossopharyngeal nerve from the posterior third of the tongue.

EXERCISES

1 Locate the external and anterior jugular veins on your own neck. Spread your thumb on one side of your neck and your fingers on the other so that all four veins are covered. Press inward gently so that you occlude these superficial veins where they cross the sternomastoid muscles. You should see all four veins bulge. Describe what you felt after 30 to 60 sec of occlusion.

   Note: Be careful to press so that you do not block the carotid arteries. You should still be able to palpate your frontal or temporal pulse.

2 List as many fully automatic bodily functions as you can. Consider only those that occur within or every few seconds. If your list were really complete you would have covered most of the motor responses of the autonomic nervous system. You would, however, include some reflexes that did not involve that part of the nervous system.

3 If equipment is available, map the normal blind spot of your partner's eyes. Your instructor will have to show you how to do this.

4 Stare fixedly at a wide, light-colored, or white surface in good but not strong light. After a few moments you will probably see *floaters,* faint little objects which usually drift downward. These are normal—actually bits of cells in the aqueous humor—and hence "media defects." Nervous patients often report them as "spots before the eyes" and get anxious about them.

5 With your eyes closed, press fairly firmly on your eyeballs. You should see faint irregular spots or stars. These are the retina's response to pressure since the only sensation the retina can transmit is sight, even though the stimulus is not light.

6 Hold your nose closed and stop breathing while tasting a cola drink, plain soda water, and cool coffee. What is the flavor? Now repeat, breathing normally. What is the actual taste of each?

7 Try to detect the odor of a small piece of onion or an open tobacco package held about 3 in from your nose while respiring quietly at the usual rate. After a few moments away from the stimulus, repeat this, but sniff. What makes the sniff more efficient?

9-2 NOSE AND MOUTH

Nose *Normal Nasal Function*   The complex turbinates within the nasal cavity break up the airflow and increase the surface with which the air comes into contact. This surface is covered with mucous membrane which is richly supplied with blood and actively secretes a watery liquid containing sticky mucus. The tears also drain down the tear ducts into the nose and further increase the water there. The nose, then, is well equipped to add water to dry inhaled air and to warm it with heat from the blood. The watery fluid and mucus also trap particles in the air, and the narrow spaces bar inhaled larger objects from passing to the lungs.

   The nasal mucous membrane is covered with microscopic, whiplike *cilia* which beat quickly in one direction with a slow recovery in the opposite. This beat is synchronized so that waves of *ciliary motion* sweep over the surface, moving in one direction the sticky mucus with its trapped particles. In the anterior part of the nose the waves move the material toward the nostrils; in other parts they sweep it posteriorly into the pharynx, where it can be "hawked up" and spit out or swallowed.

Nasal Obstruction The mechanism works very well unless the mucous membrane is damaged. It usually responds to injury—even from so simple a cause as cold air—by swelling with increased blood and then with *edema* fluid. Its glands secrete more water and more mucus, but its cilia become less effective. The result is nasal obstruction and *coryza* or runny nose.

Nasal Sinuses The sinuses, which apparently serve chiefly to lighten the facial and cranial bones, also have cilia that move secretions to and through the sinus opening into the nose. A swollen nasal mucous membrane around these openings can block them, so that fluid accumulates within the sinuses. The sinuses also are largely responsible, with the nasal cavity, for the resonance of the voice. When they are blocked off or the nose is obstructed, the voice becomes duller. What we usually call "talking through the nose" is really talking with the nose blocked shut.

Nasopharynx The nasopharynx really functions as the posterior part of the nose. Its lymphoid tissue, including the adenoids, apparently serves to protect the lungs against invading germs. Unfortunately, lymphoid tissue swells easily and in young children can obstruct the flow of air. The eustachian tube ends amid this lymphoid tissue, and any swelling around the opening can block the tube.

Mouth Breathing The mouth has tough mucous membrane which has no cilia. While moist, the oral cavity cannot add water and heat to inhaled air as the nose does. Mouth breathing, especially in dry air, can dry the pharynx painfully and in very cold air can chill the larynx and trachea painfully.

Eating and Drinking The mouth's chief functions are in eating, drinking, and speaking. In drinking, the mouth serves as little more than a passive tube. The tongue does serve as the piston of a pump when it lowers to suck liquid into the mouth, but no sucking is really necessary to pour fluid into the pharynx.

Eating solid food, of course, is a more active process. Chewing requires movement of the jaws but also of the tongue, which turns, pushes, and molds the bite during the crushing action of the teeth. Equally important, especially with dry foods such as crackers, the watery saliva flowing from the parotid, submaxillary, and submandibular glands moistens the mass. When the mass is ready to swallow, the tongue pushes it upward against the hard palate. The fauces open as the mass passes through and then close while the soft palate rises to shut off the nasopharynx, so that the mass slides through the oropharynx, pushed along by contractions of the pharyngeal muscles.

Speech In speaking, the *voiced sounds* such as the vowels are shaped and given form by the tongue, teeth, and lips. *Unvoiced sounds* like "f," "s," and "ch" are produced by the same parts as exhaled air passes over them. A person without vocal cords can say "f" but not "v," or "s" but not "z." He can only whisper. One with a paralyzed tongue can make essentially no meaningful speech sounds, and one with paralyzed lips cannot enunicate the "f," "m," "p," and other so-called *labials.*

Pharyngeal Crossing All speech requires exhaled air, and this air comes from the larynx through the pharynx. Inhaled and exhaled air from and to the nose must also travel between the nose above and the larynx. Food, liquids, and vomitus also pass through the pharynx between the anteriorly placed mouth and the posteriorly placed esophagus. Their paths then cross that of the air in the lower part of the pharynx.

If air passes into the stomach, no real harm results. If fluid or food gets into the larynx and trachea, however, the results are distressing and can even be fatal. There is therefore an elaborate mechanism to assure that air goes to the larynx and liquids or solids to the esophagus. This mechanism normally operates automatically by reflex action with each swallow.

Swallowing When the act of swallowing begins, air movement—in or out—stops. Muscles to and from the hyoid bone in the neck contract to pull the larynx upward and forward. This has two important consequences. It causes the lidlike epiglottis, which has it hinge anteriorly, to move its tip downward and close the top of the larynx. Simultaneously, the forward movement of the larynx widens the posterior part of the laryngopharynx, so that a funnellike entrance forms to the esophagus. Contractions of the pharyngeal muscles behind the food mass, and less effectively behind a swallow of liquid, slide it downward over the epiglottis, past the larynx, and into the esophagus. The throat muscles then relax, the larynx drops downward and posteriorly, the epiglottis swings open, and air can pass once more.

Everyone is familiar with "getting something down the wrong way," choking on food or liquid when these enter the larynx. This happens when some respiratory action—breathing, speaking, laughing, or coughing—is not interrupted during swallowing.

There is a greater threat when liquid is poured down the throat of an unconscious or paralyzed person whose *swallowing reflexes* are not functioning. The act of *gagging* prepares the laryngopharynx for the act of vomiting just as though the person were going to swallow. There is grave danger when an unconscious person or one without throat reflexes vomits.

EXERCISES

1 What is the source of a postnasal drip? How does the drip get to the oropharynx?

2 Breathe vigorously through your nose for several minutes. What is the sensation in your pharynx? Then pant rather vigorously through your mouth for several minutes. What is the pharyngeal sensation? What is your immediate action when you stop panting?

3 Take a mouthful of water and feel the hyoid bone while you swallow a sip. Then feel the larynx while you swallow another. While your partner's stomach is empty, place one hand on his larynx and with the other gently touch the back of his pharynx with a tongue depressor. What happens to his larynx? This is the *gag reflex*. Of what value is it in examining an unconscious or paralyzed patient?

9-3 CARDIORESPIRATORY SYSTEMS

Lungs and Airways *Processes of Respiration* Respiration involves much more than the act of breathing—the *respiratory movements*. In basic terms, respiration is the production of energy from foodstuffs, and this process must go on in every part of the body. It involves the use of *oxygen* to destroy the foodstuffs, liberate their energy, and in the process produce carbon dioxide and water. The body has other ways to produce energy and forms other chemicals in the process, but *oxidation* using oxygen is by far the most common.

Oxygen and carbon dioxide are both gases that can be obtained from or discharged into the air. Evaporated water can also be removed from the body by air. The lungs then serve as a means by which the body can obtain essential oxygen from the air and dispose of carbon dioxide along with some water vapor.

Gas Exchange The lungs themselves use only a fraction of the oxygen taken from the air. The greatest part is distributed throughout the body by the blood, which also brings most of the carbon dioxide and water to the lungs. The alveoli have exceedingly thin walls in which run the capillaries from the pulmonary arteries. Oxygen and carbon dioxide pass through the thin layers of capillary wall and alveolar wall by the relatively simple process of *diffusion*. A gas diffuses from an area of higher concentration to one of lower. So oxygen diffuses from air with its higher content into blood, which arrives at the lung with a lower concentration. The arriving blood contains more carbon dioxide than the air does, and so that gas diffuses into the alveolar air.

Lung Movements Respiratory movements simply move "used" air out of the alveoli and "new" air into them. Several factors are important in carrying out this exchange of air. The thin alveolar walls contain microscopic fibers which make the spongy lung elastic. They also secrete a detergentlike substance—a *surface-active agent*—which keeps their moist walls from collapsing and sticking together. Because of these factors the lungs tend to stay somewhat ballooned out into the pleural spaces.

These "spaces" play a significant part in expanding the lungs. Actually the pleura covering the lung and that lining the chest are in contact. At most a microscopic layer of fluid separates them, so that normally the pleural space is a potential rather than an actual one. Its presence, however, allows the lung surface to slide along the chest wall smoothly without ever pulling away from it during respiratory movements. The pleura has sensory nerve endings for pain, the alveoli do not.

Airways There are pain endings in the larynx and trachea, especially where it divides into the two major bronchi. All these airways serve two essential functions—to change the air in the alveoli and to remove material from the lungs and air passages. This removal is accomplished in three ways:

1 The tiny bronchioles and the bronchi, trachea, and larynx are all lined with mucous membrane whose glands secrete a watery lubricant containing mucus. The membrane also has cilia and these beat in waves, moving the mucus and any foreign matter it traps upward into the pharynx. The small amount usually produced is then swallowed.

2 The bronchioles also have muscular walls, and these constrict slowly one level after the other to produce a milking motion called *peristalsis*. This movement can force material upward and so provides a second mechanism for removal.

3 The third way is by coughing. A cough probably cannot move material until it reaches the bronchi, trachea, or larynx, since it depends upon the explosive rush of a considerable volume of air. The action is truly reflex—the *cough reflex*—set off by the sensation of some material in the airway. The epiglottis closes and a forceful expiration begins. Air cannot leave the alveoli, however, and so pressure increases. When the epiglottis then flies open, air rushes under pressure from the alveoli and forces the material upward along the airway until eventually it enters the pharynx.

Breathing Breathing itself is an automatic action but one which can be controlled by conscious effort. Automatic control is exercised by a center in the brainstem. This center receives nerve impulses from sensory organs which respond to changes in oxygen and in carbon dioxide in the arterial blood. If oxygen falls or if the blood becomes more *acid,* as carbon dioxide will cause it to, the center automatically increases respiratory effort.

Except during extreme exertion, the body normally uses only a small part of its ability to deliver oxygen. The resulting *respiratory reserve* is an important safety factor, since a person can survive only briefly without adequate oxygen.

The body can increase its use of the respiratory reserve in various ways. The rate of breathing can increase, and so can the depth of each breath. Only a small proportion of alveoli receive fresh air during quiet respiratory movement; deep breathing uses more alveoli and so allows more surface for gaseous diffusion. Similarly, an increased flow of blood through the alveolar walls makes for more gaseous exchange. The body can also call up reserves of *red blood cells,* which are the blood constituents carrying oxygen. In an extreme situation, blood can be shunted away from less critical areas and into vital ones which need oxygen more urgently.

There are slower processes which operate when there is a continuing high demand for oxygen. The respiratory muscles become more powerful, the lungs' capacity increases somewhat, the heart improves its ability to deliver blood, and red blood cells are produced at a higher rate. The kidneys also increase their output of carbon dioxide, which they too excrete as soluble salts.

Respiratory Defects Obviously many things can go wrong in so complicated and variable a mechanism. Probably the simplest is *obstruction* of the airway. If this occurs in the pharynx, larynx, or trachea, both lungs are affected and the extreme is *strangulation.* Obstruction of a bronchiole or even of a bronchus is not fatal but the lung beyond it collapses and becomes functionless, the condition called *atelectasis.*

Alveoli themselves can fill with fluid, as they do in pulmonary edema or pneumonia. Then too, the alveolar walls can thicken and bar gaseous exchange even though the alveoli themselves contain air.

Alveoli can be destroyed outright, leaving cavities or scars without respiratory function. They can also enlarge or join together, creating oversized air sacs. Simple geometry indicates that many small sacs will have more *surface area* than a single large one of the same volume. Thus in *emphysema* the lung volume actually increases while enlarged but less numerous alveoli develop. Even so, the surface area available for gaseous exchange decreases.

In *bronchial asthma,* the alveoli grow larger during an attack because the muscles of the bronchiolar walls contract when the patient tries to exhale. This partially traps the air and each succeeding inspiration balloons out the alveoli a little more. The ballooning in asthma and in emphysema reduces the lungs' elasticity, their ability to follow the chest wall during respiratory movement. Atelectasis has somewhat the same effect and so does *fibrosis,* the development of microscopic scars throughout the lung. This further reduces the ability to breathe.

Changes in the pulmonary circulation can cause respiratory defects. Plugging of a large pulmonary artery can result in the death of an entire lobe. Obstruction of a smaller artery promptly reduces the production of alveolar surface-active material, and the alveoli of that lung segment collapse in atelectasis.

Equally drastic at times is some impediment to the blood's return through the pulmonary vein. When this occurs, the alveolar capillaries become *engorged* and reduce the lungs' elasticity. The engorged capillaries also lose fluid which crosses into the alveoli to produce pulmonary edema.

Pleural Disturbances   An injury or disease of the lung can allow air to escape into the pleural cavity. A chest wall opening can also introduce air. When gas can enter and leave the cavity with each respiratory cycle, the resulting *pneumothorax* allows the lung to collapse to the limit of its elasticity. That lung no longer functions, but the opposite, normal one does.

A defect in the lung or chest wall that allows air to enter the pleural cavity more readily than it allows it to escape causes a *tension pneumothorax.* In this more serious condition, the lung is squeezed down by the increasing pressure, and the mediastinum with its contents shift into the opposite side of the chest. The opposite lung therefore loses some of its ability to exchange gases.

Edema fluid, pus, and blood in the pleural space produce more or less collapse of the underlying lung. Edema fluid can be absorbed and leave the pleura intact. Pus and blood, however, frequently leave scar tissue when they are resorbed. This scar, if thin or small, simply plasters the two layers of pleura together and limits the ability of the lung to move within the chest. The resulting loss of respiratory reserve is small. If the scar is thick and extensive, however, it can prevent movements of the chest wall and diaphragm, a much more serious defect.

Muscular and Skeletal Defects   Paralysis of the muscles in the chest wall and diaphragm can also interfere with these movements. While spastic or flaccid paralysis can occur, the diaphragm almost always has the flaccid type. Abdominal pressure then pushes the motionless sheet of muscle and tendon high into the thorax, further reducing the lungs' ability to function.

Even skeletal changes can impair respiratory movements. The distortion in kyphosis and scoliosis restricts the ribs' mobility, as can changes in the joints of the rib with the spine and sternum.

EXERCISES

1 If equipment is available, measure the *tidal volume* by breathing quietly into a spirometer. Then measure *vital capacity*, the total air that can be moved at a single maximal respiratory effort. The difference between the two gives a crude estimate of the respiratory reserve. What would be the result if the two were identical or nearly so?

2 If available, examine chest x-rays of simple pneumothorax, tension pneumothorax, atelectasis, and diaphragmatic paralysis. Pay particular attention to the displacement of the otherwise uninvolved parts.

3 Observe someone giving a hard cough. What is the first action you can observe? What evidence is there of increased pressure within the thorax? How long does that pressure last?

4 Breathe in and out several times through a long tube at your mouth and with your nose closed. The paper tube from a roll of paper toweling will do, a longer one is better. Now inhale without the tube but always exhale through it. Breathe more forcefully than normal. What you have done is to increase resistance in your airway with the tube. Which maneuver—inhaling and exhaling or exhaling only through the tube—was more uncomfortable?

5 Inhale and exhale repeatedly into a paper bag held over your nose and mouth. What happens to your respiration? What do you feel? You are duplicating the condition in a patient with impaired gaseous exchange.

Heart and Circulation   *Heartbeat*   Circulation of the blood, like respiration, automatically continues and adjusts to changing demands. The heart can beat without any prompting, but the autonomic nervous system largely controls its responses to varying requirements for blood.

Spontaneous and properly timed contractions of the heart depend upon a specialized part of the myocardium forming the *conduction system* (see Figure 9-1). This consists of a controlling *sinoauricular (SA) node* located in the right atrial wall, a separate *auriculoventricular (AV) node* near the tricuspid valve, and a branching *bundle* of specialized myocardium extending from the AV node along the septum between the ventricles. Branches of this bundle run just under the endocardium to the ventricular walls.

Normally the SA node rhythmically produces an *impulse* which spreads like a wave through the myocardium of the right atrium and then through that of the left atrium. When the impulse reaches it, the muscle contracts briefly in atrial systole and then relaxes in diastole.

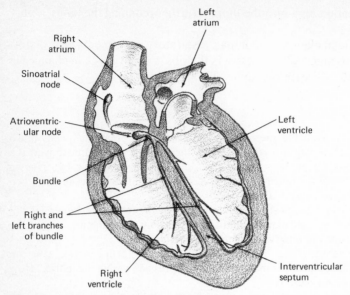

Figure 9-1   Conduction system of heart.

As it spreads through the right atrial wall, the impulse reaches the AV node. Here it is delayed for a fraction of a second and then spreads quickly along the bundle to reach the ventricular myocardium. The brief delay allows atrial systole to occur before the more powerful ventricular myocardium contracts in systole. The impulse travels rapidly over the bundle, but it reaches some parts of the ventricular wall sooner than it gets to others. The result is a very rapid, wavelike contraction that efficiently milks the blood into the aorta and the pulmonary artery.

Arrhythmias   In this normal course of events, the SA node is the *cardiac pacemaker.* The node can fail to function, its impulses may become too rapid and chaotic, or impulses may fail to spread normally over the atrium. The heart, however, has a built-in safety device. The AV node will initiate impulses and become the pacemaker if it does not receive impulses from the SA node. The ventricular myocardium itself can initiate impulses if none arrive through the AV node. These substitute pacemakers produce less rhythmic impulses than the SA node and they spread over abnormal routes, so that the resulting systole is not fully efficient.

The irregular beats introduced by a substitute pacemaker provide one cause of *cardiac arrhythmia.* Too rapid, too slow, or irregular impulses from the SA node are other causes. These SA nodal arrhythmias may be severe enough to prevent effective atrial systoles, but nonfunctioning atria do not fatally handicap the heart. Ventricular arrhythmias more seriously interfere with function and are fatal if severe. Again, the heart has a built-in safety feature. If impulses from the SA node arrive too frequently at the AV node, this node will accept only some of them. The remainder are *blocked,* and those that reach the ventricle are far enough apart to allow a slower, more effective rate.

Although the SA and AV nodes can work effectively under uniform conditions without outside influences, the autonomic nervous system and the hormones adrenalin and noradrenalin normally affect them. Nervous impulses from the sympathetic nerves and adrenalin speed the heart rate; parasympathetic nerve impulses and noradrenalin slow it. These provide the body's automatic control of the heart rate, and some drugs, particularly those mimicking actions of the autonomic nervous system, can alter the rate as well.

Cardiac Function   Within limits, the amount of blood delivered by the heart into the aorta and pulmonary artery during each minute increases as the beat quickens. The amount delivered also depends upon the volume of blood driven forward by each beat. This volume, in turn, changes with several factors. For example, too rapid a rate may not allow enough time in diastole for the ventricles to fill completely, and a reduced volume is delivered by the following systole.

A weak myocardium, incapable of contracting effectively, is a more common cause of reduced volume per stroke. The normal heart has a considerable *cardiac reserve,* the capacity for doing more work than is usually required. An increased demand, as in physical exertion, then can prompt the heart to increase its rate as well as the volume of blood delivered per beat. The heart *compensates* for the increased load put on it.

Heart Failure   A weakened myocardium can no longer meet the demands made on it. With slight weakness, exertion will make it exceed its reserve; greater weakness may make it inadequate even during rest. The heart is *decompensated* and the patient is in *heart failure.*

Under certain circumstances one ventricle may fail before the other, and for a time the patient is in right-heart or in left-heart failure. A ventricle which fails cannot move blood rapidly enough, overfills or dilates, and then no longer can empty the atrium which supplies it. The pressure rises in that atrium and is transmitted backward along the veins emptying into it. These veins distend under the pressure, but eventually the pressure rises in the capillaries drained by the veins. One result is that the watery components of the blood are forced by the pressure into the surrounding tissues. This is the source of *cardiac edema.*

When the right ventricle fails, it dilates and pressure rises in the right atrium, in the venae cavae, and in the systemic veins; that is, pressure rises in all vessels not draining the lungs. Gravity further increases the pressure within the veins and capillaries, and the lowest parts of the body are the first affected. A person who is up and about develops *ankle edema* and less obvious edema of the feet. As heart failure progresses and venous pressure rises, the edema spreads upward.

When the left ventricle fails, it dilates and pressure rises in the left atrium, in the pulmonary veins, and in the lung capillaries. These capillaries distend so that the lung becomes less elastic, respiratory movements are impaired, and gaseous exchange is decreased. Watery components of the blood leak into the alveoli to form *pulmonary edema.* Since gravity adds to the pressure, this appears first in the lowest parts, the lung bases in an upright position.

The resulting difficulty in breathing becomes worse when the patient lies down, and he may be forced to sit up in order to breathe. As left-heart failure progresses, he becomes increasingly short of breath and eventually is cyanotic as well.

Another factor contributes to cardiac edema. During heart failure, the kidneys no longer excrete salt normally. Much of the retained salt leaks from the blood with the edema fluid. This apparently forces the body to retain water, and the result is that patients in heart failure gain weight which is water rather than fat or flesh.

The patient in heart failure usually has both ventricles decompensated. As a result, the changes of both right- and left-heart failure occur together.

Hypertension Decompensation and heart failure have many causes, since they can result from anything which weakens the myocardium directly or which places too heavy a burden on it over prolonged periods. One common cause of such an increased load is *chronic hypertension.*

Several conditions can cause hypertension, but in most cases the ultimate cause is unknown. This common disease is *essential hypertension* and the problem is known to center in the smallest arteries, the arterioles.

These arterioles, lying between the arteries and the capillaries, have muscular walls. The muscle contracts, narrowing or constricting the arteriole, to shut off the blood flow in capillaries arising from it. Each body region and organ has thousands of tiny arterioles with several capillaries arising from each. Selective constriction of various arterioles is the body's way of shunting blood from inactive parts to those that most need it. This normal process helps maintain the diastolic blood pressure at the usual level, but too few arterioles constrict at any one time to raise the diastolic pressure above 90 mm of mercury.

In essential hypertension constriction occurs in a very large number of arterioles simultaneously and the diastolic pressure increases. The body's response is to raise the systolic pressure so that blood is forced through the narrowed vessels.

Pumping blood at high pressure requires more cardiac work. Initially the heart compensates and develops a thicker, more powerful left ventricular myocardium. Eventually, often after years, the load becomes too great or something weakens the overworked myocardium. It dilates and decompensation follows.

Arterial Changes Another common cause of hypertension is *atherosclerosis* or *arteriosclerosis,* hardening of the arteries. In this disease the arterioles do not constrict abnormally and so the diastolic pressure may remain well below 90 mm of mercury. Rather, changes in the walls of the arteries force the heart to increase the systolic pressure.

Atherosclerosis stiffens artery walls by replacing material that is normally elastic, much like fairly thin rubber tubing, with stiffer inelastic substances. The normally smooth lining of the artery also changes as fatty materials are laid down in *plaques* which intrude on the bore or *lumen* of the arteries. Smaller deposits of fatty material roughen the lining and make it more difficult for blood to flow over the surfaces. In smaller arteries, the rough wall may prompt a clot to form and even to *occlude* or shut off the vessel. Occlusion, if complete, deprives a body part of blood, and this *infarction* results in death of the bloodless part.

There are causes of occlusion besides arterial clots, and the infarction can occur in many parts. This *cerebral infarction* or stroke is rather common in atherosclerosis. *Pulmonary infarction* occurs for other reasons.

An artery can be narrowed so much that it is unable to deliver enough blood even though not completely occluded. The result is a relative lack of blood or *ischemia* in a part, and this is most apt to be evident when the demand for blood and its oxygen is great.

Coronary Artery Disease The changes are very common in the heart itself when the coronary arteries are atherosclerotic. Narrowing of the *lumen* or bore leads to *myocardial ischemia.* The result is very like a cramp and the pain produced is *angina pectoris,* usually a crushing sensation in the chest radiating down the left arm and into the neck if severe. It appears during exertion and is relieved rather promptly by rest.

Coronary occlusion with *myocardial infarction* often follows a period of recurring ischemia and angina. It too is usually painful, but the pain persists for many minutes even with rest, and the patient may go into *shock* with very low blood pressure.

Coronary atherosclerosis, even without symptoms of ischemia or occlusion, can deprive the myocardium of blood. This can weaken the heart enough to cause heart failure and is a common cause of decompensation in the elderly.

Aneurysms The arterial walls can be weakened by several diseases, including atherosclerosis. Usually the weak area is limited to a fairly small section of the vessel but may involve the entire abdominal aorta or a long section of the thoracic aorta. The weakened wall bulges out to form an *aneurysm*, which may be saclike or long and spindle-shaped. The danger lies in the weak wall's giving way completely, and the internal bleeding of a *ruptured aneurysm* is often rapidly fatal.

Venous Changes Arterial blood moves along in spurts, forced by the high pressure produced by ventricular systole. Venous blood flows more smoothly toward the heart, pushed along by arterial pressure forcing blood through the capillaries and sucked along by negative pressure in the thoracic cavity during inspiration. Much of its movement is from a sort of "milking" action during contractions of the body's muscles. Larger veins outside the trunk have valves at intervals along their length and these allow flow only toward the heart. Because the flow is relatively slow, clots or *thrombi* form more often within veins than within arteries. This is especially true in the legs, when bed rest deprives the venous blood of the "milking" action.

A venous thrombus can break loose to become an *embolus*, a clot that drifts with the blood flow until it reaches a vessel too small to pass. Since blood from the leg veins reaches the heart through larger and larger vessels, an embolus from there moves through the right side of the heart and enters the pulmonary artery. There it plugs a large or small branch, causing *pulmonary embolism* and infarction.

The veins' thin walls allow them to distend easily, and their valves may become ineffective. A permanently distended vein is a *varicosity*, most commonly seen as varicose veins and hemorrhoids. Less striking are networks of distended small veins in the skin of the legs.

Capillary Changes Capillaries are not only the smallest blood vessels but by far the most numerous. They connect arterioles and veins in every part and carry out all exchanges between blood and tissues upon which life depends. Pulmonary capillaries allow gaseous exchange with the air; systemic capillaries permit gaseous exchange between blood and the tissues. In this, oxygen leaves the blood and carbon dioxide enters. *Oxygenated* blood in systemic arteries is a light, bright red; venous blood is a duller, darker, slightly bluish red after it has given up its oxygen. Blood moving unusually slowly through capillaries gives up unusually large amounts of oxygen and becomes venous. This is one common cause of *cyanosis*, bluing of the lips, nail beds, and mucous membranes.

Blood can also clot in capillaries. This causes little harm if only a few are involved, but the damage is great if the clotting is extensive.

Lymphatic Changes   Lymphatic vessels have a flow in only one direction—toward the great veins and the heart. They have valves as do veins, and the lymph flow is driven by much the same forces as those moving venous blood. Lymph forms chiefly from the watery components of the blood when these leak through the capillary walls. Much of the water reenters the capillary, but some remains in the tissues until it enters tiny lymphatic vessels and is milked along toward the heart.

At intervals along these vessels the lymph passes through a sort of filter in a *lymph node.* These nodes constitute one of the body's defenses against invading bacteria and other harmful material. One response of the nodes to such an invasion is to swell, often painfully.

Lymph does not clot, but abnormal changes in the lymph nodes or blockage of the lymphatic vessels can prevent it from leaving some part. This increases the lymphatic pressure and prevents removal of water from that part. The result is *lymphatic edema,* usually more constant than cardiac edema which can come and go.

Other Changes in Vessels   The blood picks up most digested foodstuffs from the wall of the small intestine and carries it to the liver through the hepatic portal vein. During this absorption, the liver capillaries give up much of this nutrition to be stored in the liver. At other times, foodstuffs enter the blood from the liver to maintain a constant supply.

Anything—usually scar tissue—which blocks the hepatic capillaries increases pressure in the hepatic portal veins and interferes with the absorption of food. It also forces blood to bypass the liver. A few connections exist directly between the portal vein and branches of the inferior vena cava around the anus, the lower esophagus, and over the abdomen. All these dilate to form hemorrhoids and delicate *esophageal varicose veins* when the liver is badly scarred. Both of these are apt to bleed.

Blood going to the kidneys returns directly to the vena cava, but during its time in the kidney the blood gives up water, salts, and various other substances—usually waste materials. Any interruption to this flow reduces kidney function, and interference with the arterial flow to the kidney causes one form of hypertension as well.

Changes in Heart Valves   The most common defects within the heart involve the valves. The *leaves,* or effective parts of the valves, are thin but very tough. To be fully effective when closed, the leaves depend upon a tough ring of fiber around the valve opening. Disease can narrow this opening by tightening the ring or by fusing together the leaves so that they cannot fall back completely when the valve opens. This narrowing is *valvular stenosis* (see Figure 9-2).

Disease can also weaken the fibrous ring so that it distends, or the valve leaves can be so distorted that they do not form a tight fit when the valve closes. Either change allows blood to leak backward, a result called *regurgitation,* as the consequence of *valvular insufficiency.*

A significant stenosis increases the work of the heart chamber which the valve empties, since systole must force blood past the narrowed opening. Regurgitation increases the work of the chamber the valve empties because systole there must repump the blood which leaked back. An insufficient mitral or tricuspid valve also increases the work of the left or right ventricle because it must pump hard enough to deliver blood to the aorta as well as forcing blood backward into the atrium.

Each valvular lesion produces a different change in the circulation and so yields distinct symptoms and signs. To consider a single example, *mitral insufficiency* allows regurgitation into the left atrium with each

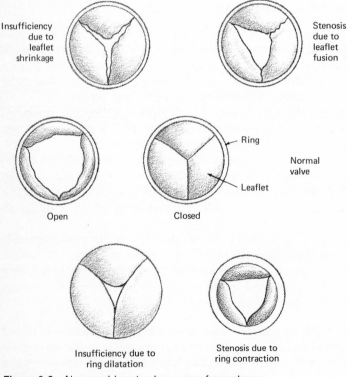

Figure 9-2   Abnormal heart valves, seen from above.

systole. On physical examination, this produces a relatively high-pitched, blowing, holosystolic murmur which often includes S_1 and S_2. It is loudest at the cardiac apex and is transmitted toward the axilla. A severe defect may also produce a palpable systolic thrill at the apex. If enough blood regurgitates, it dilates the left atrium, and the murmur can be heard over the left side of the back when this occurs.

The left ventricle increases the force of its beat in order to deliver enough blood to the aorta despite the loss from regurgitation. Its myocardium thickens in response, and the PMI may then be displaced to the left as the ventricle enlarges.

Regurgitation raises the pressure in the left atrium, and this, in turn, increases that in the pulmonary veins and capillaries. The capillaries distend, reducing the lung's elasticity and so the pulmonary reserve. The patient may then become somewhat *dyspneic,* or breathless. He usually develops pulmonary edema and rales at the lung bases.

High pressure in the pulmonary veins also forces the right ventricle to beat more forcibly, increasing the pressure in the pulmonary artery. This can lead to thickening of the right ventricular wall.

Eventually the work load may become so great that the heart decompensates. An otherwise healthy heart with only mitral insufficiency may compensate for many years and the patient's only symptoms may be easy fatigability and "palpitations."

Changes in Heart Walls The muscular septum which separates the right from the left side of the heart is not always complete. A hole in it is a *septal defect* and can connect the two atria or the two ventricles. In either place it can produce a murmur and symptoms.

Pressure is higher on the left side of the heart, so that blood leaks through an *interatrial* defect from the left to the right atrium and through an *interventricular* defect from the left to the right ventricle. This imposes an increased load on the heart and causes as well some oxygenated blood to recycle through the lungs.

The myocardium of the atria and ventricles shows other changes. An increased work load causes increased thickness and strength, a condition called *ventricular hypertrophy,* since it occurs in the ventricles. Congestive failure with myocardial weakness causes *ventricular dilatation,* a sort of generalized ballooning out of the walls. *Atrial dilatation* occurs more readily when anything raises the pressure in the thinner-walled chamber.

Localized bulging as a *ventricular aneurysm* appears when something weakens a patch of myocardium. The usual cause is myocardial infarction which, on healing, can leave a weaker area of scar replacing the destroyed muscle.

EXERCISES

1   If a model is available to show the conducting system of the heart, identify the
    SA and AV nodes with the bundles coming from the latter. Trace the course of
    the cardiac impulse over this system and explain what action occurs as the
    impulse reaches each part of the myocardium.
2   List the forces involved in moving blood and lymph through the circulatory
    system. Which two of these forces are most easily influenced for the body as a
    whole? Devise a way to demonstrate each of these.
3   In a subject whose arm has little fat, occlude the veins until they fill. If you
    look carefully on the flexor aspect of the forearm, you will see that small
    dilatations are present along the veins. Each of these is just proximal to a
    valve. Occlude the vein distal to one of these valves with your finger and with
    another "milk" the blood proximally past the valve. The blood moved past the
    valve should remain there and the vein distal to it may remain collapsed until
    you remove your occluding finger.
4   Why do the feet of normal people swell when they have been standing on them
    with little motion all day? Why does a healthy soldier faint if kept standing
    motionless at attention for a long period? What circulatory advantage does a
    patient have when he lies in bed?

9-4 DIGESTIVE SYSTEM

The digestive system reduces food to small particles, alters it chemically,
makes much of it soluble, transfers the resultant foodstuffs to the blood,
and disposes of the unused portion. It has, however, further functions in
storing foodstuffs, modifying body wastes, and removing or rendering
harmless poisonous materials. The latter functions are those of the liver.

Stomach   *Muscular Actions of the Upper Digestive System*   Food
and liquids enter the body through the mouth and traverse the hollow
digestive tract. Its muscular walls extend from pharynx to anus and, by
contracting, move the contents along.

Liquids immediately and solids after chewing are swallowed, calling
into play the muscles of the pharynx and esophagus. Characteristic waves
of muscular constriction followed by relaxation, called *peristalsis,* sweep
from the mouth toward the stomach. The stomach is guarded by the
muscular valve, the *cardia,* which relaxes and opens to receive the
contents of the esophagus. Once food is in the stomach, that organ begins
peristalsis, but a second valve, the *pylorus,* prevents immediate passage
into the duodenum. The result is a thorough churning of the stomach's
contents.

Gastric Functions and Malfunction   The mucous membrane of the
stomach contains microscopic *glands* which produce a strong acid—

hydrochloric acid—and the *gastric enzymes.* These continue the chemical breakdown of the food begun by the saliva. Normally the stomach secretes very little acid or enzymes except when it contains food. It can, however, do so, and this occurs in *peptic ulcer,* so called because one gastric enzyme, *pepsin,* may play a part in destroying some of the gastric mucous membrane.

The stomach has essentially one defense against injurious substances—the act of *vomiting* or *emesis.* Other things can cause vomiting—overloading the stomach, vertigo, even excitement. *Nausea,* the sick sensation that precedes and accompanies vomiting, can occur without emesis, and vomiting can take place without nausea.

Some air is always swallowed with food, and *carbonated beverages* release carbon dioxide into the gastric lumen. Normally the fundus contains a bubble of gas, but when this is too large, the cardia relaxes. The gas is then *belched,* or *eructated,* up the esophagus. Some of the more or less liquid gastric contents may *regurgitate* into the lower esophagus and even into the pharynx during eructation. Since it contains hydrochloric acid this material tastes sour. The cardia may also relax without discharging gas and allow stomach contents to enter the esophagus. The acid can then cause pain.

Abdominal Pain   Pain from the stomach and esophagus often has a "burning" character and, since it is felt high in the LUQ or behind the sternum, is usually called *heartburn* by patients. Sharper pains of a colicky character can arise in the stomach as well.

Colic is the pain most often arising in hollow, muscular organs—the stomach, intestines, bile ducts, ureters, and uterus. It recurs in waves seconds or a few minutes apart as the waves of peristalsis sweep along the hollow tube. When the muscles relax and the pressure in the organ subsides, the pain eases, only to recur with the next contractions, so that the pain "comes and goes."

Overdistended organs can produce a "stuffed" sensation or an aching pain, duller and more constant than colic. Such a pain is the common *stomachache,* although patients may use the term for any type of pain located in the abdomen.

Severe abdominal pain is often accompained by a characteristic sensation that is difficult to describe but sometimes said to be "sinking" or "hollow." It is often associated with nausea and is a component of *visceral pain.* The testes are originally abdominal organs and a blow to them causes visceral pain complete with "hollow" sensation and nausea.

Intestine   *Changes in the Small Intestine*   During normal digestion some food may remain in the stomach for as long as 4 hr or so. Almost immediately, however, gastric contractions move more liquid parts in small spurts through the pyloric valve and into the duodenum.

The normal duodenal contents are *alkaline* enough to neutralize the gastric hydrochloric acid or even to make the food mass alkaline. The *pancreatic secretion* with its enzymes, the bile with its *bile salts,* and the *intestinal secretion* with more enzymes are added in this region and further digest the food.

Peristalsis moves the digesting food through the duodenum, jejunum, and ileum. As the food moves along, the walls of the small intestine, especially of the ileum, absorb the digested foodstuffs, transferring them to the blood. The mass becomes a little thicker as it moves downward because the lower part of the ileum absorbs water rapidly, but it is still rather liquid when it enters the colon.

Bile, whose salts assist in the absorption of fats, contains pigments as well. These pigments normally color the stool brown. When no bile enters the duodenum, the stools are very light tannish or almost white—so-called *acholic stool.*

Gastrointestinal Bleeding   Blood entering the stomach lumen during *gastric hemorrhage* may be vomited. It is bright red if promptly expelled but is digested to a chocolate brown if it remains longer in the stomach.

The blood may, however, pass through the pylorus and be carried into the stool. Blood coming from a hemorrhage in the stomach or upper intestine is digested and appears as a black, tarry mass in the feces. Bleeding near or in the large intestine or in the rectum or anal area remains red. The normal color of the stool varies considerably with the diet, but true *tarry stools—melena—*or bloody ones almost always mean hemorrhage, as true acholic stools mean failure of bile to reach the intestine.

The liver forms bile pigments whether or not they can reach the intestine. When they cannot be secreted into the duodenum, they enter the blood and are deposited in the skin and mucous membranes. Here they produce a characteristic yellow color—*jaundice* or *icterus.* They also appear in the urine, turning it a dark brownish color.

Intestinal Movements   Once material is past the pylorus, the body usually disposes of it in only two ways—by absorbing it into the blood or by moving it along to be evacuated in the feces. This movement toward the anus can be speeded up if the intestinal contents contain potentially harmful material. The small intestine changes the character of its peristalsis, so that it moves the contents almost uniformly and rapidly toward the colon. The strength of the peristaltic contractions increases and the intestine adds water rather than absorbing it. Since the liquid contents are also hurried through the colon, they are evacuated as fluid stool or *diarrhea.* Diarrhea is often preceded by a vague burning discomfort and some colic as the food traverses the small intestine. The griping colic immediately before defecation arises in the colon.

More severe colic arises in the small intestine when there is *intestinal obstruction.* There are several causes of such obstruction, but all more or less block the passage of intestinal contents. Not all "obstruction" is due to mechanical blocking; a paralysis of intestinal peristalsis, called *ileus,* has much the same effect. As a consequence of the *stasis*—or stand-still—of the intestinal contents, gas accumulates, distending the intestine and further increasing the patient's discomfort and pain.

This pain of obstruction is colicky or dully aching. The intestine can also give rise to burning pain. One common cause of this is peptic ulcer. Since gastric acidity contributes to the formation of peptic ulcers, they occur only in the upper part of the duodenum, as *duodenal ulcers.* The burning pain is felt—as with gastric ulcers—just below the sternum "in the pit of the stomach."

Changes in the Colon   The colon receives the food residue as a somewhat fluid mass and then absorbs water, chiefly in the cecum and ascending colon. The resulting *feces* are more or less solid by the time they reach the transverse colon. Some more water is absorbed in the transverse, descending, and sigmoid colon before the feces reach the rectum as a solid mass. Throughout its length the colon moves the feces by peristalsis and, as the sigmoid and rectum fill, this peristalsis increases. This is felt as a mildly uncomfortable *urge to defecate.*

Defecation is brought about in part by peristalsis as the *anal sphincter* relaxes. The peristaltic movement is assisted by conscious contraction of the abdominal wall muscles, with the diaphragm held rigid and the epiglottis closing the larynx. This *bearing down* raises pressure within the abdomen and also in the thorax.

The colon is the prime site for colic—which takes its name from the colon. The griping pain with diarrhea is an example. Almost identical pain occurs if the colon distends with gas or *flatus.* The small and large intestine normally contain gas—some swallowed air, some produced from the intestinal contents. The colon normally disposes of this during defecation or by separately *expelling flatus.*

The feces themselves are a mixture of food residues, bacteria, and various substances such as bile pigments added by the intestines. The mucous membrane lining the gut, especially the colon, adds *mucus.* Bacteria normally grow in the colon, and complete starvation or a completely clear liquid diet does not totally stop defecation. The amount of feces is greatly reduced, since it consists almost exclusively of bacteria, but some is still produced.

The amount of stool produced normally varies with the diet, especially with the amount of indigestible tough plant fiber eaten. A diet containing no vegetables or fruits forms so little residue that the rectum may fill only every 3 or 4 days. A vegetarian diet may fill the rectum two or three times daily. The frequency of defecation then can vary widely and still be normal.

Constipation   The normal consistency of the stool is much less variable. Feces may be soft and only partially formed by passage through the rectum and anus. Or they may be firm and molded. True diarrhea is abnormal, and so is excessively hard stool that contains little water. When feces are so hard that they can be defecated only painfully and with hard straining, the patient is truly constipated. Patients often report "constipation" simply because they do not defecate daily. Constipation medically refers to the consistency of the stool, not to the frequency of its passage.

One consequence of repeatedly increasing the abdominal pressure is the venous dilatation of hemorrhoids. Passage of a constipated stool can tear the anal rim to form a *fissure*. Both hemorrhoids and fissures bleed during defecation, but the bright-red blood streaks the outside of the stool and does not mix with the feces.

Changes in the Liver   The intestine gets rid of its contents by absorbing them as well as by passing them into the feces. Since the blood from the small intestinal capillaries enters the hepatic portal vein, the absorbed material is delivered to the capillaries of the liver. The fats are an exception. They enter the lymphatic vessels and are delivered by the thoracic duct into the left subclavian vein.

The liver is equipped to remove foodstuffs from the blood, to store some of them, and to modify others before returning the products to the blood. It also removes from the blood absorbed materials which otherwise would be more or less poisonous. It changes most of these into relatively safe materials before returning them to the blood for excretion by the kidneys. The liver stores a few unsafe materials but more often secretes them into the bile, usually in modified form.

The liver is a gland and secretes *bile* chiefly as an aid to digestion. The complex *bile salts* assist in the digestion and absorption of fats. In turn, the fats in food stimulate the formation of bile and the emptying of the gallbladder.

Both the gallbladder and the bile ducts have muscular walls. Ordinarily their peristalsis produces no sensation. If, however, the cystic or the bile duct is obstructed, *biliary colic* can result. Since fat stimulates the peristalsis, the pain comes chiefly a little while after a fatty meal, especially a fried one.

One cause of obstruction is *gallstones,* which usually form in the gallbladder from the bile itself. They may cause trouble locally, but biliary colic follows when a gallstone works its way into the cystic duct or farther down into the bile duct and obstructs it.

Obstruction, if continued long enough, produces jaundice, since the bile with its pigments can no longer be secreted. Damage to the liver itself can also prevent the secretion of the pigments, so that jaundice results. In this case the stools may be less obviously acholic and the urine is less dark.

EXERCISES

1   If available, examine a series of x-rays which show the stomach after a *barium meal,* which is really a rather thick soup of material opaque to the x-rays. Identify the waves of peristalsis seen in silhouette, passage of material through the pylorus, and the barium's position in the duodenum. If the series follows the barium in the small bowel, observe its distribution there.
2   Similarly, examine films of the colon after a *barium enema.* Pay particular attention to the distribution of the remaining barium after defecation.
3   Examine a series of x-rays of the normal biliary tract and in a case of biliary obstruction. These films are made after the patient has received an opaque dye either by intravenous injection or by swallowing it. How does the dye get into the bile? What would happen if the liver were too badly damaged to function?
4   What produces the sound of a "stomach gurgling"—better called *abdominal rumbling* or *borborygmi*? What would unusually loud and frequent borborygmi suggest? What would a completely silent abdomen suggest?
5   Why question a patient about the color of his stools? Detail what you would learn from each abnormal color. If available, examine stool specimens of abnormal color.

9-5 KIDNEYS AND BLADDER

Kidneys   The kidneys' principal functions are to remove soluble wastes and surplus materials and to adjust the amount of water in the body. The kidney uses an elaborate and flexible microscopic system to do this.

Kidney Structure   This system consists of a multitude of little tubes or *tubules* packing each kidney. Each tubule begins as a tiny sac into which is pushed a minute knot of capillaries. This *glomerulus* is a filter through which water and all really soluble materials in the blood pass very freely (see Figure 9-3). Once in the glomerular sac, these blood constituents begin their passage down the long, narrow *renal tubule* that coils around before finally ending in a *collecting tubule* as urine.

The renal tubule is no passive passageway but rather a very active

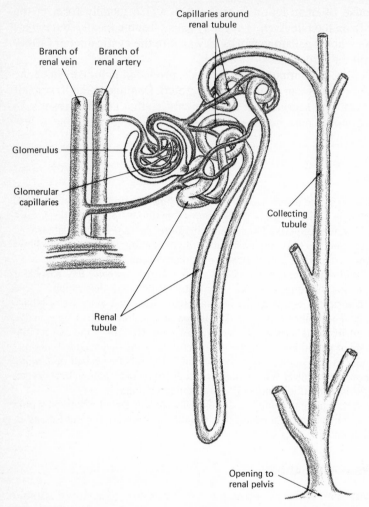

Figure 9-3 Diagram of single unit of kidney.

gland capable of removing most of the water from the forming urine. It also recaptures most of the usable materials filtered by the glomerulus, leaving waste matter dissolved in the urine. It can add further wastes as well during the urine's formation.

The blood supplying the tubule has already passed through the glomerulus. To accomplish this, the blood from the glomerular capillaries is collected by a small vein which soon breaks up again into capillaries around the renal tubule. It is then a microscopic *portal venous system.*

The formed urine is carried by the collecting tubule, which joins other collecting tubules, into the pelvis of the kidney. The *renal pelvis* is a true membrane-lined cavity lying mostly within the kidney but toward its medial edge.

Kidney Functions   When the blood contains more water than the body needs, more may filter through the glomerulus; but of greater importance, the renal tubule withdraws less water from the urine. This leaves the final urine very *dilute.*

When the blood contains less water than is optimal, the reverse occurs. Water and dissolved materials filter through the glomerulus freely, but the renal tubule takes up and restores to the blood more water than it would otherwise. The final urine then is *concentrated.*

Every soluble material, however, has a limit; more cannot dissolve in any given amount of water. If the solution becomes too concentrated, the material *precipitates* into solid form. Since it contains soluble materials which should not precipitate, there is a limit to how concentrated urine can become without causing trouble.

The kidney meets this problem by allowing enough water to remain in the urine. This will happen even if the body has a water shortage and becomes *dehydrated.* Dehydration can occur when excessive amounts of water are leaving the body as perspiration, during vomiting and as diarrhea, or in the case of massive bleeding and burns. It occurs also when various diseases produce soluble materials which require large volumes of urine to dissolve them.

The kidney actively adjusts the various salts or electrolytes in the blood and so in the body. It reduces the amount of useful salt returned to the blood if that salt is in excess, and it increases the amount put back into circulation if the blood has a relative lack of it. Obviously, in the first instance, the urine will be more concentrated even if it is of relatively large volume and, in the second instance, the urine may be relatively dilute when the volume is not increased.

The volume of urine put out is reduced by changes other than dehydration. It falls, for example, in shock, when too little blood reaches the kidney. It falls too when some disease either destroys glomeruli or renal tubules or when it blocks their function. In such situations the body can contain too much water, which forms edema even though the urine volume is low.

Kidney Stones   Overly concentrated urine can also lead to trouble. The total volume may be normal or low, and only one material may be too concentrated because the blood delivers too much for excretion. The concentrated material may then precipitate, usually in the renal pelvis, to form a *renal stone,* or *calculus.*

Urine Color   Such a stone can damage the lining of the urinary tract enough to cause bleeding. Other diseases or injury can cause bleeding in the substance of the kidney, even through the glomerular capillaries. Blood leaked into the tubules or pelvis may break down, so that the urine is a clear red solution. If the blood remains intact, the urine is red but looks "smoky."

Patients are right to be alarmed by *hematuria*—the appearance of blood in the urine. They are apt, however, to overestimate how much blood they lose. A few drops of blood will color a bladderful of urine.

The color of urine varies widely with the diet and concentration, from almost colorless when very dilute to a light orange when concentrated. Very dark brown or mahogany-colored urine means some disturbance in the body but not in the kidney itself. Most often it accompanies jaundice, where the fault usually is in the liver or biliary system.

Renal Colic   The urine usually remains unchanged after it leaves the kidney by way of the ureter. As a hollow tube with muscular walls, the ureter has peristaltic waves, and obstruction produces extremely painful colic. This *renal colic,* which is really *ureteral colic,* usually occurs when a small calculus leaves the kidney pelvis and moves down the ureter. The pain may be felt in the lower back first, but usually it travels or *radiates* around the side, down the inguinal region, and into the genitals. The stone scratching its way downward causes hematuria.

Bladder   *Urinary Bladder Functions*   The urinary bladder as a storage organ has walls that will distend when urine enters from the ureters. These walls are muscular and at the most inferior part of the bladder form a sphincter about the opening of the urethra. This sphincter remains closed as the bladder fills until the increasing tension on the walls produces the urge to urinate.

Urine is expelled when the sphincter at the bladder neck relaxes and the bladder walls contract. Urine then is forced through the urethra. Men have a second sphincter just below the point at which the prostate surrounds the urethra, and muscle fibers within the ventral part of the penis can also constrict it. Women also have muscle fibers about the short urethra, and these can interrupt the flow of urine. During urination, however, all these muscles relax to allow the urine to flow.

Changes in the Bladder   Normally urination is under voluntary control and empties the bladder before it overfills. The act also empties it so completely that only a few drops of urine remain in the bladder. If disease or injury destroys the voluntary control, the bladder empties automatically when it fills, and urination also can occur involuntarily during convulsions.

Much more often, control is lost in women with a relaxed pelvic floor. Sphincter action is impaired then, and urine leaks from the urethra during coughing, laughing, lifting, or any other action that increases pressure in the abdomen. The amounts lost are small and there is no true urination.

Women rarely have obstruction of the urethra; men get it much more often. Usually it is due to an enlargement of the prostate, but it can result from urethral narrowing or *stricture*. Typically, the bladder contracts with its usual force and the sphincters open, but only a little urine is forced through the meatus. After a little while, the stream becomes stronger, but then it tends to weaken and dribble on. This is the typical "difficulty in starting and stopping."

Both obstruction and prolapse from a weak pelvic floor may prevent the bladder from emptying completely. Bacteria grow well in the retained urine; when it is passed, such urine can cause *dysuria*—burning or smarting at the meatus or along the urethra. Changes at the meatus or in the urethra can also cause dysuria in men or women even if there is not urinary retention.

If obstruction is nearly complete or if the bladder is paralyzed, urine may distend it far beyond its normal size. This is often completely painless if it occurs slowly.

The frequency of urination normally depends upon the volume of urine the kidneys produce. It is possible, however, to urinate small amounts often and still form only normal volumes of urine during the 24-hr day. *Frequency* then does not always mean *polyuria*—the formation of abnormally large amounts of urine. Even *nocturia*—urinating at night—may be habit or due to some cause other than polyuria.

EXERCISES

1   If available, examine a normal series of timed sequential intravenous pyelograms. To make these, an opaque dye is injected intravenously. Films are then made at fixed intervals. How does the dye get into the urine? What would be the results if both kidneys were seriously damaged by disease?

2   Compare such films with normal retrograde pyelograms. These films are made by running small tubes or *catheters* from the bladder up the ureters. Dye is then forced through the catheters. What would be the result if the kidneys had little or no function? Identify the renal pelvis and ureter.

3   Reduce the amount of fluids—water, soups, soft drinks, coffee, tea, etc.—that you drink one day to about half or less your usual amount. What happens to the amount and color of your urine and to the frequency with which you urinate? The next day drink two or three times your usual volume of fluids and repeat the observations. You may feel that your kidneys are "working overtime" when you excrete large quantities of fluid. Actually, they do more work in reabsorbing water to concentrate the urine.

4 Obtain a collecting bottle of urine. Then prick your finger deeply enough so
   that it bleeds rather freely or get a small syringe filled with blood. Add the
   blood a drop at a time to the urine while you shake it. How many drops do you
   add before it is detectably pink? Before it becomes "smoky"?
5 If available, observe urine from a patient with jaundice. How does the color
   compare with normal concentrated urine?

9-6 REPRODUCTIVE TRACT

Male The male sexual organs produce *sperm cells,* suspend them in
a liquid, and deliver them into the vagina to fertilize the egg produced by
the woman. The boy begins to produce sperm and the *ejaculate fluid* at
puberty and the man continues to form them into old age.

Testicular Structure and Function Each testis contains many fine
but long, closely packed tubules. One end of this set of tubules is closed,
the other opens eventually into the epididymis (see Figure 9-4). After
puberty, the lining of these tubules continually forms millions of sperm
cells of microscopic size. Each sperm has a tiny, whiplike tail and, in the
proper liquid environment, can swim freely. The environment in the testis
and vas deferens is not proper, however, and so the sperm are passive.
Each sperm cell is, under proper circumstances, able to fertilize a human
egg.

The passive sperm are moved up to the epididymis by *cilia* and most
remain there for a fairly long time. Some are moved by peristaltic waves
in the epididymis and vas up into the prostate region. The prostate and
seminal vessels produce most of the *seminal fluid* in which sperm can be
suspended. Normally the glands store an appreciable amount of this fluid.

Erection When a man is sexually aroused, his initial obvious
reaction, *erection* of the penis, occurs involuntarily. The mechanism
involves the blood vessels, since the body of the penis consists largely of
widened spaces in which blood can collect. Each space has thin, muscular
walls and there is a tiny sphincter at its outlet into the vein draining it.
When erection begins, the walls of these *vascular spaces* relax and the
outlet sphincters contract at the same time that the arteries bring an
increased flow of blood into the penis. The result is that blood collects in
the spaces, hardening and erecting the penis. Thereafter enough blood can
pass the outlet sphincter to maintain circulation but not enough to empty
the spaces.

Less obviously, the prostate gland begins to secrete small amounts of
sticky fluid into the urethra, and the sphincter at the neck of the urinary
bladder *above* the prostate goes into a firm contraction.

Normally the erection is maintained until repeated friction stimulates

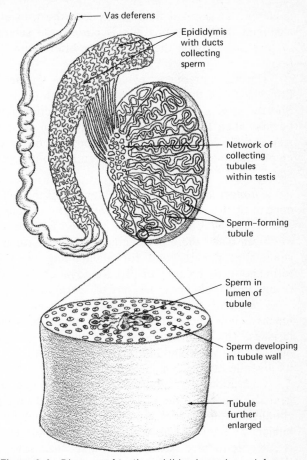

Vas deferens

Epididymis
with ducts
collecting
sperm

Network of
collecting
tubules
within testis

Sperm-forming
tubule

Sperm in
lumen of
tubule

Sperm developing
in tubule wall

Tubule
further
enlarged

Figure 9-4   Diagram of testis, epididymis, and vas deferens.

the skin of the penis. This leads to an involuntary, reflex *ejaculation.* During sexual intercourse, the stimulation is the rhythmic partial introduction and withdrawal of the erected penis in the vagina.

Ejaculation   Ejaculation, the *male orgasm,* involves contractions of the muscular walls of the epididymis and vas, forcing the immobile sperm upward. Prostatic secretion also increases but, more important, the seminal vesicles—which have muscular walls—contract and force their contents into the urethra with the sperm. This seminal fluid, secreted by the walls of the vesicles, makes up most of the volume of the *ejaculate.* In it, the sperm cells become motile and begin to swim about by whiplike motions of the tail.

The muscular walls of the urethra begin vigorous peristaltic movement as the seminal fluid pours into the prostatic portion. Since the sphincter above the prostate is closed, the semen is forced down the urethra and through the meatus in a brief series of spurts—the ejaculation.

During intercourse, ejaculation into the upper end of the vagina brings some of the sperm into contact with the uterine cervix and its os. Shortly after ejaculation, the penile erection begins to subside. This occurs when the vascular sphincters open so that blood in the penile spaces flows freely into the veins. The walls of the spaces contract as they empty and the body of the penis returns to its usual, nonerected, *flaccid* state.

Changes in the Male   Development of the sexual organs is under the control of the *endocrine* or *ductless gland* system. The testis itself is an endocrine gland as well as the source of sperm. The *male hormone* or *androgen* made there is directly responsible for the development of the genitals at puberty and for maintaining them in a functional state throughout the balance of life. Removal of the testes or *castration* then results in two changes, absence of sperm and of androgen.

Castration, either surgical or as the result of disease before puberty, blocks development of the genitals and of the secondary sexual characteristics. The resulting *eunuch* has childlike genitals, is beardless with a high-pitched voice and immature habitus, but is full size. His skin retains its juvenile fat and remains fine.

Castration after puberty removes the source of sperm while the genitals, especially the prostate and seminal vesicles, revert toward the childlike state. Sexual arousal, erection, and even ejaculation in the human are emotional as well as hormonal, and a man castrated in later life is still able to have sexual intercourse; that is, he remains *potent*. He is, however, *sterile*, since he produces no sperm. Castration before puberty causes both *impotence* and *sterility*.

Male Sterility   Sterility without impotence follows any change which blocks the delivery of sperm to the urethra. This can be mechanical, as when the vas is blocked or severed or when disease completely destroys the testicular tubules' function of producing sperm while leaving intact the production of androgens. This situation occurs also when both testes remain *undescended*, within the abdomen or inguinal canal.

Sterility can also follow removal or destruction of the seminal vesicles because ejaculation will not deliver the seminal fluid. Removal or disease of the prostate, however, does not prevent ejaculation nor produce sterility unless there is blockage of the openings from the seminal vesicles or vas.

Ejaculation is absent entirely in some nervous diseases and after the use of some drugs affecting the autonomic nervous function. Erection can be similarly impaired, leading to impotence even though the sexual organs and their function remain normal.

Changes in Potency   Impotence, however, is more often psychological. It is also relative. The sexual drive in men decreases with aging, and this normal waning may be interpreted as abnormal impotence.

The reverse condition also occurs as *priapism* or persistent erection. Usually it is unaccompanied by sexual desire. It can be painful and is always abnormal.

Normal erection followed too promptly by ejaculation almost always is psychological. Such *premature ejaculation* shortens intercourse but does not lead to sterility if the penis is in the vagina.

Spontaneous ejaculation, even without erection, occurs usually after a period without ejaculation. It commonly happens at night, often accompanied by erotic dreams, as a *nocturnal emission.* While a normal occurence, it can cause emotional disturbances in naive adolescent boys.

Female   The female sexual organs produce egg cells or *ova* periodically, transport them to the uterus—allowing an opportunity for fertilization on the way, and provide the necessities of life for the resulting fertilized egg. Ultimately they deliver the baby at birth and feed it during the early months of life. These basic female sexual functions are periodic rather than continuous, as in the male.

Ovarian Structure and Functions   The ovary is a solid organ and contains at birth all the ova that will ever be released. The organs and their ova remain small and dormant until puberty, when the ovaries enlarge and the ova begin to mature. Each ovum about to be released is contained in a bleblike *follicle* visible on the surface of the ovary. About every 26 days a mature ovum is released by rupture of a follicle on one ovary (see Figure 9-5). Two or more follicles may mature and release an ovum apiece simultaneously, providing one mechanism for twinning. The woman releases less than five hundred ova during her lifetime, as compared to the millions of sperm in each ejaculate.

Fertilization   The ovum, which is just large enough to be visible, is swept up by cilia on the funnellike end of the fallopian tube surrounding the ovary. It then begins a slow trip down the tube toward the uterus.

If intercourse has introduced sperm into the vagina shortly before or after *ovulation* or release of an ovum, sperm cells can enter the os of the cervix, passing upward through the lumen of the cervix and through the fundus and tube to meet the ovum there. At this point a sperm cell penetrates the ovum to *fertilize* it.

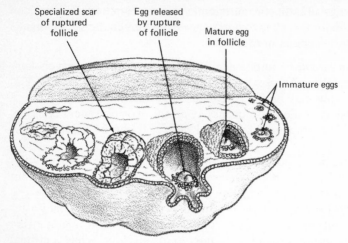

Figure 9-5   Diagram of ovary showing (right to left) maturation and release of ovum.

Uterine Function   The fertilized ovum immediately begins development into a new individual and continues its way down the tube to the lumen or cavity of the fundus. For most of each 28-day cycle, the walls of the uterus are unprepared to support growth of a fertilized egg. Once each cycle, however, the *endometrium* thickens and changes so that an ovum can develop there (see Figure 9-6). This change is so timed that the fertilized egg comes from the tube at the optimal moment and finds a receptive lining.

If no fertilized ovum arrives, the endometrium changes further and eventually sloughs off in *menstruation*. Uterine peristalsis, which can be painful (in *menstrual cramps*), moves the discarded lining through the

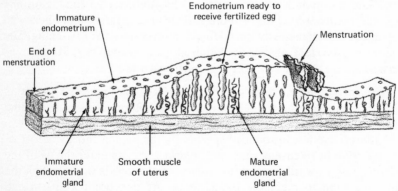

Figure 9-6   Diagram of endometrium showing (left to right) changes during menstrual cycle.

cervix and into the vagina as the *menses* or monthly period. When the lining has sloughed, it begins to build up again before the next time at which a fertilized ovum can arrive.

Pregnancy If a fertilized ovum arrives, it embeds itself or *implants* in the uterine lining, and together the developing egg and the lining form the *placenta*, or *afterbirth*, which will support the life of the developing child. This placenta is a vascular organ which keeps separate the blood of the mother from that of the child while bringing them into such close contact that gases, water, and soluble materials pass from one to the other. The *umbilical cord*, as it develops, carries blood from the child to the placenta and from the placenta to the child.

The developing baby is surrounded by a membranous sac, the *amnion*, filled with fluid. This sac bulges until it and the baby occupy almost all of the expanding uterine lumen. The placenta remains firmly attached to a portion of the wall until after the baby is born. All of this occurs in the fundus, which must undergo a rapid expansion to accommodate its developing contents. The cervix changes much less and remains constricted until shortly before birth.

Childbirth Among other changes, the muscular wall of the fundus develops as it expands. At the end of about 10 lunar months (of 28 days each) after the last menses, the enlarged and strengthened fundus begins peristaltic contractions which increase in frequency as *delivery* approaches. The later contractions are painful—the *labor pains*—and force the baby downward against the cervix.

As this occurs, the fluid-filled amnion and the lower parts of the baby begin to open the upper end of the cervical canal and move its walls aside (see Figure 9-7). As the cervix *thins,* its os begins to open or *dilate.* Some time during this process, the amnion usually breaks as the "*show of waters.*" There usually is a little bleeding, which is the "*show of blood.*"

Eventually the cervix is so thin and dilated that the baby can pass into the vagina. This ends the *first stage of labor,* which may last from a few hours to a few days. It usually is longer when the woman is bearing her first baby.

The *second stage of labor* is normally much shorter. The uterus contracts painfully every 2 or 3 min and contractions of the abdominal muscles, including the diaphragm, assist in raising the pressure against the baby. Eventually the child is forced through the vagina and its introitus, ending the second stage.

The *third stage of labor* involves the delivery of the placenta. Uterine contractions expel it into the vagina and straining to increase abdominal pressure expels it through the orifice. The fundus remains tightly con-

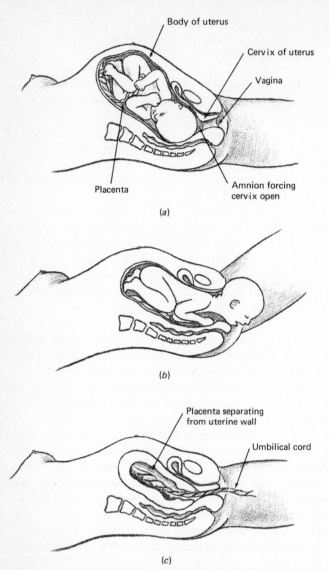

Figure 9-7 Stages of labor. First stage (above), uterine cervix being forced open; second stage (middle), head being delivered; third stage (below), separation of placenta.

tracted, so that little blood reaches the site where the placenta was attached and bleeding is slight.

After Childbirth   Over the succeeding weeks the uterus returns to its nonpregnant state, the other organs and abdominal wall resume their former positions, and the pelvic floor regains its tone. The cervix and vaginal introitus never quite return to the virginal state, however.

The breasts begin growing new glandular tissue early in pregnancy and, with the baby's birth, begin secreting milk. If the infant nurses, milk secretion will continue for months. Glandular tissue regresses only when the baby is weaned; the breasts then return to their *nonlactating state.*

Climacteric At some time between—as a rule—the ages of 40 and 50, the ovaries cease to mature and release ova. The menses often become scanty, irregular, or spaced farther apart. Finally they stop altogether— the *menopause*—while the fundus, tubes, and ovaries become smaller. During the period just before and after the menopause, properly called the *climacteric,* women usually experience one, several, or many *hot flashes.*

These hot flashes are felt as waves of warmth accompanied by flushing and often sweating lasting seconds to minutes. They may be so mild as to be barely noticeable to the woman herself or so severe that they are evident to others. Mild or severe, they are clear indications of the climacteric period, the *change of life.*

Hormonal Control The climacteric marks the end of a woman's fertility. It does not indicate the end of her active sexual life. Sexual arousal in the woman neither depends upon nor determines the release of ova. These are controlled, as are menstruation, pregnancy, delivery, and lactation by an *endocrine* or *hormonal system* that is more complicated than that in the man.

The ovary, like the testis, is an endocrine gland. It produces two female sex hormones called *estrogen* and *progestogen* which control the development and function of the other sex organs and characteristics. Together they maintain the size and cyclic changes in the uterus, including preparation to receive the fertilized ovum, menstruation, pregnancy, and labor. They are also involved in breast development and lactation.

Removal of the ovaries interrupts both egg production and secretion of estrogens and progestogens. *Ovariectomy,* the removal of the ovaries, or their failure to develop before puberty, results in a continuation of the juvenile state of the genital organs and a lack of breast development. Menstruation never appears and the woman is *sterile.*

Ovariectomy in the mature woman produces premature menopause with all its changes. After the menopause, few if any changes occur when the nonfunctioning ovaries are removed.

Female Sterility Sterility can occur from many causes. Disease of the cervix or fundus may block the passage of active sperm on their way to the ovum. Obstruction of the fallopian tubes blocks passage of both sperm and ova. Hormonal disturbances can block release of the ova, in which case the menses may become irregular or scanty. Other hormonal difficulties may leave the fundus unprepared to receive the fertilized egg at the proper time or prevent the uterus from supporting the developing child throughout the pregnancy. The latter results in a *spontaneous abortion* or *miscarriage*, but this also has other, nonhormonal causes.

Sexual Intercourse   Intercourse does not depend on hormonal changes directly. Since no obvious reaction is required of the woman, as erection is of the man, impotence does not occur. There are, however, changes in the female genitals accompanying sexual arousal. The clitoris, which corresponds to a part of the male penis, has some scant erectile tissue and does enlarge during arousal. The blood supply to the genitals increases and glands of the vulva secrete a watery lubricating fluid. Within the vagina, some fluid appears as well. Friction during intercourse does not produce a reaction like ejaculation, but the woman experiences an *orgasm* accompanied by contraction of the pelvic muscles, a release of sexual tension, and a return of the genitals to an unaroused state. The woman's orgasm may precede the man's ejaculation, follow it, or may not occur. Fertilization can occur without it if ejaculation deposits sperm in the vagina. In turn, the woman's orgasm does not depend on the release of ova from the ovaries and can occur in women after the menopause or ovariectomy.

Frigidity   Failure of the woman to experience an orgasm is called *frigidity*, but the term is also used to mean that the woman never desires sexual intercourse. In the latter sense, men can also be frigid. Regardless of which meaning is used, frigidity in the adult is usually psychological, although some diseases of the nervous system can produce it.

Abnormal Pregnancy and Labor   Just as sterility can come from any of several causes, disturbances of pregnancy and labor arise in many ways. Development of the egg can continue in the fallopian tube if it fails to move to the uterus. Such a *tubal pregnancy* eventually ruptures the tube.

The fertilized egg can develop abnormally in the uterus; so can the placenta. Both can become diseased and the placenta can detach prematurely from the uterine wall. The uterus may fail to respond to the endocrine signals and so does not expel its contents when spontaneous abortion begins. This leads to a *missed abortion* or an *incomplete* one if only some parts are retained.

In contrast, labor may begin early and lead to *premature delivery*. Much less often it may be *delayed* beyond the normal time. Both *premature* and *postmature infants* are handicapped, especially during the neonatal period.

Even when labor begins normally, its course can be abnormal. The uterus may lack the force to expel the baby or may tire during *prolonged labor.* Or it may become *spastic* and not relax between contractions. The cervix may be unable to dilate or deformities of the pelvic bones may prevent delivery. Even an abnormal position of the placenta at or near the point where the fundus and cervix join can create major problems.

Many of these difficulties can be foreseen by careful examination and history during pregnancy or even during early labor. This is one reason why *prenatal examinations* are important.

EXERCISES

1 If available, watch an educational film on human reproduction and one on pregnancy and labor.
2 What effect on reproduction and on sexual activity occurs with *vasectomy,* when the vas is tied and cut, and with *tubal ligation,* when the fallopian tubes are similarly interrupted?
3 Would removal of one ovary or one testis result in sterility? What effect would it have on sexual development if this unilateral removal were done before puberty?
4 What part of the physical examination should be done to determine whether labor is in the first or second stage? What would you expect to find in the second stage?
5 Phrase a series of questions to uncover impotence in a man. Frigidity in a woman.

9-7 ENDOCRINE SYSTEM AND METABOLISM

Glands with ducts, such as sweat and salivary glands, empty secretions onto surfaces or into the cavities of organs. The *endocrine* glands have secretions, the *hormones,* that enter the bloodstream, which carries them to other parts of the body. Some hormones affect the body generally, others cause changes in a single *target organ.*

Usually the hormones produce changes lasting minutes or days even when they are in the blood a relatively short time. They are as much a part of the body's regulating and responding mechanism as is the nervous system, but they are involved in slower, more prolonged reactions. The nervous system generally controls faster, shorter responses. The two systems not only share the control but they influence one another in intimate ways.

The body constantly carries out a multitude of chemical reactions—extracting energy from foodstuffs, building new body components, storing nutrients, and spending energy in its various activities. All these changes involving energy are grouped under the term *metabolism,* and the body must regulate them to survive. The nervous system chiefly controls the expenditure of energy in brisk reactions. The endocrine system has a wider scope, influencing the rate of energy storage and production as well as its expenditure.

Hormones from the Pituitary and Controlled by It   The small pituitary gland or *hypophysis* at the base of the brain exerts the most diverse effects among the endocrine glands. Its hormones directly influence growth of the body, its water balance, lactation, and blood pressure, as well as contraction of the uterus. Indirectly, its hormones influence metabolism by controlling the activity of the ovary, testis, thyroid gland, and the outer part or *cortex* of the adrenals. They influence indirectly other bodily functions as well.

Some pituitary hormones specifically stimulate other endocrine glands to put out their own hormones. Thus two pituitary hormones— *follicular stimulating hormones (FSH)* and *luteinizing hormones (LH)*— prompt the ovaries to produce *estrogen* and *progestogen* which, in turn, control the other female sex organs. They also control *testosterone* production as well as sperm formation by the testes.

A *thyroid stimulating hormone (TSH)* from the pituitary causes the thyroid gland to form and release its hormone into the blood. The *thyroid hormone* directly influences the rate of metabolism throughout the body. It is necessary for the normal controlled release of energy from foodstuffs and so for maintaining body warmth and vigor.

The pituitary's *adrenal cortical stimulating hormone (ACTH)* increases the production of the *cortisone* group of hormones by the adrenal cortex. These adrenal hormones influence the body's defense mechanisms against many diseases. The cortex produces other hormones, one of which controls the body's use of salt; the other is an *androgen.* Their formation, however, is not influenced by ACTH.

Body growth can proceed normally, especially during childhood, when the pituitary secretes normal amounts of *growth hormone (STH).* It directly influences the increase in size of the bones, muscles, viscera, and other parts of the body. It also indirectly influences metabolism in a more general sense.

The direct action of a pituitary hormone on *lactation* is more doubtful in the human. In any event, it causes no known disorder.

A specific effect is known for a pituitary hormone called the *antidiuretic hormone (ADH).* It directly causes the renal tubules to withdraw more water from the urine and return it to the blood. It can, under certain circumstances, raise the blood pressure.

A closely related pituitary hormone called *oxytocin* stimulates the muscles in the uterine wall to contract and begin peristalsis. It triggers the beginning of labor and of menstrual contractions. It also causes a transient drop in blood pressure.

Other Hormones   Two hormones, *adrenalin* and the related *noradrenalin,* not under pituitary control, are secreted by the central part or *medulla* of the adrenal glands. Adrenalin is the quickest of the hormones in its actions and has been called "the emergency hormone." It speeds the heart rate, raises the blood pressure, elevates the blood sugar concentration, and increases energy production.

Another pair of hormones are made by specialized tissue—the *isles of Langerhans*—in the pancreas. That organ is both a ducted gland producing digestive enzymes and a ductless gland producing hormones, the two functions being quite separate. Its two hormones have opposite actions as well.

Insulin, from the isles, is intimately concerned with metabolism. Specifically, it stimulates the use of *glucose,* a sugar, as a source of energy as well as stored energy. Both use and storage remove glucose from the blood and so decrease its concentration there.

Glucagon, the other isle hormone, increases the blood concentration of glucose. It is, in effect, an *antagonist* of insulin, and a proper balance between the two keeps the blood glucose concentration reasonably constant.

On the posterior surface of the thyroid are four small endocrine glands, the *parathyroids.* Their hormone chiefly regulates the body's calcium, the main constituent of bone. It stimulates the intestine to absorb calcium, causes the bone to release it, and prompts the renal tubule to withdraw it from the urine. Each of these effects increases the concentration of calcium in the blood.

Various other organs which are not endocrine glands make hormones as well. Some have considerable effects, but usually disturbances of the hormones accompany other evidence of trouble in the organ.

Endocrine Abnormalities   Disturbance of an endocrine gland is evident when the rather delicate balance of its hormone or hormones is upset. The result is a specific abnormality of metabolism.

Endocrine diseases arise in either of two ways: the organ produces too much hormone—*hypersecretion*—or too little—*hyposecretion.* The specific effects are fairly predictable from the hormone's actions. Castration produces hyposecretion of androgen and the changes which follow affect the genitals and secondary sex characteristics under that hormone's control. Hypersecretion of androgen causes less evident changes in a man, but in a woman or a child the result is *masculinization.* The voice deepens, the features coarsen, a beard and body hair develop, and the clitoris or child's penis enlarges. The menses cease and the breasts regress.

Hypersecretion of estrogen or of progestogen in the woman causes menstrual disturbances, usually irregular or heavy menses. Hyposecretion is the state after menopause or castration. Estrogen in a man causes growth of the breasts, a feminine distribution of body fat, and a tendency of the internal sex organs to return to the juvenile state. It does not, however, cause homosexuality.

Too active secretion of the thyroid gland, *hyperthyroidism,* typically steps up the general metabolism. Heat production increases; the patient feels and is warmer than normal. He tolerates cold unusually well and is uncomfortable in warm surroundings. He eats more than normally but uses the food rapidly and stays thin. He moves quickly, feels nervous, has a fine tremor, and sleeps poorly. He is overalert and may be jumpy or emotionally unstable. His heart rate is rapid and his systolic blood pressure elevated. He is constantly in "overdrive."

Hypothyroidism is typically the opposite. The adult patient is "slowed down," moves slowly, thinks slowly, tends to sleep much and eat little. He feels chilly and prefers the room warmer than most. His heart rate is slow, his systolic pressure low, his skin cool and coarse, his hair scant and dry. He seems placid and dull. Characteristically his eyelids are puffy and his face looks edematous. This is not true edema, however, but *myxedema.*

An untreated hypothyroid infant becomes a *cretin*—mentally deficient, stunted, coarse-featured, potbellied, and lethargic. He usually has a myxedematous, heavy-lidded face and may have a *goiter* or enlarged thyroid gland.

Hypoinsulinism is probably the mechanism of true *diabetes mellitus.* As the body cannot use glucose, its blood concentration rises and the glucose begins to appear in the urine. Here it must be diluted, hence less water is absorbed and *polyuria* results. As water is withdrawn from the blood, the patient becomes increasingly thirsty and drinks large amounts of water. His appetite may decrease and he does not obtain the normal amount of energy from his food. He begins to lose weight and feels weak. If untreated, he may go into coma and die.

If he lives long enough, the patient may develop changes in the peripheral nerves; abnormalities of the optic nerve or retina may cause blindness. His disturbed metabolism can lead to atherosclerosis and to changes in the renal glomeruli.

Hyperinsulinism is much rarer. The patient develops hunger, becomes increasingly jittery, and unless he eats may go into coma and convulse, since the brain depends on glucose for its energy.

Hyperparathyroidism causes only vague symptoms, such as weakness and weight loss, until enough calcium is withdrawn from the bones to make them brittle. *Hypoparathyroidism,* with a resulting low blood calcium concentration, causes muscle spasms, especially in the forearms and hands, a condition called *tetany.*

Hypersecretion of the adrenal medullary hormones produces symptoms and signs similar to those of hyperthyroidism. The blood pressure is usually high and the blood glucose concentration is elevated. The patient often has episodes of severe symptoms lasting only minutes. Hyperthyroidism, on the other hand, comes on slowly and is chronic. Hyposecretion of the adrenal medulla by itself does not produce recognizable signs or symptoms.

Hypersecretion of the adrenal cortex classically produces changes called *Cushing's syndrome,* a syndrome being a collection of signs and symptoms. The patient becomes weak with loss of muscle mass, and he develops characteristic fat deposits. His cheeks become puffy, so that he has a typical round *moon face,* and his trunk becomes fat, especially about the shoulders, to produce a *"buffalo hump."* He bruises easily and streaks of thinned skin appear on the hips, thighs, and lower abdomen. He often develops diabetes and hypertension. He may become psychotic. Women show changes induced by androgen as well.

Hyposecretion of the adrenal cortex classically causes *Addison's disease,* with weakness, weight loss, and darkening of the skin. The blood pressure is low and so is the blood glucose concentration, sometimes with symptoms like those of hyperinsulinism. Usually the patient complains of loss of appetite, nausea, vomiting, and diarrhea.

The pituitary gland can fail as a whole and so present a general metabolic disturbance including hypothyroidism, lack of androgen or of estrogen and progestogen, and Addison's disease. To these are added the effects of hyposecretion of the pituitary hormones acting directly on the body. The reverse situation, an overproduction of all pituitary hormones, does not occur. Individual hormones can be hypersecreted, however.

Hypersecretion of the growth hormones before puberty produces a true *giant.* Hypersecretion after puberty causes the disease *acromegaly,* with gradual growth of the jaws, hands, and feet. The facial features coarsen as the skin thickens and the nose grows. Long wrinkles deepen and the lips become fuller. The voice deepens in both men and women and both men and women develop an unusually "husky" appearance. This is heightened by kyphosis and slight bowing of the legs. On physical examination, the teeth are wide set, the tongue is large, and the viscera are increased in size, especially the liver and heart.

Despite the appearance of strength, the patient often is rather weak and the hand feels doughy despite its size. Acromegaly is frequently accompanied by progressive blindness, which is produced mechanically by the enlarging pituitary. The enlarging gland squeezes the optic nerves which pass near it, progressively constricting the visual fields.

Hyposecretion of growth hormone before puberty causes *pituitary dwarfism*. The individual remains childlike, small, and without pubertal development of the genitals or secondary sexual characteristics. Not all undersized children are dwarfs, and pituitary dwarfism is usually unrecognized until the age of puberty. Lack of growth hormone is not evident when it develops in the adult.

There are several kinds of dwarfism caused by different defects. In addition to cretins and pituitary dwarfs, there are hereditary forms with normal hormones. One of these somewhat resembles the pituitary dwarf but becomes a miniature, sexually mature adult. True pygmies probably arose from such individuals. A more common condition is the *achondroplastic dwarf*, who has a normal head and trunk but much shortened arms and legs.

Hypersecretion of the antidiuretic hormone is not recognized, but hyposecretion produces *diabetes insipidus,* in which the urine volume is much increased. The patient drinks large amounts of fluid to replace the lost water or he becomes dehydrated. The symptoms resemble those of diabetes mellitus, but the cause is very different and the glucose metabolism remains undisturbed in diabetes insipidus.

EXERCISES

1 If available, examine briefly a patient with untreated hypothyroidism and one with hyperthyroidism.
2 A patient reports an increased urinary output and high fluid intake. What questions would you ask him?
3 What questions would you ask to help distinguish between hyperthyroidism and hyperadrenalism? Between Cushing's syndrome and hypersecretion of androgen in a woman?

9-8 NERVOUS SYSTEM

The functions of the nervous system are more complex than those of the endocrines. It is possible, however, to consider its functions as (1) sensing changes, (2) causing actions, and (3) controlling these responses. Most disturbances of the nervous system involve all three components, but the symptoms and signs can be sorted into these three functional categories.

Sensation   *Sensory Functions*   The special *senses* include those of sight, hearing, smell, and taste. The more generalized senses can be grouped into the following categories: the *exteroceptive,* which detect changes from outside the body; the *interoceptive,* which feel changes deeper within the body; and the *proprioceptive,* which orient the body with respect to its surroundings while detecting movement and the position of body parts.

Exteroceptive sensation is characteristic of the skin and mucous membranes in direct contract with the surroundings. These senses are touch, or *tactile sensation;* temperature, or *thermal sensation;* and *superficial pain.*

Interoceptive sensations are more vague and less localized. They include sensations of *deep pain,* such as colic or visceral pain; of *fullness,* which is felt in hollow organs—the stomach, colon, and urinary bladder; and of *engorgement,* which usually is associated with increased blood supply, particularly in solid organs.

Proprioceptive senses are largely centered in bones, joints, and muscles, although the sense of balance mediated by the inner ear is also proprioceptive. Apart from this are the sensations of *stretch* or *tension* felt in the muscles, tendons, and ligaments, usually without conscious awareness; of *pressure;* of *deep pain* as in fractures or injured muscles; and of *vibration.*

These three groups of senses are simple insofar as they do not involve directly the higher centers of the brain. The higher centers combine and interpret the simple senses, usually without conscious control. It is possible, then, to consider as *complex senses* the *localization* of sensations on or within the body; *recognition* of the shape, texture, and weight of objects; and even *identification* of numbers or letters traced on the skin. The senses of body *orientation* in space and of *motion* are also more complex. Somewhat simpler is a sense called *two-point discrimination,* by which a person tells when he is touched at two adjacent points rather than only one.

Each of these complex sensory functions involves two or more simple senses. Body orientation, for example, includes sight, vestibular sensations, stretch sensations from muscles, tendons, and ligaments, pressure on the parts contacting a surface, and often touch as well.

The number of sensory impulses coming to the brain at any one time is more than the conscious mind can handle, and so much of a person's response is unconscious. The brain has still another mechanism to protect against being overburdened or distracted by sensations. It can *extinguish* awareness of a sensation. Perhaps the clearest example is the extinction of smell, so that an odor does not remain detectable. Much more frequent is the extinction of touch, which prevents a person from being constantly aware of his clothing or of his hair where it touches his skin.

Sensory Disturbances   Disturbances of sensation occur in only a limited number of ways. The sensation may be felt more keenly than normal; this is called *hypersensitivity*. It may be dulled in *hyposensitivity* or lost completely in *insensitivity*. There may be spontaneous sensations without any stimulus or provoking change, a symptom called *paresthesia*. This occurs most often with the sense of touch and is usually unpleasant, described as "ants crawling on the skin" or "pins and needles." Less common are *dysesthesias* in which one sensation is felt as another, so that touch may give a sensation of warmth or cold may be felt as pain. *Phantom* sensations, as when the patient complains of the awkward position of an arm which has been amputated, may be a dysesthesia.

Itching is not an independent sensation. It is the mildest form of one kind of superficial pain, a sort of minimal burning pain.

Defects in sensation can occur anywhere in the nervous system, from the local area where the disturbance is felt to the cortex. Each kind of simple sense depends upon a sense organ, usually microscopic, but large in the case of special senses such as the eye. The defect may be in this sense organ, as when it is destroyed by injury.

The usual sense organ sends its impulses to the central nervous system by way of a nerve and its dorsal roots which enter the spinal cord (see Figure 9-8). A defect of nerve or root can destroy sensation, reduce it, or distort it. This occurs when a person injures his ulnar nerve by hitting his "funny bone" and experiences transient paresthesias as well as pain, or when his leg "goes to sleep." A defect in a peripheral nerve or in a spinal nerve root produces a characteristic distribution of the sensory disturbance or loss. Usually more than one simple sense is lost in that area. These results are most clearly seen when a nerve or root is cut or torn.

The dorsal or spinal sensory ganglion may be the location of a defect. It is involved, for example, in *shingles,* or *herpes zoster,* a rather common disease. Shingles usually involves a limited band of skin extending, most often on the trunk, from the spinous process around to the midline in front. Burning pain begins to appear in this band—pain which increases to true hypersensitivity with some dysesthesia. The patient may experience severe pain when someone blows gently on the area. One sign of shingles is the appearance of small vesicles with red halos around them, but the hypersensitivity to pain is what distresses the patient.

Some sensory impulses pass up the spinal cord to the brainstem and thence to the cerebellar hemispheres. Defects within the cord can interrupt these pathways, sometimes in very specific ways. This occurs because fibers carry the sensory impulses upward, and the fibers of certain senses run side by side within the cord. A *localized defect*, then, will alter these associated sensations and not others. Since proprioceptive

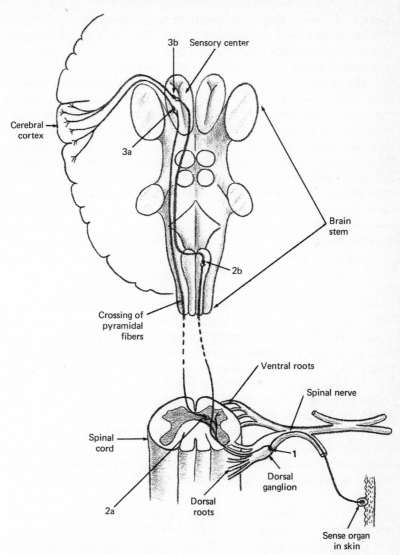

Figure 9-8 Sensory pathways to brain. Numbers 1, 2a, 3a are one chain of nerve cells along pathway, numbers 1, 2b, 3b are along different pathway.

fibers run together, there may be loss of the sense of position, motion, and vibration, with some loss of touch but with all other senses intact. Pain and temperature similarly are associated, but tactile sensation is chiefly carried by fibers traveling alone.

Localized defects occur within the cord in several diseases. One is *multiple sclerosis*, which can produce insensitivity to touch alone in an area or to pain and temperature alone. These insensitive areas usually regain sensation after several weeks or months, but other defects commonly appear later. These may also be transient.

The brainstem contains *sensory centers* which can route the impulses to the cerebellum or cerebrum, can modify and coordinate sensations, and can initiate responses to the sensory impulses. Generally impulses from proprioceptive sense organs are directed to the cerebellum, which also receives fibers from other organs that detect position and motion. Interoceptive impulses go chiefly to brainstem centers which control automatic bodily functions, and exteroceptive impulses ultimately find their way to the cerebral cortex, where the sensation is perceived. Some fibers carrying interoceptive and proprioceptive impulses ultimately reach the cortex also, since a person can be aware of posture, motion, and visceral sensations.

The brainstem is a compact area with many fiber tracts and centers close to one another. It is common, therefore, to have more than one function involved in a single defect. Since most cranial nerves have centers there, a defect can involve their functions as well as those of fibers from the spinal cord. Motor, in addition to sensory, functions are usually impaired, and the resulting difficulties are apt to be widespread. Because motor difficulties are more obvious than sensory changes, it is easy to overlook abnormalities of sensation in brainstem defects.

The cerebrum is the point at which awareness of sensations occurs and where the centers for many combined sensations are found. Difficulty in localization, recognition of shape and texture, or two-point discrimination suggests a *cerebral sensory defect*. This is especially true if the defect is unilateral but fairly widespread over that side. Very complex sensory disturbances such as the loss of the ability to understand words which are heard clearly point to defects in the cerebral cortex.

Motor Functions The motor functions controlled directly by the central nervous system are those involved in muscle movements which can be voluntarily controlled. Some of these movements proceed automatically, as does breathing, but can be altered directly and voluntarily.

Motor Defects Disturbances of muscular movement can occur anywhere in a long chain of control and reaction. Obviously a defect in the muscle itself can interfere with movement, as it does in any injury such as a strain or charley horse.

Each microscopic muscle unit has a special tiny area where the motor nerve joins it. This *neuromotor junction* is the point at which the motor impulse prompts the muscle unit to contract. A defect in this junction can disturb the motor control, and this indeed occurs in a rare disease, *myasthenia gravis*, where fatigue sets in so rapidly that the patient may be able to keep his eyelids open only a short time.

   The motor fibers reach the neuromotor junction by traveling from the central nervous system in the ventral nerve roots and out the peripheral nerves (see Figure 9-9). The severing of a ventral root or nerve then

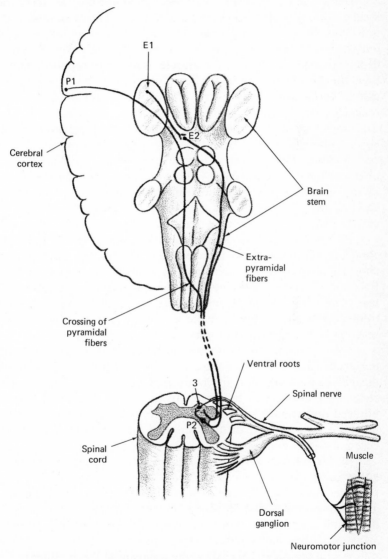

Figure 9-9 Motor pathways from brain. P_1 is pyramidal cell, P_2 is second nerve cell along pyramidal pathway. E_1 and E_2 are nerve cells in extrapyramidal pathway. 3 is final motor nerve cell in spinal cord.

interrupts the motor impulses and so paralyzes the muscles. The fibers arise within the spinal cord or brainstem near where the motor root emerges. Any defect at this point has much the same effect as does destruction of the motor root. Such a defect, in fact, accounts for the residual paralysis in *poliomyelitis.*

Defects in the *spinomuscular area,* including muscle, nerve root, and local cord region, share certain characteristics. The weakness or paralysis is usually confined to one or a few areas such as an arm or a leg. The muscle has either a loss of tone or is completely *flaccid* and flabby, depending on how much of the muscle or its nerve supply is damaged. In time, the muscle loses bulk. Earlier, it often shows fine, shivering motions called *fibrillations.* Movement, of course, is impaired and the local reflexes are reduced or absent.

Obviously the brain sends motor fibers to the local levels in the spinal cord. Otherwise there would be no voluntary control and no fine coordination of movements. Clinically the motor fibers from the brain can be divided into certain groups—*pyramidal* fibers from the cerebral cortex, *extrapyramidal* fibers from the brainstem, and *cerebellar* fibers from the cerebellum. All these groups are closely interrelated, but each presents certain characteristics when defective.

Pyramidal defects cause generalized weakness and partial rather than complete paralysis of the affected part. The muscles are maintained in contraction and so are *spastic.* The reflexes are hyperactive and the Babinski reaction is present when a leg is spastic. The muscles do not waste and show no fibrillations. There are no abnormal movements like tremors, but an attempt to make a simple movement may result in the reaction by a large group of muscles.

The pyramidal fibers show one characteristic of considerable importance. They travel from the cerebral cortex through the central part of the hemisphere and into the brainstem. In the lower part of the brainstem, they cross over to the opposite side of the spinal cord as they proceed downward. As a result, the left cerebral cortex controls movements of the right side of the trunk and the right arm and leg. The right cerebral cortex controls the left side.

In a *stroke,* or *cerebrovascular accident,* an artery of the brain is either occluded or it bleeds, or both. This commonly occurs where the resulting defect involves the pyramidal fibers of one cerebral hemisphere. The stroke victim often becomes unconscious and in this early stage is flaccid all over. As he begins recovery, he develops the symptoms and signs of a pyramidal defect, with spastic paralysis and hyperactive reflexes on one side. This side is the opposite of the cerebral hemisphere that is damaged.

A right-handed person has a motor center for speech in the left cerebral hemisphere. Fibers from this center pass very near the pyramidal fibers on that side, so that a left-sided cerebrovascular accident commonly produces right-sided paralysis and *aphasia* or loss of speech. Aphasia does not accompany left-sided paralysis with the cerebrovascular accident in the right hemisphere. The exact opposite is true for a left-handed person whose speech center is in the right hemisphere.

Many times a frank stroke is preceded by one or several transient episodes called *little strokes* which may last only minutes or a few hours. In these, pyramidal symptoms may appear on one side, the patient reporting that his hand or leg becomes stiff or clumsy. He may have some transient paresthesias or numbness on the opposite side and may be briefly aphasic.

Extrapyramidal defects present still another picture. There is generalized weakness and partial paralysis, but this paralysis is *rigidity* rather than spasticity. Such rigidity is characterized by slow contraction and slow relaxation of the muscles. The face is almost expressionless and blinking is infrequent. The handclasp is one of slow, gradual pressure and a sort of dragging release. It is so characteristic that it is diagnostic.

The muscles do not waste or show fibrillations and the tendon reflexes can be normal. There is, however, abnormal movement. This is a rhythmic, swinging, rather slow and quite coarse tremor at rest. It is reduced or disappears momentarily when the patient uses his extremity in a voluntary movement. The hands at rest may have a rhythmic motion of the thumb and fingers which is well described as *pill rolling*. The most common of these disturbances is due to *Parkinson's disease.*

Other extrapyramidal diseases are uncommon. They produce other abnormal movements rather than a rhythmic tremor with abrupt, jerky motion or continuous writhing of one or more parts.

Cerebellar defects cause no paralysis, true weakness, or muscle wasting. The muscles do show reduced tone and the reflexes are diminished. The most striking effect is in the movements which show poor coordination, the condition called *ataxia*. This may be evident only during motion when each act seems broken up into many poorly controlled parts. The movement cannot be stopped precisely and so misses its target or overshoots it. The ataxia may be apparent at rest as a series of random, uncoordinated movements. Tremor, if present, is absent at rest but appears on voluntary motion and grows worse as the motion proceeds, the so-called *intention tremor.*

Tremors do not always come from nervous system defects nor do all irregular, purposeless motions. Weakness and fatigue cause trembling when a motion is made, and pushing a normal muscle to extremes of exertion produces a rapid, fine tremor in it. Most people have experienced one or two random jerking motions or a brief episode of tremor, especially as they fall asleep. None of these indicates a nervous system defect, nor does the fine tremor of hyperthyroidism.

Elderly people often have trembling hands without other evidence of nervous difficulty. This *senile tremor* tends to be coarse and rhythmic, resembling that of Parkinson's disease but less extensive. Often, however, the senile tremor at rest grows worse on motion so that it is also an intention tremor.

Convulsions   Convulsions can be considered the extreme of tremors and always indicate a serious defect. They may occur, especially in infants, as a result of fever or other nonnervous conditions. In general, however, convulsions are evidence of a defect in the cerebral cortex. Whatever the cause, the convulsion is massive, disorganized motor activity.

Epilepsy is the commonest cause of recurrent convulsions. A typical *grand mal* seizure, as it is called, often follows a day or two of warning symptoms when the patient feels a change of mood or some rather vague, bizarre uneasiness. Immediately before the attack he commonly has an *aura,* an abnormal sensation such as a "hollow feeling" in the epigastrium, a characteristic odor, peculiar taste, flashes of light, or tinnitus.

Within minutes or seconds the seizure begins with an involuntary, harsh, screaming *epileptic cry.* At the same time, the patient loses consciousness and falls, often injuring himself as he does so. He then goes into a *tonic contracture* or spasm of all his muscles with his head back, his back arched, his legs extended, and his arms flexed. He is not breathing and becomes cyanotic.

After a minute or so in this tonic spasm, the patient relaxes and then goes into another briefer spasm. Relaxation follows and then another spasm. This *clonic stage* can last for many minutes, the spasms gradually becoming weaker and farther apart. During the clonic stage the jaw opens and closes in spasm so that the patient may bite his tongue to ribbons. At the same time the spasms are forcing expiration, expelling saliva mixed with air from the mouth. This is the "frothing" or "foaming at the mouth." The patient also urinates and defecates during many seizures.

Typically the patient lapses into deep, snoring sleep as the clonic stage subsides. He may seem to regain a dazed consciousness and wander about disoriented and confused. When he finally regains consciousness some hours after the attack, he usually is bewildered and remembers nothing of his seizure.

Any one seizure may lack parts of this typical picture. There may be no warning period, no aura, or no clonic stage. The attack may be prolonged or very brief.

There is one type of epilepsy in which the patient has different but characteristic seizures. This *Jacksonian type* begins with a tonic stage, followed by a clonic stage in some one part—a hand, the face, the tongue, or even a single finger. From that part the spasms may spread or *march* regularly up the arm or leg, from face to neck, and eventually over the entire body as a generalized grand mal seizure. The march may be confined to the original side of the body or even to the first part affected. There may be a very rapid or relatively slow progression and the patient may or may not lose consciousness.

Obviously the sensory parts of the nervous system are involved in the aura of an epileptic seizure. The tonic and clonic stages, however, arise in the motor centers of the cerebral cortex. The Jacksonian seizure indicates a more localized defect in the motor cortex on the side opposite to that on which the seizure begins. This defect can be the delayed result of a head injury which occurred weeks or months before the first seizure.

Complex Nervous Functions   Sensory and motor defects often occur together or follow one another in diseases of the central nervous system. Such defects can also be associated with evidence of disturbances in the parts of the brain concerned with emotions, intellect, memory, and personality. During recovery from a stroke, for example, a previously stable, well-adjusted, placid patient may become highly emotional with outbreaks of temper, weeping, and agitation. This occurs especially when the vascular defect involves those parts of the brainstem concerned with emotions.

Vascular changes, especially impaired circulation due to atherosclerosis, may affect only the higher centers without producing motor or sensory difficulties. The changes then are those seen in true senility, in which the *intellectual functions* decrease. Personality changes may follow without any acute episode such as a stroke.

Some of the most serious diseases of the nervous system have as their earliest manifestation only headache. This can be extremely mild and variable at first, with nothing to distinguish it from the run-of-the-mill, more trivial headaches which arise outside the skull and which are much more common. A headache that indicates a serious condition is, however, more apt to be constantly present even if slight.

Autonomic Nervous System   *Autonomic Functions*   Disturbances of the central and peripheral nervous systems are much easier to detect and characterize than are those of the autonomic nervous system. The chief controlling centers of this system lie in the brainstem, which directs most unconscious, automatic activity of the body. The sensory side of the autonomic system deals with interoceptive sense and chiefly sends its fibers along with those of the other senses to the central nervous system. The motor fibers of the autonomic system, however, supply glands and such *involuntary muscles* as those in the heart, blood vessels, and viscera. They do not send impulses to the *voluntary muscles,* which are controllable at will.

The autonomic system usually supplies a double and opposing nerve supply to the parts it controls. These two components, the sympathetic and the parasympathetic systems, have opposite effects and provide a balance of control. Thus sympathetic impulses cause the pupil to dilate and parasympathetic impulses cause it to constrict.

Similarly, sympathetic impulses provoke the salivary glands to secrete only thick, ropy saliva; parasympathetic impulses produce thin, copious saliva and tears. In the digestive tract the parasympathetic fibers carry impulses prompting glandular secretions, increasing muscular tone and peristalsis, and relaxing the sphincters.

Sympathetic impulses speed the heart's rate, increase its output of blood, and augment the conduction of impulses through the AV node. Parasympathetic impulses do just the opposite. Sympathetic impulses also constrict the blood vessels; hence their total effect is to increase the blood pressure.

Parasympathetic impulses increase the tone of the urinary bladder wall, increase its motility, and bring about the contraction which empties it. Simultaneously they relax the sphincter at the bladder neck during urination.

It is possible to recall the effects of the sympathetic nervous system by considering them as preparing the body to fight or as akin to fright. The dilated pupils, dry mouth, arrested digestion, increased heart action, elevated blood pressure, and inactive urinary bladder all prepare a person to meet an emergency.

The parasympathetic system, in contrast, prompts the activities more associated with a relaxed conduct of the body's routine business. Copious saliva, increased digestive activity, decreased heart action, and urination are all components of such relative relaxation.

Autonomic Defects   Defects of the autonomic nervous system can be suspected when there is disturbance of any function controlled by it. This is especially true when there is other evidence of nervous system defects. It is obvious, however, that many other conditions can produce the same signs and symptoms without demonstrably disturbed autonomic control.

EXERCISES

1   Using a pin and with the subject's eyes closed, press it lightly on the pulp of his fingertip. Ask him to describe precisely the spot where you touched. Then

repeat the maneuver on his back about the level of the shoulder. Can he localize the stimulus at one spot as well as he can at the other?

2 Determine just how much pressure you must apply to the pin to produce a painful sensation on the side of your finger. Then move the pin a very small distance and repeat this. Keep this up until you know how close together the pain sense organs are in that part. Then repeat the same on the point of your shoulder. Does it require the same pressure to produce a painful sensation here as on the finger? Are the pain sense endings equally spaced in the two areas? Do the areas itch after you finish pricking them?

3 Squeeze your Achilles tendon until you produce pain. Is this deep pain as sharply localized as skin pain? Does it have the same quality?

4 Stand on one foot for several minutes. This will make you aware of proprioceptive sensations involved in balancing. At the moment you touch your other foot to the ground, you will be aware of pressure as a component of balance. Now, still standing, read aloud and rapidly. Are you aware of pressure sensations from your feet as you read or has your nervous system extinguished the sensations?

5 Put your two palms together with your elbows flexed and abducted. Press your palms together as hard as you can. Observe the tremor of effort and describe it.

6 If available, watch a film or observe patients with various motor defects. Try to decide in each case which defects are involved—spinomuscular, pyramidal, extrapyramidal, or cerebellar.

9-9 MUSCULOSKELETAL SYSTEM

Bones and Joints The bones are living organs which undergo changes as long as life lasts. Most of their substance is nonliving mineral contained in a fibrous framework, but the tough, living covering on the surface and the central *marrow* or *medulla* is tissue capable of forming and destroying bone. There are living components even within the "solid" bone, so that the mineral not only gives strength to the skeleton but serves as a storage depot.

Cartilage covering the articular surfaces of the bones at joints is, if anything, more inert than the bone. It contains little mineral but forms a smooth, somewhat springy surface that makes movement easier even when the body's weight forces the moving surfaces together.

Since the articular cartilages must always be moist in order to glide smoothly and since cartilages need some foodstuff and oxygen, the joint is surrounded by a synovial membrane. This vascular membrane forms the joint fluid which lubricates and supplies the cartilage with its metabolic needs. The total amount of fluid is normally very small even in a large joint.

Slick surfaces would let one bone slip completely away from the other at any joint unless the two were held together. Ball joints like the shoulder and hip are held in position by a tough fibrous *capsule* outside the synovial membrane. This capsule, attached around each bony part of the joint, is loose enough and flexible enough so that rotation can occur but tough and tight enough to keep the bones from slipping out of position or *dislocating.*

Round or flattened fibrous strands or *ligaments* also bind the two joints together. They are so arranged that they allow motion through the full range in the normal directions but do not allow much movement or play in other directions.

Even capsules and ligaments are not enough to stabilize most joints, however; the associated muscles help. Stabilization is usually increased by a muscle ending in a tendon on one side of the joint. This tendon then inserts on the bone which forms the other side. These tendons may be cords or flat and sheetlike. They are essentially like ligaments but attach muscle to bone rather than bone to bone.

The intervertebral joints are somewhat different, although they too have a capsule attached around the edges of the adjacent · vertebral bodies. This capsule is backed up by ligaments running across the space. The difference from other joints lies within the capsule. Here there is a ring-shaped, tough fibrous pad between the vertebral bodies and a central very soft, jellylike *nucleus* which acts as a cushion between the bodies. Together the ring-shaped pad and the nucleus make up the *intervertebral disc.*

The processes of the vertebra's neural arch are bound together by ligaments, and the entire neural canal which they form is lined by what amounts to a continuation of the capsule around the intervertebral discs. The nerve roots leave the neural canal by passing through this fibrous lining.

Bone Changes   Bones become brittle when their mineral content is decreased below a certain amount or when a part of the bone is destroyed locally by a disease process. Several conditions produce generalized demineralization and brittleness. Hyperparathyroidism can do so, as can a long-continued diet deficient in calcium, the principal mineral. Much more common is the demineralization that accompanies aging, especially in women. This can lead, among other fractures, to partial slow collapse of one or more vertebral bodies with abnormal curvature of the spine.

A more localized demineralization occurs in "disuse." The bones of a part give up calcium if the part is not used. A flaccid arm, for example, will have demineralized bones. Patients who are bedridden for months or years can have such generalized and extensive demineralization of disuse that their bones fracture easily.

Arthritis   More people, however, suffer from *arthritis.* This is a general term for painful joints. Injury to the cartilage, ligaments, capsule, or synovial membrane produces *traumatic arthritis*. Germs growing in the joint cause *infectious arthritis*, and allergies can produce *allergic arthritis*. Other diseases produce other forms of arthritis as well. The two most common types of arthritis—*osteoarthritis* and *rheumatoid arthritis*—are both called "rheumatism" by patients.

Osteoarthritis almost universally accompanies the aging process. It occurs most often in the weight-bearing joints—the spine, pelvis, hips, legs, and feet—of obese people and those who have carried heavy loads. This suggests that it may result from wear and tear, but it also appears in the shoulders, arms, and hands, and heavy labor is not a necessary prerequisite.

Typically an osteoarthritic joint is stiff and painful but not red or hot. The pain is most felt when the joint is first moved after it has been immobile for some time. Use then "loosens up" the joint, the stiffness decreases, and the pain may disappear. If the joint is used too long, the pain and stiffness return and may be relieved by rest.

Patients with osteoarthritis "feel the weather" because the stiffness and pain often disappear for days, weeks, or months, only to return in damp weather. Overuse of the joint can precipitate the pain in any arthritis, but osteoarthritis frequently foretells the weather by reappearing or getting worse even before a damp spell begins.

Stiffness limits the motion of osteoarthritic joints, but there may be mechanical limitations as well. The disease is accompanied by a thinning or disappearance of articular cartilage, so that bone surfaces come in contact. The bone there becomes very hard and smooth, so that motion is still possible. It is not so easy as with cartilage and often is accompanied by audible gritting or grating.

The bone shows another reaction. Projections grow out around the joint, and these too may limit motion. In the fingers, these bony projections appear at the distal joints, where they are readily palpable as *Heberden's nodes*.

Osteoarthritis limits motion and may distort the joints somewhat, bowing the knees, angling the fingers, or causing "lumpy" joints as the projections form. It is not, however, a truly crippling disease which completely immobilizes joints.

Rheumatoid arthritis can do that slowly or rather quickly. Typical rheumatoid joints are hot, red, and quite swollen as well as stiff and continually painful. The joints also have an increased amount of fluid and are tender to pressure. If untreated, they frequently fuse and become fixed. This *fusion* produces a characteristic pattern in the fingers. They are stiff and straight but are flexed at a right angle at the metatarsophalangeal joints. The fingers also swing rigidly toward the ulnar side, away from the thumb.

The main point of attack in rheumatoid arthritis is the synovial membrane. The joint cartilages are destroyed and the bone beneath does not become smooth. Rather, it roughens and fuses with the bone opposite it to form an immovable union.

Rheumatoid arthritis attacks in episodes lasting weeks, months, or years if untreated. There may follow a long period free of further symptoms and then a recurrence. Almost always several joints are involved in any one episode and almost any joint can become arthritic.

A disease limited to the spine, called *rheumatoid spondylitis,* resembles rheumatoid arthritis but differs from it. Spondylitis is both painful and crippling. Untreated, it leaves the spine fused into an anterior curvature which permanently doubles the patient over.

Back Pain   Most back pain is not due to spondylitis. This very common symptom, especially *low back pain,* is usually not due to arthritis at all, particularly in younger persons. It appears in obese people, pregnant women, persons wearing badly fitted shoes or individuals who maintain a faulty posture. In most instances it probably results from poor body mechanics and is really muscle pain.

One relatively common cause of low back pain is more significant and can occur in young as well as in older adults. This is due to a *ruptured disc* or *herniated nucleus.* As the names indicate, it occurs when the fibrous ring of the intervertebral disc tears and the nucleus passes through it to the edge of the intervertebral space. The ring ruptures in its posterior part and the nucleus may tear the capsule so that it protrudes into the spinal canal.

Usually this rupture involves a lower lumbar intervertebral space. At this level the spinal canal contains the roots of the lumbar and sacral nerves, and these roots form part of the sciatic plexus which gives rise to the sciatic nerve.

When the herniated nucleus presses on the nerve roots, pain is felt not only in the lower back but down the back of the leg along the course of the sciatic nerve. From this comes *sciatica*—the old name for the pain. If the pressure is long continued or severe, the root is injured and there is weakness and wasting, especially in the calf muscles. This is a spinomuscular defect and so the ankle jerk is diminished or absent. Hyposensitive areas can also appear on the lower leg and foot.

Herniated nucleus also appears in the cervical area where it involves the roots of the brachial plexus. The symptoms and signs then appear in the arm.

Other conditions cause difficulties that are identical to a ruptured disc and some are much more serious. The ruptured nucleus, however, often returns to its proper position with bed rest alone and the condition clears up. It may then return, usually after some exertion such as lifting, or driving a golf ball. Often the patient reports several such episodes before he seeks care.

Bone Diseases   Bones too are subject to specific diseases that do not directly involve joints or demineralization. In one such disease there is formation of extra, spongy bone just beneath the membrane covering the bone's surface. This is especially noticeable along the front of the tibia, which becomes prominent and somewhat curved to produce a *saber shin*. The same patient will often have a prominent forehead with an indistinct knob or boss on either side of the frontal bone.

In children, the bony processes where tendons attach sometimes separate from the shaft. This is especially apt to occur at the insertion of the patellar tendon on the upper anterior part of the tibia.

Muscular Disorders   The muscles themselves are fairly tough. Their chief function, of course, is to produce movement by contracting, but they are also a source of body heat. This is most evident when a person is chilled and shivers to produce heat. The rapid, fibrillating contractions do not give effective movement but they do raise the body temperature by warming the blood passing through the muscle.

The muscles are uncommonly the seat of diseases. Much more often, pain in the muscles is due to overuse. While this is familiar after heavy exercise, especially when a person is "out of condition," it occurs also without exercise. This is seen in *splinting,* a very common response to a painful joint or injured part. To ease the pain, muscles which move a painful part go into contraction, holding the part more or less rigid. This splinting rather effectively prevents pain from an arthritic joint or a torn ligament. It also overworks the muscles involved, and in time they begin to ache. The patient then reports pain in a part not directly involved in the true defect.

Tension headaches arise in the same way. They really are cramped, painful muscles in the back of the neck, and the pain usually radiates from the occiput up over the head. The tension may be completely emotional, but it can also result from a long day's drive with the head held rigidly upright as the driver watches the road.

True *cramps* are more painful than splinting or the ache of tension. They are involuntary, prolonged contractions of one or more muscles and almost everyone has experienced them at one time or another. Usually the onset is sudden and the hard, knotted muscle remains contracted until it can be induced to relax.

Cramps usually arise within the muscle itself, but they can be caused by excessive motor impulses from central nervous system disease. They may reflect increased irritability from generalized disease, as they do in hypoparathyroidism. Impaired circulation that deprives the muscle of oxygen can make cramping more likely. Usually it is either simple fatigue and the accompanying metabolic changes in the muscle or a sudden excessive contraction in an unguarded movement that causes the cramp.

EXERCISES

1 If available, question and examine a patient with a herniated lumbar nucleus. Pay particular attention to the history of repeated attacks and what precipitated them. Try straight leg raising as part of the examination.
2 If available, question and examine a patient with common low back pain. Pay attention to the symptoms, how they began, and what makes them worse. Try straight leg raising.
3 If available, examine an unstable knee and one with extensive osteoarthritic changes. How do they differ? Why?
4 Put a blood-pressure cuff around your upper arm and inflate it above the systolic blood pressure. Now with that hand squeeze a rubber ball vigorously. What is the result? As soon as the effect is obvious, release the pressure completely. How long do the changes last? What does this show about the role of circulatory changes in muscular symptoms?

9-10 BLOOD

Composition and Function of Blood   Blood is usually described as a liquid, but this is only partially true. It can easily be separated into two parts—one fluid, the other solid. The solid part consists of millions of microscopic *red blood cells* or *erythrocytes,* a smaller number of *white blood cells* or *leukocytes,* and many fewer small fragments called *platelets.* The straw-colored fluid, the *plasma,* is a complex solution which clots rather promptly unless it is changed to prevent this. The clot or *thrombus* begins to contract after it forms, and as it does a clearer, straw-colored fluid, the *serum,* separates from it.

The erythrocytes, although called red blood cells, are not complete cells. Under the microscope they are yellow-orange discs, pinched in on either side. Since they lack a *nucleus,* the term "cell" is not really accurate. They are highly specialized because they contain the colored *hemoglobin,* which is the body's main means of transporting oxygen from the pulmonary alveoli to the tissues.

The leukocytes are true cells complete with nucleus, and they contain no hemoglobin. Their function, then, is not oxygen transport. Rather, they are one of the body's principal defense mechanisms against foreign intrusion in the form of bacteria, viruses, and the like, as well as any foreign tissue introduced into the body. There are various types of leukocytes, some capable of surrounding and engulfing foreign matter, others able to make and release special chemicals. Among these latter are *antibodies,* complex substances which are able to combine with foreign chemicals and render them harmless or to assist in the destruction of bacteria and viruses.

The platelets are very small pieces of cells, fragile and without nuclei. Their function is to assist in the formation and shrinkage of a thrombus or clot.

Clotting The principal ingredients of the clot are, however, dissolved in the plasma. Here they exist in a delicate balance which keeps them in solution unless something disturbs that balance. Usually this occurs when a blood vessel wall is opened, in which case the thrombus forms to plug the hole. Clot formation or *thrombosis* can, however, occur within the vessels whenever the lining of these vessels or the heart becomes abnormal. Anything that stops or slows the circulation for a long period makes thrombosis more likely.

A thrombus within a blood vessel can plug it off or *occlude* it completely or only partially. If the intravascular thrombus is soft, all or part of it may break off and float away in the bloodstream as an *embolus.* This is carried through the vessels until it plugs one of them and causes *embolism.*

Plasma Functions Besides the clotting components, the plasma carries gases, water, foodstuffs, salts, wastes, hormones, and all other essential materials throughout the body. Among these blood components are the *plasma proteins* which, with the salts, play an essential role in keeping enough water in the blood. The capillary walls let water and many dissolved materials pass from the blood into the tissue spaces. The blood pressure even assists in forcing the water out through the thin walls. If this movement went unchecked, the blood would become too thick to circulate.

The check is the plasma proteins. They cannot pass through the capillary walls and in a sense they pull water back through the walls into the blood. This keeps the plasma fluid, but it does not recapture all the water and dissolved materials. Some enter the tissues and are used there. Some remain in the spaces until they encounter and enter the lymphatic system.

When too much water leaves the capillaries, when not enough reenters the blood, or when the lymphatics cannot drain away enough, water collects in the tissue spaces as *edema.* When the excess collects in the abdominal cavity, it is called *ascites.* When it collects in the thoracic cavity, it is called *pleural effusion* or *hydrothorax.*

Abnormalities of Blood *Hemorrhage* Blood, like all parts of the body, is subject to defects. It is complex enough to be defective in many ways. The simplest defect, perhaps, is blood loss, or hemorrhage. If this is massive and sudden, there is a deficiency of all the blood components. The decreased blood volume results in low blood pressure and *shock;* the loss of erythrocytes and their hemoglobin causes a generalized lack of oxygen in the tissues; the reduced water available dries up the tissues; and the body defenses are weakened. Loss of clotting materials may even impair the blood's ability to plug injured vessels.

If the patient survives the hemorrhage, replacement of the lost substances begins immediately. Water is drawn from tissues and from the intestine to replace volume, the liver—which makes plasma proteins—begins to form them rapidly, the clotting substances are replaced, and new blood cells begin to appear. The body has reserves of leukocytes in the lymph nodes, organs, and bone marrow, and they quickly release these cells into the blood. The marrow promptly replaces platelets as well. There are some reserves of erythrocytes in the spleen and marrow, and they too are released. They cannot make up an adequate number, however.

Erythrocytes are produced in the bone marrow and must be filled with hemoglobin to function. It requires time both to develop the erythrocytes and to make hemoglobin, which contains iron. Especially if the body's iron stores are low, the replacement of lost hemoglobin lags behind all the other replacements.

Anemia This explains why repeated, smaller hemorrhages do not produce the same changes as massive bleeding. The body can often replace all the lost materials except the hemoglobin and erythrocytes. The result is *anemia,* a lack of these two components. Since the hemoglobin gives the blood its red color, the mucous membranes and nail beds appear pale and the skin of white patients does as well. Lack of oxygen-carrying capacity deprives the tissues of that essential gas and the patient is weak and listless.

Hemorrhage, acute or chronic, is only one cause of anemia. A continued low intake of iron prevents hemoglobin production, as does a generally deficient diet. Liver disease and renal failure also interfere with hemoglobin formation. A defective marrow has a similar result. This defect may be in the marrow itself or in specific substances that it requires to form fully mature erythrocytes.

There are diseases in which hemoglobin or the erythrocytes are destroyed too rapidly by the body itself. Unlike the hemoglobin deficiency anemias, these destructive *hemolytic anemias* often release hemoglobin which the liver then converts into bile pigments. The result in severe hemolytic anemia is jaundice accompanying the findings of the anemia itself.

Other Erythrocyte Defects The reverse of anemia also occurs; the body forms more erythrocytes and hemoglobin than normal. One result is *plethora*, the condition of too red a face, too scarlet mucous membranes and nail beds. An excess of erythrocytes can be a disease in itself, but it is also one protective response to reduced respiratory capacity in severe lung disease.

Erythrocytes and hemoglobin may be imperfectly formed, as they are in *sickle cell anemia*. Usually defective erythrocytes are destroyed too rapidly and anemia results. Abnormal shapes may cause the erythrocytes to jam in the capillaries rather than gliding through them. The resulting multiple microscopic emboli can cause pain and deranged function in many organs.

Leukocyte Defects Leukocytes are less often deficient in number than are erythrocytes and the effects are more subtle. The patient may feel normal but be subject to severe infections, particularly in the pharynx. Usually, however, some other condition, chiefly anemia, accompanies this reduction of leukocytes.

With many infections, leukocytes normally increase in number as the body defends itself against invasion. When the invasion clears, the number returns to normal. *Leukemia* is, however, a very different condition, a disease in itself. The leukocytes are not only greatly increased in number but also abnormal. The patient often has few symptoms until the rapidly forming white cells crowd the marrow so that erythrocytes cannot form and anemia results. The lymph nodes where other leukocytes form may also enlarge and cause symptoms, or there may be clotting disturbances.

Clotting Defects A deficiency of platelets, whether appearing by itself or as the result of leukemia, seriously interferes with clotting. The deficiency usually shows itself by the appearance of multiple petechiae and purpuric areas. These areas of bleeding into the skin and mucous membranes may resemble macules with their dilated capillaries. On pressure, however, a macule blanches as the blood is forced from the capillaries into the veins; petechiae and purpuric spots remain colored because the blood cells are outside the vessels. A few diseases and injury cause an increased number of platelets, but this rarely produces signs or symptoms.

Clotting difficulties more commonly arise because of changes in the plasma clotting mechanisms. A number of diseases and defects can upset the delicate balance and result in deficient clotting or in abnormal coagulation of the blood. Liver disease, low blood calcium, vitamin deficiency, severe injury, and inherited defects, including *hemophilia*, can all produce bleeders. In these conditions, prolonged bleeding from rather minor vascular injury is more characteristic than are petechiae. The bleeding may be superficial, and thus visible, from the skin or mucous membranes of the nose, mouth, and rectum. It may be into the gastrointestinal, urinary, or female genital tract. Or bleeding may be into muscle, internal organs, synovial spaces, or body cavities. The patient may notice the continued bleeding, of course, but the symptoms and signs of chronic hemorrhagic anemia may appear first, especially with gastrointestinal hemorrhage.

Increased clotting activity is less common and, when it occurs, causes intravascular thrombi and embolism. Most such thrombi are due to changes in the vascular walls, however.

EXERCISES

1 With a glass tube about ¹/₄ in in diameter and with smooth edges at both ends, suck up the skin on the palmar side of your forearm. You can get enough suction with your mouth to pull the small skin area well up into the tube. Maintain this suction for 5 min or so. When it is released, you should find a few petechiae. Near this point, slap your forearm repeatedly with one or two fingers. The area should redden as the capillaries fill with blood. Now press on the reddened area and over the petechiae. A glass slide is best, but you can use your finger if you look immediately when you release the pressure. Can you tell the difference between petechiae and dilated vessels?

2 Examine, if available, a white patient and a black patient known to be anemic. Look for changes in the skin, lips, conjunctivae, oral mucosa, and nail beds.

3 Prick your fingertip or earlobe with a sterile *stilette* or blade after you have wiped the area with alcohol or acetone. Be sure to let the area dry. The stab should be deep enough to produce a drop or two of blood without pressure. Let one drop fall on a glass slide where you can watch it clot. Note the time of the stab and, after getting the drop on the slide, touch the wound lightly with a piece of filter paper or blotting paper. It should pick up a drop of blood. Touch the area to a fresh spot on the paper every 30 sec. Then note how long it takes for the clotting to prevent the paper from picking up any blood. This is the *bleeding time* as tested in patients. Meantime, examine the clotting of the blood on the slide and watch later as the clot retracts. To do this, you must keep the slide in a very moist place or it will dry before it retracts.

4 If available, examine a tube of blood that has been prevented from clotting and then spun in a centrifuge. The bottom red layer is composed of erythrocytes, the white layer atop it of leukocytes and platelets, and the liquid layer above of plasma. Also examine a tube of clotted blood drawn an hour or more earlier. Look at the character of the clot and of the serum. Test the consistency of the clot by poking it with a small rod or stick. Is the mass fragile or tough?

9-11 SKIN

Skin Functions The skin has important functions, most of them readily apparent. It protects against sharp and blunt objects, friction, injurious chemicals, light, and drying. In areas where motion is needed, it provides a smooth surface, cushioning hair, and lubrication. In contrast, its ridges increase friction where grip is necessary.

The skin receives varied stimuli and is one of the principal sense organs. It is, as well, a highly active tissue, especially in regulating the body temperature. The skin's blood vessels can dilate to bring overheated blood near the cooler surface. And the skin surface gives up heat in three ways: it loses some by *radiation* much as a light bulb radiates heat; it delivers some to cool air moving across its surface by a process called *convection;* and—primarily—it cools by *evaporation.* It evaporates chiefly sweat, which the skin itself secretes as a dilute salt solution.

When the body temperature is too low, the skin also reacts. Its blood vessels contract, reducing the delivery of warm blood. This in itself cuts down heat loss by radiation and convection. The skin also stops sweating and so almost eliminates heat loss by evaporation.

The layer of fat in the deeper part of the skin passively limits heat loss, as any other insulating material would. It also stores foodstuffs and assists in a more subtle function of the skin, sexual attraction and personal recognition.

Skin Defects These multiple functions allow many defects to appear in the skin due to local or generalized disturbances. The skin's exposure to the surroundings and its reactivity make it vulnerable to various assaults. Its visibility makes patients aware of any changes, so that symptoms related to it are common.

Disease arising in the skin or lesions produced by generalized disease often appear first in one local area. The defect may then spread outward from this *pilot lesion.* This is usual in diseases of the skin itself; the defects are more apt to appear in separated areas at about the same time when due to generalized or systemic disease. There are, however, exceptions to both these statements.

A lesion undergoes a series of changes whether or not it spreads. There may be worsening, an improvement, or both may occur together. One condition may be present for a rather brief period as an acute stage, only to be followed by a quite different condition as the chronic stage.

The *acute stage* is more apt to show certain signs. Fiery redness, pus formation, local edema, and sharp pain usually are acute. A dusky redness, true hardness, fissures, duller pain, and, of course, scarring usually indicate that a defect is more *chronic.*

Classification of Defects Dermatologists speak of *primary changes,* which include macules, papules, nodules, vesicles, pustules, and petechiae as well as *bullae* or large blebs, wheals or urticaria, tumors, and ecchymoses. Some of these may be acute, others chronic. *Secondary changes* are exudation or weeping of serum, crusting or scabbing of the exudate, scaling, fissuring or cracking, excoriation or scratching, *atrophy* or thinning, and scarring. These are more apt to occur in chronic conditions.

Other changes are usually chronic but do not follow acute defects. These special changes include *comedones* or blackheads, *milia* or whiteheads—the small, chronic, superficial white globules that appear where the skin is normally thin—larger cysts, calluses, *telangiectases* or collections of small, dilated superficial veins, and *lichenification.* This latter is a firm or hard raised area with a flat, usually roughened surface which may fissure or scale. It can, if small, be called a *plaque.*

The texture, thickness, oiliness, and moistness of the skin vary from one part of the body to another. The structures within the skin—*hair roots, sweat glands,* and *oil glands*—also vary, as do the underlying structures. It is to be expected that some diseases are more likely to appear or even to be confined in certain areas. For example, *acne* attacks the face, neck, chest, and shoulders, areas where oil glands are numerous and large. It is, therefore, important to determine just where any abnormalities first appeared, to what areas they have extended, and where they are when the patient is seen.

Itching Localization is also important in describing itching. The symptom may be limited to one small spot, as it is with a mosquito bite, or it may cover a larger but still limited area as in sunburn. It may also be generalized and cover all the skin, as it is apt to do in liver or kidney disease.

Itching varies from the mild, transient sensation that follows release of pressure, as when a tight belt or underclothing is removed, to a severe, persistent, maddening state. Patients may prefer pain to itching and scratching may be an unconscious, reflex effort to convert the one to the other.

The symptom may appear before any change can be seen. It may mark healing, often replacing the pain of an acute abnormality, as it does in sunburn. Almost anyone with severe itching will scratch himself hard enough to produce excoriations. The excoriation is seen as a line of tiny scabs where the nail has broken the skin. This sign indicates itching even in a comatose patient.

EXERCISES

1 If possible, examine the skin of patients with various skin diseases. For the various diseased areas, describe accurately and with the correct terms the changes you see. Try to identify which changes are acute and which are chronic, which are primary and which secondary.

2 What is your own reaction or response in the presence of a person who is scratching constantly? Does this indicate anything about the role of the mind as a possible cause of some skin trouble?

Chapter 10

The Pathological Basis

Pathology includes all that pertains to the study of disease except its diagnosis and treatment. There are extensive descriptions of each disease, with the changes it produces during life and those found after death. In these varied abnormal conditions, however, certain more or less generalized reactions occur repeatedly. It helps in examining patients to know the nature of these pathological reactions.

To understand their nature, it is necessary to know something of the microscopic structure of the body. Complex as it is, this structure too embodies certain generalizations.

10-1 THE MINUTE STRUCTURE OF THE BODY

The basic microscopic unit of body structure is the *cell*. Very similar cells and their products grouped together form *tissues*. Tissues of various types are firmly associated to form *organs*. Organs of related functions are grouped together as *systems*.

Cell Structure   Each typical cell, regardless of its shape, has a *nucleus* which is separated from the remainder of the cell by a *nuclear membrane* (see Figure 10-1). Within this nucleus is the fundamental

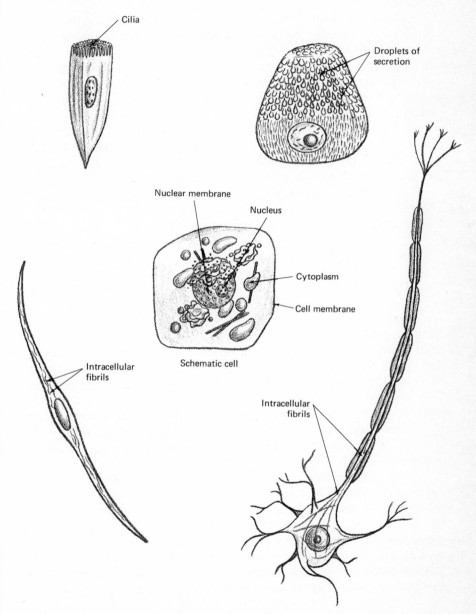

Figure 10-1   Typical cell (center) and some cell types.

genetic material which directs chemically the cell's activity. Many cells retain the capacity to duplicate this genetic material, and when they do, the cell can divide to produce two cells, usually two that are almost identical.

Around the nucleus and forming the bulk of most cells is the *cytoplasm*, surrounded by a *cell membrane*. Everything entering and leaving the cell must pass through this membrane, which is by no means passive; it actively controls what can enter and leave. The cytoplasm, the workshop of the cell, contains minute structures which carry on the cell's metabolism. Other cytoplasmic structures provide the mechanism to perform its specialized functions as a component of the body.

One such function for certain cells is the production of specialized *extracellular fibers*. The fibers in cartilage and bone contain and are embedded in salts and other substances which are laid down by the cells and which give these tissues their characteristics.

Cells vary enormously in size and appearance as well as in function. These characteristics are so typical for any one type of cell, however, that they are readily recognized by a trained person.

Tissue Structure   When these typical, similar cells group together to form sheets, clusters, or large masses, they are recognizable as a tissue (see Figure 10-2). Some tissues are almost exclusively composed of cells, as is glandular tissue, muscle tissue, or *epithelium*—the outer cells of the skin and the inner cells of the hollow organs. Other tissues contain relatively few cells but considerable extracellular fibers, salt deposits, or other material. One chief function of these cell-poor tissues is to bind body parts together, and they are collectively called *connective tissue.* They include such dense fibrous tissue as tendon, ligament, and sclera as well as bone and cartilage. Another form—*loose connective tissue*—is fibrous, but the fibers form a relatively open network that allows movement in several directions. This loose connective tissue throughout the body forms a flexible cement that holds other tissues together and in place.

Nervous tissue may resemble fibrous tissue, especially when nerves form tough cords. It is, however, more cellular than fibrous, because the minute *fibrils* that help make it tough are *intracellular.* Nerve cells characteristically have a cell body that sends out very fine but very long cytoplasmic processes within which run the fibrils. Most nerve cell bodies lie within the brain, spinal cord, or ganglia in the head or trunk. The nerve endings in the toes include processes that arise from spinal cord cells at the anatomical level of the upper lumbar and lower thoracic vertebrae.

Organ Structure   Each organ is composed of several types of tissue bound firmly together (see Figure 10-3). The intestine, for example,

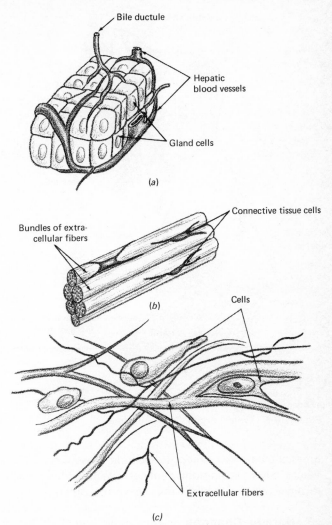

Figure 10-2 Typical tissues; cellular tissue of liver (above); dense connective tissue of tendon (middle); loose connective tissue (below).

has an epithelial lining resting on loose connective tissue. This tissue layer contains blood vessels, small nerves, and glandular tissue whose secretions empty into the gastric lumen. Outside the loose connective tissue are several layers of involuntary muscle bound together by more loose connective tissue and surrounded by still another outer layer of the same connective tissue.

Blood vessels within organs run through loose connective tissue which allows free passage of water and dissolved materials. Most of the

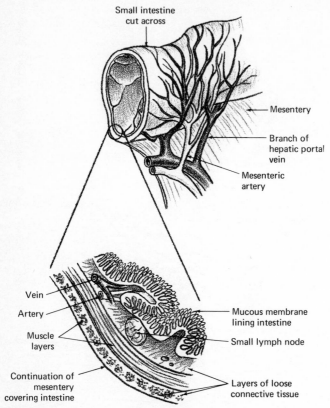

Figure 10-3 Typical organ. Small intestine.

extracellular space, then, lies within loose connective tissue, and this is where edema commonly collects. White blood cells also pass freely through this tissue when they leave the capillaries.

Normal Changes Cells, tissue, and organs constantly change. Some cells die and are replaced by division of nearby cells. Cell division occurs throughout the body of the growing infant and child, but it occurs locally in the adult as well, especially in the skin, mucous membranes, bone marrow, and lymph nodes. Nerve cells are exceptions, since they do not divide and can never be replaced when they die or are destroyed. Their long, fibril-filled processes can, however, grow again from the cell body if they are cut.

It is in this changing normal scene that disease appears, worsens, regresses, or progresses. Pathological processes, then, occur side by side with the normal course of events.

EXERCISES

1 If available, examine sections of tissue under the microscope. Sections of pancreas, tendon, loose connective tissue, stomach wall, and skin are good examples. In making the sections, killed tissue is cut into very thin slices and stained so that cells, fibers, etc., are more easily seen. The nucleus of the cell stains blue, the cytoplasm generally pink. Fibers are usually pink as well. Look at each slide without a microscope and then at the small illuminated area when the slide is under the microscope. You see only a small portion of this lighted area at any one time through the microscope, which gives you some idea of how small the cells and fibers really are.

2 In the microscope, identify cells and their nuclei. Note the resemblance of the cells within any one tissue. Then, in the stomach and skin, note how the various tissues together form a single organ.

3 Blood vessels are rather easy to identify because of the erythrocytes in them. Notice how the smallest capillaries as well as the larger vessels are surrounded by loose connective tissue even though this may be rather scanty. Notice too that none of the cells is really very far from a capillary.

10-2 ABNORMAL GROWTH AND DEATH OF BODY PARTS

Growth Defects　*Failure to Grow*　Perhaps the easiest pathological change to understand is *hypoplasia,* the failure of a tissue or organ to grow to full size. The extreme form is *aplasia,* in which the organ or tissue fails to grow at all, but this rarely occurs. Hypoplasia and aplasia may involve only part of the tissue in one organ, or they may involve an entire organ or limb. The cells usually look normal even under the microscope, but there are fewer than normal cells, fibers, and other tissue components. There will, of course, be no cells or tissues in true aplasia, as when a baby is born with a finger missing.

Most hypoplasias and aplasias are *congenital,* present at birth; some hypoplasias appear during development. When the genital organs fail to develop, for example, they are hypoplastic in adult life.

Overgrowth　*Hyperplasia* is the reverse; the number of cells increases beyond normal but each cell remains of normal size, appearance, and function. Somewhat more cell divisions occur than usual, or they continue for a longer period. Often hyperplasia is the body's response to a need for greater function of a part. For example, the blood-forming tissues of the marrow become hyperplastic after a hemorrhage.

Hypertrophy is a somewhat similar response in tissues with cells that do not divide readily. Each cell gets larger than usual, but there are not more of them than normal. This occurs in muscle—in the voluntary muscles of athletes during training, in the heart muscle during chronic hypertension. Hypertrophy, like hyperplasia, is a response to increased demand; the two processes may occur together, as they do in glandular tissue like the liver. Both changes can appear in some diseases, however, even though there is no increased demand.

Withering Atrophy marks a reversal—a loss of tissue, both by the disappearance of cells and by their growing smaller or by a decrease in fibers and other tissue components. Cells that die are destroyed and replaced in the usual course of events. When they die without replacement, their number decreases gradually. Cells that remain alive may shrink in size and content. Either change brings about a loss of function.

Some atrophy, like some hypertrophy and hyperplasia, is normal. The breasts enlarge to feed the infant and then the glandular tissue decreases or atrophies when nursing ceases. It atrophies even more at the climacteric. Indeed many of the changes of aging are atrophy, as is apparent in the thinning skin.

Atrophy often is a consequence of disease; a muscle becomes *atrophic* when deprived of its nerve supply. It may also occur as the primary disease; the brain can atrophy without other disease. It may arise because of factors that are from outside the body; the wasting of starvation is atrophy.

Degenerative Diseases Atrophy occurs along with hyperplasia and hypertrophy in one major category of diseases, the so-called *degenerative diseases.* These include osteoarthritis, when atrophy of the joint cartilages is accompanied by hyperplasia in the bony processes around the joint and by a form of hypertrophy in the smooth, dense bone under the wasted cartilage. Atherosclerosis or arteriosclerosis is another degenerative disease that combines in the same arterial wall a complex of atrophy, hyperplasia, and hypertrophy.

Degenerative diseases can involve atrophy alone; in hemorrhoids and varicose veins, the vessel wall is weakened. Male-type baldness is a degenerative condition due to atrophy of the hair roots.

At times, degenerative diseases include the laying down of abnormal materials in atrophic tissue. Fatty substances and calcium salts are deposited in the atrophic connective tissue as arteriosclerosis develops. Cataracts of the senile type are due to deposits of fats and other substances in atrophic parts of the lens.

Tissue Death Atrophy appears when cells die off without replacement and the normal rate of cell death may even be increased somewhat. There is, however, no mass destruction of cells. The rapid death of large numbers or all the cells of a tissue, organ, or part does occur in *necrosis.* Associated structures such as fibers or mineral deposits in bone may persist apparently intact for some time during necrosis, but they too eventually disintegrate and are removed or replaced.

Poisonous substances and infections can cause necrosis, as can direct physical injury, burning, or freezing. More often, interference with the blood supply kills the tissues. An embolus in an artery, for example, deprives cells of oxygen and food. As a result, these cells die, producing an area of necrosis called an *infarct*. This is why coronary occlusion is said to cause myocardial infarction and an embolus in the pulmonary artery causes a pulmonary infarct. Death of a large mass of tissue is often called *gangrene* as well as necrosis.

While they may sound rather similar, atrophy and necrosis are rarely confused clinically. Atrophy of the skin thins it and makes it vulnerable; necrosis of the skin produces an ulcer.

Necrosis is clearly abnormal. The body—if the patient lives—must repair, replace, or remove the necrotic area. Some parts, like the liver and skin, can *regenerate* to a considerable degree as cell divisions restore necrotic areas. *Replacement* by scar occurs when regeneration cannot occur completely or at all, as is true in the myocardium and lung. *Removal* may be as dramatic as the dropping off of a gangrenous toe, or it may consist of walling off the necrotic area in a *capsule* of scar tissue. Localized fat necrosis can be walled off under the skin and the mass is felt as a tumor.

Abnormal Growths   *Neoplasms* constitute another very different set of tumors. They are new growths which differ from regeneration, hyperplasia, and hypertrophy in that they grow beyond some rather indefinite "normal limits." They can be said to show unrestrained proliferation or growth and, when large enough or superficial enough, can be seen or felt as masses. If untreated, some continue to increase in size.

Neoplasms are conveniently divided into two categories: *benign* and *malignant.* There is, however, some overlap between these two and in some instances it is hard to say whether a neoplasm is wholly benign or somewhat malignant.

Benign Tumors   *Benign neoplasms* commonly consist of cells that closely resemble those of the normal tissue from which they grow. They contain blood vessels, nerves, and connective tissue much like normal tissue, but usually most of the cells are of one type. Almost always there is a clear edge or boundary about the mass of neoplastic cells, and often connective tissue forms a fibrous capsule around the tumor. Some cells will continue dividing in a normal fashion, but not very many, and the cells can carry out normal functions, as when an endocrine cell tumor produces a hormone.

The really distinguishing feature of benign neoplasms, however, is that they grow where they arise. They extend only by expanding and so produce damage chiefly by pressing upon the surrounding structures.

Malignant Tumors *Malignant neoplasms,* also called *malignancies* or *cancers,* differ from benign tumors in important respects. Their cells are not identical with those from which they came, although in *differentiated tumors* there may be a clear resemblance. *Undifferentiated malignancies* often contain cells so changed that it is difficult or impossible to recognize their origin. Usually many of the cells, even in differentiated tumors, have abnormal nuclei, or a single cell will contain more than one nucleus. Cell divisions typically are numerous, but they too are abnormal, so that the two cells formed often differ from one another. This difference between cells of the same origin is another characteristic of malignancy.

The tumor usually but not always grows in a disorganized fashion, often with few or no blood vessels to nourish it. It has no capsule and the malignant cells invade the surrounding normal tissue, whose vessels supply most of the oxygen and foodstuffs. The poor blood supply sooner or later fails to sustain the central areas of the tumor as it grows, and these areas then become necrotic.

Malignant tumors, unlike benign neoplasms, spread by processes other than simple expansion. Their cells *infiltrate* locally by invading normal tissue, and they can also reach distant areas of the body to form secondary tumors or *metastases.* Metastases develop when malignant cells enter the bloodstream and are swept along to lodge in a new place and begin spreading there. In addition to this bloodstream embolism, malignant cells may enter lymphatic vessels and be carried to the next lymph node, where they form a metastasis. This, in turn, may free cells which are carried to the next node. Metastatic spread also occurs by a third mechanism when the neoplasm reaches the surface of an organ in the chest or abdomen. Cells then can break from the tumor and, carried by gravity or by movement of the organs, *implant* on the lining membranes of the cavity.

Some malignant tumors form metastases early, when the primary neoplasm is still small. Others metastasize only later. Similarly, some malignancies grow locally by invasion much more rapidly than others. In general, however, growth is more rapid than that of any benign tumor.

Cancers apparently harm the patient in several ways. Their growth destroys normal tissue in addition to producing pressure disturbances or obstructions. Their necrotic centers have a tendency to bleed, and invasion of a larger blood vessel by tumor can cause severe hemorrhage. Many malignancies cause symptoms of fatigue, lassitude and malaise, and signs of weight loss, even to almost complete wasting away. Others produce anemia and various functional disturbances.

Malignant tumors have a variety of names, each specifying the type of cell from which it arises. There are, however, two large general categories and two smaller groups whose general names are important.

Types of Malignant Tumors   *Carcinomas* are malignant neoplasms arising from epithelial cells, usually of the skin, mucous membranes, or glands. *Sarcomas* arise from connective tissues—including cartilage and bone—or from muscles and blood vessels. Usually two other conditions are grouped with the sarcomas—the *leukemias* and the *malignant lymphomas*, arising in the bone marrow and lymph nodes.

One smaller group consists of malignant neoplasms arising from nervous tissue for which there is no general term. The other small group comprises the *malignant mixed tumors* which have both epithelial and connective tissue cells.

The skin, like other parts of the body, has neoplasms. A common benign one involves fat cells growing within a capsule. The tumor grows slowly and does not spread, although there may be more than one on the patient. Malignant tumors also arise in the skin, and some metastasize even while still small. Others spread only locally. A fairly large, malignant skin carcinoma often becomes necrotic and forms an ulcer, as would any other necrotic skin lesion.

EXERCISES

1 If available, examine briefly patients who show superficial hypoplasia or aplasia, as of an ear or mandible; hyperplasias, as in the breast during pregnancy and lactation; hypertrophy, as in the heart of a patient dying with chronic hypertension.

2 Compare the relative volume and physical characteristics of the skin and muscle of an aged or debilitated patient with those of a normal young person. In the skin, try to define which tissues are atrophic. In the muscle, compare the changes in the tendons with those of the muscle itself. Which of the two shows greater evidence of atrophy?

3 If available, examine closely the consequences of necrosis in skin ulcers or other superficial lesions such as burns. How does the body rid itself of necrotic tissue in this instance? What happens to necrotic tissue after a crushing injury of the thigh?

4 If possible, examine as an example a benign skin neoplasm. Pay particular attention to the history of its growth and, on physical examination, to its boundaries, movability, and appearance.

5 Examine, if possible, a malignant skin neoplasm, noting the same characteristics. In addition, examine the lymph nodes along the lymphatic vessels draining the part. What would you expect to find as characteristics of a node containing a metastasis? Does the patient show these?

6 Examine locally the malignancy in any other available patient who has one. If you examine several, note the variability and the ease with which the mass can be confused with other findings.

10-3 INFLAMMATION

Acute Inflammation The most widely known basic process in pathology is *inflammation.* Everyone experiences it to some degree at times, from the neonatal period to senility. And this is not surprising, since it is the body's defensive response to a wide variety of threats to health. A patient may say that his eye is "inflamed" when in fact it only shows some vascular dilatation. The medical term is more precise.

Inflammation may be *acute* or *chronic,* depending upon its duration, but the tissue changes involved gradually blend from one form into another. The precise type of tissue change can be named and often the location and cause are given as well. The medical word ending of *-itis* means inflammation of some sort, so that "conjunctivitis" means inflammation of the conjunctiva and "dermatitis" means inflammation of the skin. Noninflammatory conditions are given the ending *-osis,* so that a "dermatosis" is a noninflammatory skin disorder.

Localized Acute Inflammation A localized acute inflammation of the skin, tonsils, or joints has certain characteristics which can be seen on examination. They are most evident as the inflammation becomes full-blown but some are present at any time during the course. There are really five characteristics—*heat* and *redness, pain* and *swelling,* and *disturbed function.* Heat refers to local warmth, and pain may be present only on pressure, so that it really is tenderness. It is easy to remember these because they occur full-blown in severe sunburn, where the disturbed function is the loss of temperature control.

Each of these signs and symptoms has its roots in the body's defenses. A disturbed organ or part begins its defensive reaction by *vasodilatation.* As the capillaries become engorged, they deliver more warm blood to the area, producing the "heat" and "redness." Engorgement itself may be painful, and water with dissolved materials promptly leaks from the capillaries into the intercellular spaces, causing swelling and increasing the pain. Furthermore, part of the tissues' reaction liberates chemicals which, among other actions, stimulate the nerve endings for pain. Pain, engorgement, and edema all interfere with normal function.

The increased blood supply to the damaged area assists the body's defenses in several ways. It brings in leukocytes and the protective antibodies of the blood. It also carries away chemicals which may damage tissue and spreads other chemicals which initiate beneficial reactions in distant parts of the body.

Leukocytes, when they arrive in the capillaries of an inflamed area, first adhere to the walls and then force their way between the lining cells. Once in the intercellular space, they move toward the injured area, drawn by chemicals from the damaged cells or other leukocytes. Their actions in the area depend upon the cause of the damage. In a simple, clean cut, they begin breaking up and removing killed or severely injured tissue cells as well as any erythrocytes outside vessels. In an infection with bacteria, some begin engulfing the invading bacteria. These invaders may be destroyed by the leukocytes or they may kill some of the white blood cells as well as tissue cells. When this occurs, the dead cells form pus. In some infections bacteria grow within cells, including leukocytes, without killing them immediately. The result is a much more complicated and often chronic infection, one cause of chronic inflammation.

Healing When the inflammatory response successfully removes invading material or when the injury is simple and small, acute inflammation leads to rapid healing. This process involves the division of surviving tissue cells, such as epithelium, which have the càpacity to divide. The connective tissue cells also divide and replace lost fibers, thus binding or "knitting" the tissues. New blood vessels bud off from old capillaries and extend into the healing area to restore its circulation. The redness, warmth, swelling, and pain subside as the healing progresses.

Larger but still simple wounds and infections or those occurring in tissue which cannot divide and regenerate heal in a different fashion. Lost tissue then is replaced by a more active response of the connective tissue, which forms dense masses of fibers. These masses are the *scar.*

Healing is different again when the damaged tissue contains material that the leukocytes cannot remove. If this material is pus or bacteria growing within cells, the connective tissue may form a dense *capsule* which prevents further spread. This encapsulated area is an *abscess* if deep, a *pustule* if on the surface. Eventually an abscess either ruptures and discharges its contents, as pustules often do, or it slowly contracts and becomes converted to a mass of scar tissue.

Connective tissue similarly encapsulates any *foreign matter*—wood, glass, or even dead bone. If the body can destroy the matter, it does so slowly. Otherwise the foreign substance may remain encapsulated and, if it is irritant, produce chronic inflammation around it. Even foreign liquid, such as an oil, can be encapsulated to give a *sterile abscess.*

This process of acute inflammation is common on the skin. Acne shows the stages through healing very well. An abrasion such as a scraped knee demonstrates some aspects even better. Hemorrhage followed by coagulation here is part of the initial reaction. If the wound is not infected, removal of the scab when healing has begun uncovers a pink, moist, rather lumpy area in the center. New epithelium can be seen as a thin sheet growing in from the edges. The central area is *granulation tissue,* one form of regenerating connective tissue. When this overgrows somewhat, as it sometimes does, it is called *exuberant granulation* or *proud flesh.*

Granulation tissue with its newly forming capillaries is fragile and bleeds easily in small local areas. It also is moist with interstitial fluid or exudate and may "weep" rather copiously. As it dries, the exudate, often mixed with some blood, forms a *crust.*

The advancing epithelium eventually covers normal, healthy granulation tissue. At first thin, it gradually thickens to its usual toughness when healing is complete. If the injury is deep, extensive, or infected, the granulation tissue may thicken and toughen into a scar, which may or may not be covered by epithelium of nearly normal appearance.

Internal Inflammation Inflammation within the body is basically the same process as on the skin, but one or another characteristic may be prominent. It is possible to speak of *exudative* or *serous inflammation* when fluid is poured from the inflamed surface of the pleura, pericardium, synovial membrane, or peritoneum. In *fibrinous inflammation,* the inflamed surface in these areas is covered with a thin clot. Such fibrinous inflammation produces loud pleural and pericardial rubs. Frank bleeding from inflamed areas marks *hemorrhagic inflammation.* An outpouring of mucus, as in the common cold, is part of *catarrhal inflammation.* The presence of pus marks *purulent inflammation.*

Generalized Inflammatory Changes The acute inflammatory reaction may remain a local one, especially if the area involved is small and the reaction not very severe. There may, however, be a general or *systemic inflammatory reaction* secondary to the local inflammation. One result is fever, which can be produced by several mechanisms depending on the cause of the inflammation. Another symptom is weakness and lassitude or *malaise,* a general, vague feeling of being unwell if not outright ill.

A somewhat different form is the acute *generalized inflammation* that occurs with some acute infections which spread widely in the body. This is particularly true of many viral diseases but can occur with certain bacterial and fungal infections. Here there may be many simultaneous local inflammatory responses in widespread areas. Measles, for example, inflames the eyes, pharynx, skin, and sometimes the lower respiratory tract or the meninges covering the brain.

Chronic Inflammation Chronic inflammation represents in many ways delayed healing of acute inflammation, but it has certain distinct characteristics. It often starts as an acute process, but it may never show the five typical characteristics. On the skin, the redness tends to be less fiery, more dusky, or even a violet color. The area is only slightly if at all warmer than the surrounding skin, swelling tends to be hard, and there may be little or no tenderness. Function is disturbed, however. Internal lesions have corresponding characteristics.

The evident differences between acute and chronic inflammation stem from the changes in the tissues themselves. In the chronic condition, the capillaries are no longer conspicuously filled with blood, although there may be considerable edema. The leukocytes leaving the capillaries are of a different type, less prone to liberate pain-producing chemicals, and there is considerable growth of connective tissue in the interstitial spaces. Indeed, regenerating connective tissue mingles intimately with dying cells and leukocytes. Regeneration by division of surviving cells is slow and may also occur near dying cells. The impression is generally that the repair is barely keeping up with the continuing damage.

One common result is the accumulation of granulation tissue in masses called *granulomas*. These granulomas may, in time, be encapsulated by scar tissue, or they may become necrotic. Some of this necrotic tissue can become thick like cheese, a process that occurs in tuberculosis.

Chronic inflammation, like acute inflammation, can produce systemic changes. These may include fever, usually slight or intermittent, weakness, malaise, and generalized wasting.

EXERCISES

1 Describe in correct terms the full course of a single acne lesion as an example of local inflammation.
2 Describe in correct pathological terms the course of events when a fairly deep splinter is neglected; when a knee, elbow, or chin is abraded; when a new shoe rubs a heel.
3 Trace the local and systemic changes of the 3-day common cold, describing the evidences of inflammation.
4 Name the five characteristics of inflammation and give examples other than the above.
5 Name the special types of inflammation in which some one characteristic is prominent.
6 Distinguish both by symptoms and signs and by pathological changes between acute and chronic inflammation. How would you distinguish between them in skin lesions?

10-4 INFECTION

One of the most common causes of pathological changes is *infection*. Almost without exception the infecting, living matter is too small to see with the naked eye, warranting the name of *microorganism*. The name of the particular microorganism is one usual way of specifically designating an infection, as in "streptococcal sore throat." At times the infection bears a specific name of its own, as does "measles" or a "boil," and local infections are also described by their location, as "tonsillitis." The infection may be acute or chronic or even *recurrent* and, since most cause inflammation, the type of pathological change may be included in the name, as it is in "chronic purulent tonsillitis."

Disease-producing Microorganisms Infecting microorganisms fall into several natural groups with many subgroups, and each bears an individual name as well. The major groups are usually given as four: (1) *viruses*, (2) a group of very small bacterialike microorganisms called *Rickettsiae*, (3) *bacteria*, and (4) *fungi*. All the microorganisms are small, but the above list goes from smallest to largest.

Viruses and the *Rickettsiae* live exclusively inside living cells of the body. Bacteria and fungi may be similarly *intracellular*, but often they live and divide outside the cells. Obviously all can survive outside cells and can pass from one person or *host* to another.

It is usual to consider some infections as *communicable, contagious,* or *"catching."* Other infections do not pass easily from one person to another and some can develop only when a part of the body has been injured. These are *noncommunicable infections.*

Viruses Scientists divide the viruses into subgroups, in part depending on their size. In general, viral infections are contagious and any *susceptible* person in contact with an infected patient can get the disease at some stage in its development. Several childhood diseases are viral— *measles, German measles, chickenpox,* and *mumps,* for example. So are other diseases as common in adults as in children: the *common cold, influenza,* and *smallpox* fall in this group. All these are quite contagious. *Viral hepatitis* and *poliomyelitis,* on the other hand, are less contagious. All these *systemic*—generalized—infections are acute, although viral hepatitis may become chronic or recurrent.

The best-known chronic viral disease is *warts,* although the lesion hardly resembles that of most viral infections and it produces no systemic symptoms. Most acute viral infections do cause systemic reactions with more or less fever—usually rather low-grade—and considerable malaise, muscular aching, and weakness.

Rickettsiae The *rickettsial diseases* are fewer in number and less common than viral infections. The best-known in the United States is *Rocky Mountain spotted fever* which, like other rickettsial diseases, is generalized and produces considerable systemic symptoms. These diseases are not contagious and are carried from person to person by biting ticks and mites.

Bacteria   *Bacterial infections,* in contrast, are numerous and varied. One common division of the causal microorganisms is into *gram-positive* and *gram-negative bacteria,* depending upon how they can be stained for microscopic examination. Diseases caused by gram-positive bacteria include many *pneumonias, boils* and *carbuncles,* most *tonsillitis* and severe *pharyngitis, scarlet fever, diphtheria,* and many *wound infections.* Obviously some of these are local, some more generalized infections, some contagious and some not, some producing severe systemic symptoms and some not.

Gram-negative bacteria cause such varied diseases as *gonorrhea, dysentery, typhoid fever,* and many *renal infections.* Some produce only local disorders, but others cause highly symptomatic, generalized diseases.

Another group of bacteria, called *acid-fast* because of their reactions to stains, cause *tuberculosis* and *leprosy.* Still another group includes the microorganism involved in *syphilis* and other less common diseases.

Fungi   The *fungi* differ from bacteria in several ways, one being that the microorganism often contains more than a single cell; bacteria are one-celled. The most common *fungal disease* in the United States is one form of *athlete's foot.* Some other fungi can, however, spread throughout the body.

Animal Parasites   In general, bacteria and fungi are plantlike. Rather simple, small animals can also cause disease. Most of these diseases are tropical and occur only rarely in the United States.

Some of these animals, usually called *parasites,* contain only one cell. They cause *malaria* and the dysenteric disease called *amebiasis.* Other parasites are *worms* and include *hookworms* and *tapeworms,* which can infest the human intestine. Such parasitic diseases are properly called *infestations* rather than infections.

Infections   *Transmission of Infections*   Infecting microorganisms, especially viruses, can be inhaled after they have been sprayed into the air by coughing, sneezing, or talking. Many invaders enter the body from dirty hands or by being swallowed in food and water. Some bacteria penetrate the skin, especially through wounds, and some are transmitted during sexual intercourse. The latter, including gonorrhea and syphilis, are *venereal diseases.* Some viruses, *Rickettsiae,* and parasites are carried from person to person by the bite of mosquitoes, other insects, mites, and ticks.

Defenses against Infection   The body defends itself against invasion by bacteria and fungi in part through an acute inflammatory reaction which probably also affords some protection against viruses. Another defense plays a larger part, however, against viruses and many bacteria.

This defense, the *immunological response,* depends upon the body's ability to form chemical protectors. In its simplest form, this response begins when certain leukocytes come into contact with a virus or with poisonous chemicals called *toxins* produced by some bacteria. Leukocytes produce, and liberate into the blood, chemicals called *antibodies*— or *antitoxins* if they form in response to toxins. The antibodies can interfere with the spread of viruses and neutralize toxins and so assist in overcoming infection.

Immunization   The leukocytes that form antibodies never return to their original state even after the infection is cured. They remain able to form the particular antibody very rapidly and effectively if the body is again infected by the same microorganism. This is one very common form of *immunity* to an infection and provides the basis for intentional *immunization.*

Fortunately, some microorganisms can be artificially modified so that they no longer cause disease but still provoke leukocytes to produce antibodies. *Vaccination* against smallpox and other immunizations against measles, German measles, poliomyelitis, whooping cough, and typhoid fever as well as some other infectious diseases make use of such modified microorganisms. Immunization against some other diseases including diphtheria and tetanus uses a modified toxin to force production of antitoxin, since toxin rather than bacteria themselves causes the trouble in these infections.

Course of Infections   The course of infections varies with many circumstances, but in general it follows a certain pattern. The infection starts when disease-producing microorganisms enter the body and begin to multiply. At first there are too few to cause symptoms or signs. This *asymptomatic* interval is the *incubation period* and the disease may be contagious during it. There follows a *period of symptoms,* usually mild at first but slowly or rapidly increasing as the disease reaches its peak. The patient generally remains contagious during this period but the body is defending itself with increasing efficiency against the infection. The defenses may prove inadequate and then the patient dies. If the defenses are sufficient, they begin to overcome the infection, so that the patient rapidly or slowly recovers. At some point in this process the patient almost always becomes noncontagious as the microorganisms disappear.

The defenses may not eliminate all the microorganisms even though the patient recovers. If the microorganisms remain deep within the body, the patient is no longer contagious but the continuing infection may later produce a relapse or recurrence of symptomatic disease. If the microorganisms remain where they escape from the body, the patient can pass on the infection and is a *carrier,* a contagious person without symptoms.

The body's defenses against parasites operate in much the same way as they do against bacteria or fungi. Mature hookworms and tapeworms remain within the intestine, however, as chronic infestations. They produce little obvious disease, although hookworms can draw enough blood from the intestinal wall to cause anemia.

EXERCISES

1   Vaccination against smallpox causes two types of reaction. On the first vaccination, nothing is seen for 4 days or more; then a small papule appears and gradually enlarges until it becomes a sizable vesicle surrounded by a large inflamed area. On subsequent vaccination, a papule appears earlier, forms a small vesicle in a small inflamed area, and then promptly subsides. Explain the difference.

2   What is the meaning of *epidemic, endemic,* and *sporadic* as used to describe diseases? Which of these must involve contagious disease?

3   Will a patient who has a contagious disease and is an accurate reporter always give a history of contact with a person who has that disease? Why or why not?

4   Communities often have small epidemics of the common cold. During such an epidemic a patient complains of a stuffy, runny nose and sneezing. What questions would you ask to help decide whether he represents a new case in that epidemic?

5   Viral hepatitis is not highly contagious yet there have been epidemics within groups of heroin addicts. Why should such groups be prone to have them?

6   Some infectious diseases confer a lifelong immunity against a second attack. Some give only partial immunity. Some immunizations—often called *inoculations*—give almost total protection against the disease for a long time, others are less effective. Look up the duration and extent of protection after a natural attack as well as the course of the disease after inoculation for the following diseases: smallpox, diphtheria, tetanus, typhoid fever, whooping cough, poliomyelitis, and influenza. (A textbook on pediatrics is a good source.) How does this information help in taking a history?

7   What information about a patient's life is it important to elicit in order to decide whether he may have a parasitic disease? Why is it important in today's world?

8   What information is important in determining whether a patient may have a venereal disease? What is the best way to elicit this part of the history?

10-5 ALLERGY, HYPERSENSITIVITY, AND AUTOIMMUNE DISEASES

The body's defense mechanisms themselves cause the group of diseases called *allergy.* The production of antibodies against microorganisms and toxins involves interaction with foreign substances that threaten a person's well-being. The body can also produce antibodies and locally heightened defenses after contact with other substances as well, even though these are only plant pollen, house dust, or a bee sting. A patient can react similarly to chemicals such as medicines or plastics and to animal products like serum. The reaction may be basically protective, but it is so strong in some persons and under some circumstances as to threaten a person's life when he later has contact with the same or similar substances.

Allergy is often referred to as *hypersensitivity,* but the latter term covers more conditions. In general, a hypersensitive patient reacts with symptoms to something that does not really disturb the majority of people. This unusual reaction may be allergic, but it may also be congenital or hereditary. Albinos who lack pigment in the skin and most very fair redheads are hypersensitive to sunlight and burn very readily. There is also a hereditary, chemical abnormality in the erythrocytes of some people, usually blacks, which makes them hypersensitive to certain chemicals, including some drugs. These conditions involve no immune mechanisms.

Severe Allergic Reactions   *Allergy* is a general term for the state in which a patient has an inappropriately great immune response to a substance called an *antigen.* This antigen, which may be any of a wide variety of substances, characteristically causes no detectable reaction on first contact or even on a second. One very potent antigen is injected horse serum, which is sometimes used to provide a patient with antibodies against a specific disease. The first injection or a series of injections given over a short period produces no ill effects. Another injection after an interval of weeks, months, or even years often causes one of several reactions depending upon the antibodies formed against the serum itself.

The most serious reaction occurs within seconds or minutes after injection and is called *anaphylaxis.* This is a severe shock state which can kill promptly if untreated. A very similar reaction called *anaphylactoid shock*—because it resembles anaphylaxis—can follow reinjection of a variety of substances including penicillin. Anaphylactoid shock can also occur after the sting of a bee, wasp, hornet, or other insect.

A less threatening reaction—*serum sickness*—appears from several days to 2 weeks after reinjection, a second ingestion, or occasionally after an initial contact. It is systemic and variable with fever, joint pain, abdominal pain, enlarged lymph nodes, and skin eruptions. A skin eruption, on the other hand, may appear alone within hours after injection or ingestion of an antigen.

Common Allergies   Much more common and benign allergies are *hay fever,* appearing in the fall, and *rose fever,* in the spring. There are related allergies in the summer and all are due to wind-borne *pollen* of various plants. Typically they recur at the same season in any one patient, with itching, tearing eyes, profuse watery nasal discharge, and sneezing. The conjunctiva and nasal mucous membranes are inflamed but, despite the name, there are really no systemic symptoms such as fever.

Bronchial asthma also may be an allergic response either to airborne antigens like pollen or ingested or injected ones. Many attacks of asthma, however, are triggered by emotional upsets and some are associated with infections or other nonallergic conditions.

A variety of local skin reaction, including hives or *urticaria* and *eczema*, can occur as the result of allergy. Some antigens such as poison ivy, plastics, and cosmetics usually provoke inflammation at the point of contact. Others can produce lesions at a greater distance from that area.

The pathological changes in allergy are varied but often are inflammatory, as in hay fever and many skin reactions. For this reason the symptoms and signs may suggest infection and only a careful history will give a clue as to the cause.

Autoimmunity A separate group of diseases is usually included among those caused by abnormal immune reactions. These so-called *autoimmune diseases* apparently arise when the body develops defensive reactions against some of its own components. The disorders are inflammatory and most are uncommon or rare. A rather common one is *rheumatoid arthritis*.

EXERCISES

1 What questions would you ask to discover whether a patient is likely to have or have had allergies? Give your reason for each question.
2 A patient complains of difficulty in breathing. How would you determine whether it is due to acute obstruction of the bronchioles? If you decide that it is, how would you try to discover what triggered the attack?
3 Patients sometimes will say that they are allergic to some food such as spinach, which they dislike, a troublesome cousin, or even a distasteful idea. Is this allergy? Why or why not?

10-6 NUTRITIONAL DISORDERS AND INTOXICATIONS

Nutritional Disorders Since the body carries out so many chemical processes and depends upon some of them for life, it is not surprising to find chemical disorders among the diseases. These disorders can divided into those produced by chemicals taken into the body and related to the processes of metabolism.

Undernutrition   Malnutrition occurs when a person does not get optimal amounts of food containing the proper chemical balance. An adequate diet must contain *proteins, fats, vitamins* and *minerals,* and sufficient *carbohydrates* as well. Since the latter—the sugars and starches—are cheap foods, they are most likely to be eaten. Protein and fat are more expensive and therefore more likely to be deficient, especially since protein of vegetable origin can be incomplete—lacking some of the essential components. It is unlikely that anyone who gets a daily, reasonable serving of meat, fish, or fowl, as well as an egg and a glass of milk, will be deficient in protein or fat. Growing children, pregnant women, and lactating mothers require more protein than other healthy people. Similarly, patients with severe acute systemic diseases and chronic wasting diseases require more protein as well as more food in general.

The essential vitamins and minerals can be obtained in large part from the meat-egg-milk component. When a person also eats fresh fruit or fruit juice, green leafy vegetables, and vegetable salads daily, he is unlikely to be malnourished unless he has a disease that increases his need for vitamins and minerals. A person must, of course, get enough total food intake to supply his body's need for energy and to maintain normal weight.

Undernutrition causes serious damage, especially during infancy and childhood. The child not only fails to grow at a normal rate but, if seriously undernourished, is stunted mentally as well. Adolescents and adults withstand undernutrition much better, but if it is severe or prolonged, it can produce disease.

The general wasting of starvation is readily evident, but the loss of resistance to infection and to injury is less apparent when the protein intake alone is inadequate. Vitamin deficiencies to the point of disease are uncommon in the United States, but lack of any particular vitamin produces a specific disorder. These disorders are chiefly degenerative in type, as in *night blindness* or in *scurvy,* but some are inflammatory, as is the dermatitis of *pellagra.*

Mineral deficiencies include anemia from lack of iron and weakening of bones from a low calcium intake. More dramatically, a lack of adequate salt when a person perspires very heavily can cause weakness and

ous malnutrition occurs most often in certain
atients with other diseases and the extremely
addicts often eat too little to be well nourished.
those with no teeth, risk *protein deficiency.*
refuse to eat a reasonable diet and may develop

nutritional problems. Food faddists with fixed, erroneous ideas of what to eat rather often become malnourished.

Overnutrition   *Overnutrition* is even more common than undernutrition in the United States. It accounts for almost all *obesity*. Overconsumption of some vitamins can cause disease, especially in infants and children. This occurs when a person receives vitamin preparations in addition to the diet, and then only when parental enthusiasm or faddism leads to the intake of much larger than normal amounts. Overconsumption of calcium in milk or as medicine may contribute to the formation of kidney stones, but this is unusual.

Intoxications   *Alcoholism*   Overconsumption of alcohol is a form of chemical disease. Basically alcohol causes medical difficulties in three situations. *Acute alcoholism*—drunkenness—depends chiefly on drinking too much too fast. Alcohol is a *sedative* that depresses the nervous system, but its first impact is on the cerebral cortex. As this effect dulls the restraints of the higher centers, the person usually becomes livelier if not more physically active. Larger amounts taken in a short period depress the cerebellum and lead to incoordination. More still affects the brainstem and produces unconsciousness or coma. Such a "dead drunk" person is not far from fatal depression of the respiratory centers.

Chronic alcoholism results from drinking too much over too long a period. The effects of the alcohol are complicated by those of malnutrition in most instances and by the repeated accidents and exposure to which the alcoholic patient is prone. The consequences of alcoholism are essentially degenerative and are commonly seen in the liver, which is partially destroyed. This is followed by some regeneration and much scar formation within the liver to produce *hepatic cirrhosis*.

Degenerative changes also occur within the brain and peripheral nerves, due in part perhaps to deficient nutrition. In some patients changes in the myocardium lead to heart failure, and the degenerative alterations in the skin are well known.

To such changes can be added *gastritis*, inflammation which leads to nausea and vomiting. There may also be hemorrhage with bloody vomitus and tarry stools. Cirrhosis can lead to even more severe gastrointestinal bleeding because it interferes with the hepatic portal circulation.

The third set of problems for alcoholics are really *withdrawal* difficulties which appear when the chronic alcoholic abruptly stop drinking. The headache and lassitude of the hangover after an acute of drunkenness rarely is serious. Withdrawal in the chronic alco often a medical emergency. Apparently mild withdrawal sym tremor, lassitude, and malaise may suddenly develop into severe epilepsy-like convulsions.

The more severe withdrawal disorder, *delirium tremens*, or DTs, is widely recognized as a complication of chronic alcoholism. Many people believe that it is a manifestation of drunkenness, but it most often appears when the consumption of alcohol is reduced or stopped *after* an episode of drunkenness. The patient may first become increasingly restless and sleepless, irritable and jumpy. A coarse tremor of the hands, tongue, and face appears and the patient becomes delirious, with confusion, disorientation, and hallucinations. These hallucinations are usually bizarre and visual, frequently of animals—"pink elephants" for example. The patient is very active and disruptive, fearful, and restless. He often has a fever and rapid pulse.

DTs seem particularly apt to occur when the patient has trauma, an operation, or an acute infection such as pneumonia. Initially the symptoms can be mistaken for complications of such a condition. Untreated DTs can last from 2 to 10 days, sometimes complicated by convulsive seizures. The untreated patient very often dies, especially if his general condition is poor.

Other Intoxications Barbiturates are also depressant drugs—"downers"—and overdosage or acute intoxication causes sleepiness followed by deep coma. More dangerous, the respiration is markedly depressed, and the patient can become cyanotic without developing a flushed face, as he would in acute alcoholic intoxication.

Barbiturates can be abused acutely or chronically, but the signs of chronic barbiturate intoxication are not clear cut. If severe enough, the overuse produces physical and mental sluggishness, but the real danger comes during withdrawal.

The withdrawal changes resemble those in delirium tremens, with initial restlessness and anxiety. Somewhat later—usually after a day or so—a tremor appears, with twitching and jerking of the arms and legs. These usually lead to epileptic seizures and then a period of sleeplessness. A day or two later the patient becomes delirious, with visual hallucina-
tion, disruptive behavior, and fever as the usual pattern.
prolonged period of sleep, but untreated
withdrawal.
ost related drugs are also depressants, and
on sleep or coma. They are respiratory
of death. The pupils are pinpoint in size and,
on, strongly suggest the cause.
on—is marked by abrupt changes in mood
mptoms of withdrawal, with restlessness,

runny nose, malaise, and hostility. Eventually the patient becomes undernourished and often he develops secondary complications, particularly local infections and viral hepatitis if he injects the drug.

Withdrawal from heroin and related drugs is uncomfortable, with restlessness, nervousness, disturbed sleep, repeated yawning, and runny nose. Within a day these become more severe, and vomiting, diarrhea, and abdominal discomfort occur. The patients usually exaggerate the severity of their symptoms, but the risk of serious difficulty or death is slight.

The *amphetamine* group of drugs, in contrast to the preceding ones, are *excitants*—"uppers"—which acutely produce restlessness, talkativeness, and heightened reactions. They also cause anxiety and sometimes hallucinations or delusions. The pupils are dilated and the systolic blood pressure rises.

Chronic abuse is almost always accompanied by undernutrition, often severe because the drugs reduce the appetite. The patient is apprehensive, restless, and unable to sleep. He has a fine tremor and jerky movements, with enlarged pupils and hypertension. He may develop delirium with hallucinations and often paranoid delusions.

Withdrawal causes few symptoms except sleepiness and a great sense of fatigue. Occasionally the patient becomes depressed.

Cocaine produces an almost identical acute, chronic, and withdrawal picture. Very large doses of caffeine can cause similar acute reactions except that delirium does not occur. All these stimulant drugs in overdose resemble hyperthyroidism, which tends to produce its changes much more slowly.

Hallucinogenic drugs, including *hashish, marijuana, LSD, peyote,* and related drugs, are so named because they produce vivid hallucinations in large enough doses. The more potent drugs—LSD and DMT, one of its chemical relatives—cause a truly psychotic state in which the patient may consider himself capable of any feat. As a result, he may kill himself by "walking on air" out a high window. He is usually disoriented and—"on a bad trip"—extremely frightened. There are, however, no signs that specifically indicate the cause of the disorder.

The intoxicated patient may present a very confusing picture when he takes several drugs simultaneously. It is usually more important to determine what he has taken than to try to determine the cause by physical examination.

The same procedure is in order when the patient has taken an overdose of any medication or ingested anything that may be poisonous. All drugs in overdose produce undesirable chemical changes and functional disorders. These may also be caused by ingestion of poisonous plants, by the bites of poisonous snakes and spiders, or by the stings of poisonous insects or fishes. The changes are so many and so variable that the history of exposure to poisonous substances becomes of greatest importance.

EXERCISES

1   An obviously poor, undernourished, disheveled 35-year-old man appears with pneumonia. He is treated and begins to recover promptly, with a fall of fever and general improvement. On the second night he becomes increasingly restless and wants reassurance that everything is going to be all right. He is noticeably trembling and his pulse is rapid. What questions would you ask? Why?

2   What questions would you ask in evaluating the usual diet of a 76-year-old woman who lives alone and is obviously too thin? Of a 16-year-old, chubby girl whose mucous membranes look pale? Of a 200-pound, 36-year-old housewife? Of a robust 27-year-old man with an inguinal hernia?

3   A 27-year-old hospital attendant admits that she has managed to get and take about five times the usual dose of a barbiturate daily for the last year "to calm her nerves." She "swore off" yesterday and now doesn't feel well. What questions would you ask her? What are you considering as a likely course of events? What will you watch for?

4   The medicine cabinet is found unlocked and a 21-year-old hospital orderly is found very soundly asleep in the linen room. What questions would you ask and what observations would you make?

5   A distraught mother arrives with her 3-year-old son who looks well enough except that he is crying. She announces that he has "poisoned himself." What questions would you ask?

10-7 METABOLIC DISEASES

Disturbed metabolism is a chemical abnormality whose cause arises within the body. Many metabolic diseases are endocrine in origin; diabetes mellitus due to relative lack of insulin, hyperthyroidism from excess thyroid hormone, and masculinization of girls who produce too much androgen are examples. Besides these endocrine abnormalities, there are disturbances in metabolic processes not under endocrine control.

Gout   Probably the most widely known of these is *gout,* a disordered metabolism or excretion that results in excessive amounts of *uric acid* in the blood. Uric acid salts normally stay in solution in body fluids, but they are not very soluble. As the concentration rises, small, needle-shaped crystals form in tissues, especially in and around joints. These are highly irritating and are also deposited in cartilage and tendons, where they form an encapsulated nodule called a *tophus.*

The first sign of gout often is an inflamed, painful joint at the base of the great toe. This *gouty arthritis* disappears in a few days or weeks and later recurs more and more often, involving more and more joints. Tophi typically occur in the cartilage near the top of the external ear with little inflammation.

When uric acid salts precipitate in the renal pelvis they form kidney stones, usually small and multiple. Recurrent bouts of renal calculus may be the only evidence of gout.

Inborn Errors   There is a familial tendency to have gout, but it is less marked than in a group of hereditary diseases often grouped as *inborn errors of metabolism.* This group includes *sickle cell anemia* and other less common anemias where the body forms abnormal hemoglobins.

Many of the "inborn errors" appear in infancy or early childhood, where the first sign is a failure to grow normally. The symptoms vary greatly depending upon which metabolic reaction is abnormal. None is a common disease but many are fatal.

A more common hereditary disease of children, *chronic cystic fibrosis,* is sometimes considered an inborn error of metabolism. It affects essentially all ducted glands, most importantly the pancreas, the mucous glands of the respiratory tract, the salivary glands, and the sweat glands. Affected children have a chronic cough, some wheezing, thick sputum, and repeated respiratory infections. They early develop signs of chronic obstructive pulmonary disease with hyperresonance and diminished breath sounds. Even in the absence of pulmonary disease, they may have chronic diarrhea with foul-smelling stools, abdominal cramps, and abdominal distention. Their symptoms are usually made worse by fatty foods but carbohydrates are tolerated much better. The intestinal disorder results in malnourishment and stunted growth. To this may be added the liver scarring of hepatic cirrhosis.

Defects in Protein and Fat Metabolism   Chronic cystic fibrosis only occasionally first appears in young adults, but other metabolic disorders appear at any age. Some affect the formation of blood proteins. Antibodies may be reduced or absent, so that the patient is prey to infections. Other abnormalities in protein metabolism occasionally produce clotting difficulties, including bleeding tendencies.

Metabolic difficulties in the use and transportation of fats are more common than those involving proteins. This is not simple obesity due to overeating and the patient may be thin. Rather, there is an abnormal increase in certain fats carried in the plasma. Some of these abnormalities are associated with early and severe arteriosclerosis, and some produce yellowish plaques of fat in the superficial layers of the skin, often around the eyelids.

Salt and Water Defects   The body's salt metabolism is regulated so that the input of salts into the blood, extracellular fluid, and cells carefully balances the output. The balance of salts, including those derived from carbon dioxide, determines how *acidic* or *alkaline* the blood is and adjusts this value to a very narrow range. If the balance of salts or the alkalinity—usually called the *pH*—of the body fluid and cells is much altered, the consequences are serious. Since the salts are in solution, the amount of water in the body is also very important.

Abnormal salt metabolism and disturbances of water balance occur usually as a result of other disorders. When the kidneys fail, for example, they may excrete too much or too little of certain salts. Pulmonary disease causes retention of carbon dioxide and so disturbs the salt and pH balance. Excessive sweating, diabetes mellitus, diabetes insipidus, and extensive exudation in burns increase· water loss and can lead to dehydration. Congestive heart failure causes water retention and abnormal salt balance. Several endocrine disorders, chiefly those of the adrenal cortex and the parathyroids, upset the salt balance more subtly. So do extensive vomiting and diarrhea, which also cause water loss.

Salt and water *imbalances* produce some of the symptoms and signs of the diseases causing them and if uncorrected can be the mechanism of death. Minor changes can be detected only by laboratory tests, but more severe ones can be suspected from the history or physical examination.

Water *retention* increases the body weight and often reduces urine output. When retention is severe enough, edema appears, usually at the ankles, around the eyes, or at the lung bases. *Dehydration* shows itself in a dry tongue and mucous membranes. Later the skin loses its normal turgor; the eyes and facial tissues appear shrunken.

Sodium and *chloride retention* accompany edema. Too low a blood sodium concentration usually occurs when salt is lost by vomiting or diarrhea or when excessive sweating leads a person to drink water without taking in salt. The patient becomes progressively weaker, tired, and sometimes confused. He can then lose consciousness.

Low blood *potassium* usually accompanies other diseases or the use of drugs to increase urine output. The patient feels progressively weaker and eventually may become paralyzed. He may have abdominal distention and a weak pulse as well. Too high a blood potassium causes no recognizable symptoms or signs despite the fact that it is a serious condition.

Too high a blood *calcium* level may be chronic, as it is in overdosage with *vitamin D,* hyperparathyroidism, and in other diseases. This leads to abnormal calcium deposits, especially in the kidney tissue, and to the formation of kidney stones. The patients usually are constipated and feel weak, with little appetite. They may also have emotional symptoms and mental disturbances that make them appear neurotic.

Too low a blood calcium level occurs with lack of vitamin D, in hypoparathyroidism, and in some other diseases. In children who lack vitamin D, the typical skeletal changes and stunted growth of *rickets* appear. Adults often show no symptoms or signs until those related to acute changes appear.

These acute changes appear in overreactive muscles. When fully developed, this overactivity leads to the spasms called *tetany,* in which the hands flex at the wrists with the fingers straight but bent, as a whole, in toward the palm. The feet bend downward and the face may be fixed, with the corners of the mouth drawn downward. Almost all muscles may be spastic, including those of the larynx, and ultimately convulsions can occur. It is possible to uncover the tendency toward spasm before it occurs spontaneously. The best test is to tap the face just in front of the external auditory opening. If the tendency exists, the facial muscles on that side go into spasm. The typical spasm of the hand can be produced by stopping circulation to the arm with a blood-pressure cuff.

Abnormalities in the blood pH are both produced and corrected by changing the respiration, since carbon dioxide plays a large part in its regulation. Thus the pattern of respiration provides a clue to the pH.

When the pH shifts to the acid side—the condition called *acidosis*—because of some deranged function not involving the lungs, the body reduces its carbon dioxide content by increasing the rate and depth of respiration. In the reverse situation, called *alkalosis,* not due to changes in pulmonary function, there is much less effect on normal respiration. It may, in fact, decrease slightly, but the body still requires oxygen, so that respiration must be maintained to supply it.

Acidosis can result from the lungs' inability to get rid of carbon dioxide. This *respiratory acidosis* occurs in severe lung disease such as chronic obstructive bronchial disease, pneumothorax, or when the respiratory centers are depressed by alcohol, barbiturates, or heroin. The existence of such conditions suggests respiratory acidosis.

Respiratory alkalosis results from overbreathing, which reduces the blood carbon dioxide level below normal. This does not occur during exercise, because the body is producing excess carbon dioxide, nor during acidosis, when the body already has excess carbon dioxide. It does occur during *hyperventilation* from emotional causes. As a result, the patient feels lightheaded and "dizzy" without vertigo, becomes weak, and may faint. Since a low carbon dioxide level depresses the blood calcium, the patient may show tetany or be found to have the facial or hand signs of impending tetany.

EXERCISES

1 A 37-year-old man's chief complaint is an inflamed, aching left great toe which he does not recall injuring. What questions would you ask as a start toward deciding whether this could be gout?

2 What questions would you use if you suspected that a 2-year-old girl had an inborn error of metabolism?

3 A 23-year-old laborer is brought in at 4 P.M. in August because he has become weak and somewhat confused after digging in the sun all day. What are your questions and immediate observations?

4 A 58-year-old known diabetic man who has refused treatment is brought in comatose. Uncontrolled diabetes causes acidosis. You can also smell alcohol on his breath but the odor is not strong. What observation will give you a clue as to whether he is in acute alcoholic stupor or diabetic coma? What is the functional basis for a decision?

5 An 18-year-old girl waiting to be seen for some unknown complaint has been sitting quietly for 30 min and then is seen breathing very hard, sitting rigid in her chair with her hands bent at the wrist, fingers extended and bent toward the palm. What is the likely cause of her immediate difficulty? On what grounds can you say this?

10-8 PSYCHOSOMATIC DISEASES

Some diseases arise from mental or emotional causes rather than being *organic diseases* of anatomical, chemical, or infectious origin. The *nonorganic diseases* include some psychoses, psychoneuroses, and the *psychosomatic diseases* which produce chemical or anatomical changes rather than being caused by such changes.

As psychosomatic disease can produce organic disorder, so organic disease very often alters the mental state. Few persons approach an operation without anxiety or remain free of depression during a painful chronic illness. All diseases have *psychic* (mental) and *somatic* (organic) components, but the psychosomatic diseases represent a distinct group.

Mixed Psychosomatic and Organic Disturbances Many psychosomatic disorders present symptoms and signs that can also arise from organic causes. They are particularly intermingled with allergic disturbances; both emotions and antigens can provoke similar reactions in the same patient. Only careful questioning then gives a clear lead to the underlying cause.

The skin, for example, can react with urticaria or eczema to specific antigens or to emotions. Eating shellfish makes some patients break out with hives, but anxiety about examinations can cause the same lesions. Allergy to cosmetics can produce eczema; so can an unhappy marriage.

Respiratory and Cardiac Symptoms   Bronchial asthma, specifically contraction of the bronchiolar muscles, is often triggered by the patient's emotional turmoil when faced with an unpleasant situation. Identical attacks occur due to pollen allergy, animal dander, or even exposure to cold.

Hay fever is a typical pollen allergy and is called *acute allergic rhinitis.* There is a similar chronic condition called *vasomotor rhinitis,* which is not confined to the pollen seasons. Some patients with vasomotor rhinitis seem truly allergic; others have symptoms on an emotional basis, especially when there is prolonged tension in an unpleasant situation.

In contrast, true hyperventilation with its consequences, including tetany, seems always to be psychosomatic. It occurs most commonly during an *acute anxiety attack,* when the patient also has trembling, tachycardia, and sighing with sweaty, clammy palms and considerable fear of impending disaster. These attacks can come in any setting and may even wake the patient from a sound sleep.

Tachycardia results from a variety of organic conditions including shock and violent exercise. It can also be purely emotional in origin, as it is in stage fright. In the same way, dyspnea may be organic or the result of being startled.

Gastrointestinal Disorders   Peptic ulcers are among the best-known psychosomatic diseases. Tense, conscientious, worrying, resentful people, usually thin and active, are most apt to develop gastric or duodenal ulcers. Ulcers also occur, however, as a complication of severe burns, alcoholism, and excessive hormone from the adrenal cortex. Patients with these causes often do not fit the personality pattern of the typical person with psychosomatic ulcer.

Similarly, tense, worried people develop frequent attacks of indigestion, constipation, diarrhea, and even the more serious *ulcerative colitis,* which involves frequent watery, bloody stools. All these symptoms occur in organic disease as well, even though the patient is a relaxed individual.

Headache and Backache   *Migraine* is clearly psychosomatic and predictably occurs in neat, meticulous, ambitious persons often called *obsessive-compulsive* or put into the "achiever" group. The attack characteristically comes when such a person relaxes—on weekends, for example. Often a period of increased activity and alertness precedes the attack, which begins with a brief period of seeing bright spots, flashes, or lines. There follows an excruciating headache—usually on one side of the head and lasting hours or a few days—which leaves the patient exhausted.

Migraine is a vascular disorder. Prior to the headache, the arteries to the head constrict. The reduced blood supply to the retina probably causes the visual symptoms. The constriction is followed by dilatation, flooding the vessels of the head with blood, and at this stage the headache occurs.

Another kind of psychogenic headache has a direct organic counterpart. Anything which forces a person to hold his head rigid for a long period produces aching neck muscles. These muscles attach to the skull at the occiput and the ache centers there but spreads, as a dull pain, to include the entire head. A person often holds his head rigid when he drives, when he does paper work, when he has osteoarthritis of the cervical vertebrae, or when he is emotionally taut. This, then, produces what is sometimes called a *tension headache*.

In a similar way, splinting of back muscles occurs farther down the vertebral column. Some backaches of this sort are clearly psychosomatic, others are obviously organic.

Patients with Psychosomatic Disorders   There is nothing imaginary about psychosomatic diseases or about the mental state that produces them. Patients may be unaware, however, of the emotional strains involved in such everyday situations as entertaining the boss, meeting mortgage payments, or taking examinations at school. Many people with psychosomatic disturbances cope with tense situations better than their associates and are fundamentally productive and well-adjusted. It is doubly important to gain the confidence of such patients and to question them intelligently in order to uncover the true cause of their difficulties.

EXERCISES

1   Given a tense, nervous patient who complains of recurrent headaches, map out a course of questioning to uncover possible emotional causes.

2   A patient has admitted during the history taking to an extramarital affair. Subsequently the spouse appears with evidence of a peptic ulcer. What questions would you ask this second patient in attempting to uncover possible psychic factors?

3   A 45-year-old woman who has had a 10-year course of recurring bouts of painful rheumatoid arthritis has almost no crippling deformity. She begins another and more severe recurrence of the disease. She gives evidence of being very anxious, cries frequently, insists that the disease will kill her this time and that she will welcome death. What questions will you ask her about her emotional state? Why ask any? Do you suspect psychosomatic disease?

4   A 23-year-old woman who has just come home after delivering her first baby complains that she has twice wakened during the night and sat up in bed with increasing difficulty in breathing. What questions would you ask?

5   A 12-year-old boy comes in with inflamed, weeping eczema of both hands. What questions would you ask him? What would you ask his mother? Would you question him only when his mother was in the room? If you did decide to ask him something when you were alone, how would you get the mother out of the room?

6   A 26-year-old Iranian secretary newly arrived in the country speaks almost no English. She makes you understand that she has a headache and lays her hand carefully over the left side of her head to indicate where it is. What observations would you make and what questions could you ask to get some idea as to whether she has migraine?

INDEX

Commonly used Latin and Greek plurals are given in parentheses behind the singular form of the terms. Page references in *italic* indicate illustrations.

AAL (*see* Axillary lines)
Abbreviations, use of, 88
Abdomen, 66–72, *67*, 83, 185–193
  anatomy of, 282–296, *283, 286, 288, 290, 292, 295*
  distention of, 187
  fluid in, 187–188, 239
  hernias of, 186
  mass in, 70, 83, 188–189
  muscles of, 185, 187, 351
  in nontraumatic emergency, 248
  pain in, 349
  quadrants of, 66, *67*
  regions of, 185, *186*
  rumbling in, 353
  tenderness in, 188, 239
  trauma in, 238–239
  variation in, 319–322, *321*
Abortions:
  in obstetrical history, 228
  types of, 366
Abrasion, 28, 407–408
Abscess, 407, 409
  sterile, 407
Absorption:
  in colon, 351
  in renal tubule, 355
  in small intestine, 350
Acetabulum (acetabula), *283,* 284, 306, *307, 309,* 323, *323*
Achilles tendon (*see* Tendon)
Acid:
  in blood, 422–423
  gastric, 349
  hydrochloric, 349

Acne, 394, 407
Acromegaly, 371–372
Acromion, 274–275, *275*
ACTH, 368
Acute illness, 128
Adenoids (*see* Tonsils)
Adnexum (adnexa) of uterus, *77,* 204–205, *204*
Adrenal cortical stimulating hormone (ACTH), 368
Adrenal gland (*see* Glands)
Adrenalin, 341, 369
Adult diseases, questions about, 13
Affect (*see* Emotion)
Aging, 319, 322, 324, 384, 385, 402
Air conduction, 139
Air sac (*see* Alveolus)
Alcoholism, 125, 416–418, 425
Alkalinity, 422–423
Allergy, 413–415, 424–425
Alveolus (alveoli), 44, *45,* 335–338, 388
Amphetamine intoxication, 419
Anaphylactoid reaction, 414
Anaphylaxis, 414
Androgen, 360, 368–371
Anemia, 390–391, 404, 413, 416, 421
Aneurysm:
  arterial, 184, 192, 344
  rupture of, 344
  ventricular, 177, 347
Angina pectoris, 343
Ankle, 79, 210, *310,* 312–313, *313,* 323
Anomaly, 325–326